MW01057186

IF PROBLEMS TALKED

The Guilford Family Therapy Series
Michael P. Nichols, *Series Editor*

Recent Volumes

If Problems Talked
Narrative Therapy in Action

Jeffrey L. Zimmerman   Victoria C. Dickerson

Afterword by Karl Tomm

The Guilford Press
New York   London

© 1996 The Guilford Press
A Division of Guilford Publications, Inc.
72 Spring Street, New York, NY 10012

Jeffrey L. Zimmerman and Victoria C. Dickerson are coauthors of this
book, making different, but equal, contributions in its creation.

Printed in the United States of America

This book is printed on acid-free paper.

Last digit is print number: 9 8 7 6 5 4 3 2 1

Library of Congress Cataloging-in-Publication Data

Zimmerman, Jeffrey.
    If problems talked: narrative therapy in action / Jeffrey L.
Zimmerman, Victoria C. Dickerson.
        p. cm. — (Guilford family therapy series)
    Includes bibliographical references and index.
    ISBN 1–57230–129–5
    1. Storytelling—Therapeutic use. 2. Metaphor—Therapeutic use.
I. Dickerson, Victoria C. II. Title. III. Series.
RC489.S74Z55   1996
616.89′14—dc20   96-31853
                                                          CIP

Acknowledgments

We especially thank the following people.

From both of us:
  Cheryl White, for encouraging us, like she has so many others, to take ourselves seriously and to write about our own ideas. Michael White, for introducing us to these ideas, which have resonated with us in our lives, our interests, and our desires. David Epston, who delights in our delight in writing.

  Our narrative community, Janet Adams-Westcott, Gene Combs, Jill Freedman, Melissa Griffith, and "Griff" Griffith, of which we have been a part since 1988/1989, and from whom we continually learn and with whom we continually grow.

  Stephen Madigan, our colleague, friend, and late-night discussant. John Neal, who we have been able to count on to comment on our writing and with whom we collaborate in thinking and teaching. And more recently our friendship and ongoing collaboration with Bill Lax, Sallyann Roth, and Kathy Weingarten, who also made helpful comments on earlier drafts and continue to inspire us, prod us, and laugh with us.

  Kitty Moore, our editor, who took seriously our playfulness. Lisa Berndt, who embraced some difficult tasks, freeing us to do this writing. All those at Bay Area Family Therapy Training Associates, who managed without us over the last two years, and continued their work.

From Vicki:

Jeff Zimmerman, who, through his own creativity, reminded me of the creative version of self that I prefer. Brandy Caroline Belvel, my goddaughter, who reminds me that it's all just perspective, and unfailingly makes me laugh.

From Jeff:

Vicki Dickerson, for joining in this vision and using her strength to help move things forward. Stephanie and Meg Zimmerman, for the love they give and things they teach. D'Ann Whitehead, my partner in life, who shows me love when I most need it. Rhoda and Leonard Zimmerman, for their pride. The "Dead" and all Deadheads, for freedom.

Contents

PART III. BRINGING IT ALL BACK HOME

PART I

If Problems Talked

CHAPTER 1

This Is Not Kansas

THE TIMES THEY ARE A-CHANGIN'

Bob Dylan's song "The Times They Are A-Changin'" became the rallying cry of a generation; it signified an ushering in of a new world. The new, "multiple" set of realities would affect all our ways of thinking and performing, and all the arenas in which we think and perform (e.g., politics, religion, movies—and, yes, therapy). Indeed, as Walter Truett Anderson (1990) has compellingly documented, "reality isn't what it used to be." (See also Kenneth Gergen, 1985, 1991.) How do we write a book that reflects this so-called "postmodern" understanding? How do we convey some complicated and very different ideas? Can we do this in new and creative ways that are more consistent with the ideas themselves? Can we write a book about how to think about and address problems in so-called "psychotherapy" without using conventional, academic forms as our primary style?

If in the modern era we were consumed with the way things are—that is, with essences and absolutes and truth and analysis—we are now more interested in how they might be. We are concerned with possibilities and various points of view and their effects. In writing about truths, it was easy to be consistent with certain ways of thinking; one states truths in direct ways. In writing about how people construct meaning from their experiences, it makes sense to us to do so by generating experiences for people, so that they can take part in the ideas instead of just having the ideas presented to them. Our therapy involves experiences and asking questions to create meaning. We hope this book will do the same thing—create experiences and raise questions about them.

3

In the film *Forrest Gump*, Forrest's mother tells him, "Life is like a box of chocolates." This now-famous comment becomes a metaphor for the way Forrest sees the world and approaches life. It defines who Forrest is and what he does. What if if his mother were to say instead, "Life is like a den of rattlesnakes"? This would have quite a different effect on the way Forrest understands himself and presents himself to the world. Forrest would, in fact, be a different person, and the world would know him in quite different ways. We believe this applies to psychotherapy as well. The metaphors therapists use shape their clients' view of themselves and their view of the problems for which they seek help. These metaphors shape the therapists' view of the same things. They even shape therapists' view of what a therapist is and the forms therapy and the therapist are supposed to take.

Just as Forrest Gump is a device to take us though a history of our generation (in a postmodern way—through interviews of various "realities"), we use certain devices in this book to make some points about different views and their effects, and about our work in general. These devices don't represent reality either, but they are consistent with the metaphor we use in our therapeutic work.

HOW DOES THE SONG GO?

Our first device is to present some fictionalized snippets of the lives of three clients, each from the point of view of a different therapy experience each client might have had. Their therapists were clearly influenced by a different metaphor about what a problem is, and therefore about what therapy should address. We also talk to you, our readers, and raise questions about the possible effects of coming from these different therapeutic vantage points. We follow all of this with a fictional panel discussion, "debating" and (we hope) demonstrating the origin of these points of view. None of this is representative or inclusive of any view; they are just bits of ideas done in playful ways. At various points we, the authors, speak to you. (We will say more about this later.) There is one last device at the very end of the chapter—we want to warn you that he tends to be obnoxious, but then problems often are. Enjoy!

HOW CAN YOU BE IN TWO PLACES AT ONCE AND NOT BE ANYWHERE AT ALL?

Story 1

Susan came home from work bone-tired. She heard the phone ringing, so she ran up the stairs, pushed open the door, and grabbed the phone—just as it stopped. "This is how my day has gone," she thought to herself. "I'm 35 years old and still putting up with too much junk." She had had that thought a lot recently.

Susan was particularly irritated because she had had a fight with her boss. "Why can't I control myself?" she wondered. Susan reflected on her difficulties with men, both at work and in her personal relationships. "Personal relationships—that's a fake," she thought. "What I do best is make people mad at me. It's going to be one of those nights," she decided. "Those nights" happened a lot when the house was empty.

"Maybe I'll call someone—that could turn things around." But who? Most of the time when Susan called someone, it was her sister, which rarely led to her feeling better. Her therapist had helped her realize that she had always been competitive with her older sister. Her own rather significant feelings of incompetence, along with the kind of jealousy all siblings feel, had fueled this competition. She'd been glad when her therapist, after identifying these jealous feelings and tracing them back to their origins, had said that this is how things work in most families. Susan's mother agreed with Susan's therapist. She frequently said that she knew she had spoiled Susan by trying to spend more time with her. She did this because Susan's older sister had done so well, and, as her mother, she felt guilty. Mom had come to understand all this through her own therapy.

Susan was dreading therapy this week. Usually she was able to make herself feel okay about her appointment, because she knew it was good for her. Her therapist was a nice person, and she trusted him enough—most of the time—to dump stuff on him. But after the fight at work earlier in the day, and her date with Fred over the weekend, she knew she would have to admit defeat in some of the areas she'd been working on. "I have been doing so well at controlling myself," she thought. "Why did I have to blow it?"

Susan's therapist had helped her see what a hurt and angry person she was, and how she alienated people through her anger—anger left over from her upbringing. Susan did feel angry sometimes, but was usually able to hide it. Most of the time she didn't know what she felt. She really did want to be responsive to the people in her life—her friends, her boss, Fred, even her parents (sort of). Her therapist said her anger came out when people got too close, and so she got them to reject her out of fear. Susan wasn't sure of this, but she was sure that if she saw her therapist and tried not to talk about what happened this week, it would just get him going about her lack of trust. Susan really did want to get better, but sometimes it all seemed too much to listen to. She just wasn't in the mood for the usual feedback on things that put others off. Sometimes she just wanted to say, "Don't bug me today," and not hear back something about her mother.

While Susan was in the middle of making dinner, the phone rang again. It was her friend Ellie from work. When Susan heard Ellie's voice, she realized she had no desire to talk with her. "Maybe I *am* just a cold bitch," she thought. Of course Ellie wanted to talk about the "incident" at work. "How do things get around so quickly?" Susan wondered.

"I can't believe you said that to him," Ellie scolded. "Do you want to lose this job, too?"

"My mother says I just have to learn to shut up," Susan replied. "I think my therapist agrees with her."

"That's good advice," answered Ellie. "When the boss says something to me, I figure he's right and I should just shut up."

"I wish I could be one of those women, you know, who smile and say 'Thank you,' the ones that men really appreciate," Susan said, half wistfully and half kidding. "I'm not made like most women. Maybe if I work harder in therapy, I'll get straightened out."

When Susan got off the phone, her dinner was ruined. Tears filled her eyes. She wished she was normal and not a problem. She told herself she wouldn't complain about therapy any more, and she would work hard to overcome her destructiveness and her deficiencies. She sometimes wondered if there was really any hope.

Story 2

When Betsy arrived home, her mother was waiting for her at the top of the stairs. She wondered if they would end up having one of their heated discussions. She wasn't in the mood for that tonight. She'd had a really hard few days.

"Yoo-hoo," her mother called. "I made dinner—something special for you because I thought you needed cheering up. Come join us."

Betsy remembered that in their last family therapy session, the therapist had questioned Betsy's relationship with her mother. He'd asked her dad what he thought of her relationship with her mom. As usual, Dad didn't have much to say, and the therapist didn't push it. Instead, he turned back to Betsy and asked her about why she thought her mom was still doing all that stuff for her. Before therapy Betsy had thought her mom was just being a mom—you know, helpful. Now she realized that her mom was "overdoing it" and might have reasons of her own for this.

Betsy wasn't sure what she wanted. If she asked to be left alone and went to her room, she would feel some relief. It was also less likely that she and her mom would fight. But then she would be lonely, think too much, and hurt her parents in the process. She imagined that was what her therapist would want her to do—be more independent of her parents.

When she came in the front door, her father was sitting in his favorite chair, reading as usual. "Hi, dear. How was your day?" he said, looking up from his magazine and smiling at her.

Betsy's father always said those same words when she came home from work. Ever since he'd retired, he seemed to have little else to say. Come to think of it, before he'd retired, he hadn't said that much to her either. He'd just talked a little about his work. Their therapist was trying to get her mom to talk less to her and more to her dad. Getting Mom and Dad to talk together about family matters—now that would be some feat.

Betsy's mother came into the room and said, "Let's all eat together tonight, like a normal family."

"But Mae...." (Betsy had decided she was supposed to call her mom by her first name.) "I thought we weren't a 'normal' family. I thought you decided we were 'dysfunctional.'"

"Well," Mae said, "between those shows we watch on TV and that therapist we all had to go to because *you* were having problems, what else am I to think?"

Betsy felt herself getting really angry. "First of all," she said, "it was the therapist's idea that we *all* come. I just wanted help for the problems I was having with my relationships. Second of all, according to him, if you and Dad would get your act together, maybe you'd leave me alone and I'd be better able to connect with others."

Mae was really hurt. As parents, she and John had done everything she thought they were supposed to do. She had worked very hard with both her girls to give them everything they needed. Her mother had done the same for her. Now she was finding out in therapy that she had been doing *too* much, and that this had actually hurt Betsy. What was more, these problems had been going on across the generations. Sure, she'd fought some with her mother, didn't everyone? But Mae had no complaints about how she had turned out. She looked over at John, but acknowledged to herself that he would be no help. He had never said much to her or to Betsy, and now not in therapy either.

"Betsy," she said. "Your father and I are trying to talk more. You know our therapist thinks if we do this, maybe you would be able to connect more with others."

"I know you're trying," Betsy replied. "I just get so frustrated. I want our relationship to be better. I want to be closer to you and to others. It's just so hard."

"Don't worry, dear." Mae said. "We'll work all this out. I'm sure we'll learn what we're supposed to learn—to give each other more space and have the kind of closeness your therapist thinks we should."

Secretly, Mae wasn't too sure, though. There seemed to be such a long way to go, and it had gone the way it had for so many years. If only John could . . . but she knew, deep down inside, it was up to her to make all the relationships better. With help, she was willing to keep trying.

IS THERE ANYBODY OUT THERE?

The Authors Speak

Before we go on to Story 3, we'd like all of you to say what you think. We are leaving a blank space for you to think it in. We've started the "conversation" for you with examples. (We imagine you could think about whatever else you want instead.)

QUESTION 1: How are you thinking about Susan?

READER 1: She is possibly borderline and definitely needs boundaries supplied to her.

READER 2: She needs to be cared for, not confronted.

READER 3: There is a lot of anger and demandingness.

READER (YOU): _____

QUESTION 2: What effect(s) might these descriptions have on how she thinks about herself?

READER 1: She would know she's fragile and needs help.

READER 2: However, needing more care doesn't mean she's a bad person.

READER 3: If she sees these things, then she could begin to control herself.

READER (YOU): _____

QUESTION 3: What effect does such knowledge have on the way you believe you need to respond to her?

READER 1: I would prepare for inevitable acting out.

READER 2: Well, I'd give her the care and nurturance I know she needs.

READER 3: Perhaps I'd get her to attend more accurately to others.

READER (YOU): _____

QUESTION 4: How are you thinking about Betsy?

READER 1: She has not been given enough independence.

READER 2: I think she has been very smothered.

READER 3: She has no room to assert herself.

READER (YOU): _____

QUESTION 5: What effect(s) might these descriptions have on how she thinks about herself?

READER 1: She can see that the damage was caused by her parents.

READER 2: Well, she can blame her family rather than herself.

READER 3: I think she might realize she was just caught in a bind.

READER (YOU): _____

QUESTION 6: What effect does such knowledge have on the way you believe you need to respond to her?

READER 1: I would allow her to begin to set her own limits.

READER 2: I'd see the family.

READER 3: I'd begin to push her to make her own decisions at home.

READER (YOU): _____

THIS IS NOT KANSAS

Story 3

On her way home from work, Ann decided to stop at Joe's. She really wanted to discuss something with him, despite their disagreement of a few days ago. This was a big step for Ann—feeling she had the right to ask something of Joe.

Ann began to feel **guilt** and **anxiety** attack her as she made her way up to Joe's. **Guilt** and **anxiety** were trying to talk her out of going there. Ann laughed to herself when she realized she was thinking this way. There was a time when **guilt** and **anxiety** would overwhelm her. Now she saw them as somewhat separate from herself. They still caused her a lot of discomfort, but she was beginning to be able to manage them. Seeing them as things—as created by the problem—was a new development in her therapy sessions. It was a really odd way to think, she acknowledged to herself, but she really liked how it felt.

Ann had gone to therapy complaining about problems with relationships. She had shared with her therapist the range of feelings she experienced around others—anger, depression, guilt, anxiety, and so on. Her therapist had asked her about the effect of these feelings, and she'd told him that she had begun to doubt herself. Her therapist began to talk about the problem as ***self-doubt.***

Ann recalled how she began to really notice the effects **self-doubt** was having on her life. It was interfering with her ability to communicate to those she cared about; it made her feel bad; it stopped her from getting what she wanted; and it prevented her from using her talents and abilities. When it grabbed her, it often shut her down. Sometimes she ended up exploding when it constrained her for a long period of time. Her therapist noticed that after she did this, it attacked her with **guilt.** Ann was beginning to catch onto **self-doubt**'s tactics and was thinking about how she, Ann, preferred to respond to things.

When Joe answered the door, he was surprised to see Ann. He wasn't sure Ann had forgiven him for what he said to her the other day. He was glad she was there, as now he would have a chance to apologize for the effects he'd had. He'd realized, after she left, that she had interpreted his remarks in a way he did not intend—as closing off space for her opinions. It was this kind of process that was being addressed when he occasionally attended sessions with Ann and her therapist.

"Hi, Ann. Thanks for stopping by," Joe greeted her.

"It's okay that I'm here, then," Ann said apologetically. "I wasn't sure."

"Yeah. I'm sorry about the other night," Joe said, greatly relieved to have a chance to say so. "When you got angry and left, I realized that something I said must have given you the message that what you thought was unimportant."

Ann smiled and felt really good inside. She wasn't completely sure what to make of what had happened. *Self-doubt* tried to tell her it was her problem. But then she remembered that often *self-doubt* was dependent on **lack of entitlement**—a thing that affected many women. **Lack of entitlement** tries to tell women they should give up what they want or think for what men want or think. When **lack of entitlement** was operating on Ann, she ended up feeling disconnected and/or frustrated and angry. It was a turning point for Ann when her therapist helped her notice that she did have her own ideas and wants and was sometimes able to put them out to herself and to others. He asked her what allowed her to do this, and she said, "Strength of will." She imagined that she used that same strength of will to fight **lack of entitlement** and **self-doubt,** and to be able to come today and ask Joe's opinion about something that had happened at work.

"Thanks, Joe," Ann finally answered. "I appreciate hearing that. It's good to know you are on my side. I really came to talk with you about another problem. I just wanted confirmation I was going on a good track."

Joe felt really good that Ann was able to trust him so soon after their disagreement. He knew she was working on figuring out what kind of person she wanted to be—with him, at work, with her parents, and with herself. He was ready to listen to any developments she wanted to share. He really liked the person she was being with him, even though at times it forced him to remember that his experiences as a man often influenced him to respond in ways he didn't like.

"It's good to see you taking charge of these problems," he said. "I know it's what you want."

"I'm feeling a lot stronger," Ann stated. "No problem will keep me down any more."

The Authors Speak

This is a different kind of story. We're wondering what you think about it.

QUESTION 7: How are you thinking about Ann?

READER 1: She's working hard to fight some tough problems.

READER 2: She's able to take care of herself.

READER 3: I see her beginning to stand up to cultural restrictions.

READER (YOU): _____

QUESTION 8: What effect(s) might these descriptions have on how she thinks about herself?

READER 1: She would notice her own strength and knowledge.

READER 2: It might feel empowering to her.

READER 3: She would be able to set her own direction.

READER (YOU): _____

QUESTION 9: What effect does such knowledge have on the way you believe you need to respond to her?

READER 1: I'd let her set her own pace.

READER 2: I would wonder about all the ways she is caring for herself.

READER 3: I'd support her in taking charge.

READER (YOU): _____

The Authors Speak

Here is what we hope you've noticed so far (because it is our experience that these ideas are important to this work):

1. There are multiple points of view about clinical situations.
2. They shape what each of us notices, who we see, the questions we ask, and the language we use.
3. Each point of view has *real effects* on us and the lives of people who consult with us.

A PANEL DISCUSSION
WE'VE ALWAYS WANTED TO HEAR

Next, we are presenting what we hope is a humorous and entertaining way to discuss the very complicated theories that inform the therapists' approaches in these stories. We hope you can bear with it. Our experience is that the material is hard to "get." We have tried to put it in a palatable form, rather than to present it as straight theory in a didactic manner. Many people who have attended our workshops have shared with us how difficult it is to grapple with this theoretical material, especially in the forms that have previously been available. So we have tried to review just the critical ideas, and to do so in a form that is different from anything we have written about or read about before.

We have compared three points of view in an effort to help you flesh out distinctions (our Batesonian friends would be pleased to hear about their influence here). We mean no offense in our caricatures of the panel members. We just wanted to make this part a bit more fun to read and

experience. We have picked "Otto Freudian" to represent individualizing, pathologizing psychologies—his comments reflect a wide range of
analytic and neoanalytic work. We have similarly picked "Virginia
Batesonian" to represent family work, and "Jerome Foucaultian" to
represent social constructionism and postmodern views.

We can describe all these points of view as radical in their own time.
Freudian theory fought against repression but was limited by the culture
it was created in, so that Freudians ended up inadvertently replicating
the culture. Today the theories seem almost provincial. Batesonian
theories evolved in a particular time and can also be seen as consistent
with and/or limited by their cultural era. Others (therapists) took these
ideas and applied them to family work in a multitude of ways, more or
less consistent with the ideas. In retrospect, structural family therapy may
have had an oppressive effect for women, if as a result of therapy they
ended up going along more with their husbands. In this way, the challenges of family therapy also turned into inadvertent replications of the
culture. A Foucaultian reactive radicalism seems to stand out in today's
world; these ideas have been a major influence on narrative work. These
ideas also reflect the current culture and its postmodern viewpoints. It is
likely, though, that years from now, when the culture has moved on and
these radical ideas have long become part of the mainstream, there will
be new points of view that will pay attention to the limitations and blind
spots of the current work (Foucaultian) we now find so salient.

One more thing: You might ask why we have to use any of this new
theoretical language (some call it "jargon"). We use it not to mystify but to
demystify, so that you can read other theoretical material in this area a bit
more easily. Also, the new language does capture the thinking in a more
precise way. We hope you will be interested in learning this "foreign
language." If you've ever had the experience of learning another language,
you know how it helps you relate to and appreciate the local culture better.

Part 1

MODERATOR (MOD): The first question I'd like to pose has to do with the
    questions addressed to the readers. Why do you think the authors
    are asking these questions?

OTTO FREUDIAN (OF): We would need to explore the vicissitudes of each
    author's unconscious mental life to answer such a question.

VIRGINIA BATESONIAN (VB): You see *that* because that's your point of
    view. (And besides, I wouldn't go near these authors' mental life.)

OF: What do you mean? I see it because it is there. The importance of
    the unconscious cannot be underestimated. Our work proves this!

VB: It is "there" because you interpret what you see along the lines that your ideas allow and not along other lines. You pay attention only to certain aspects and only in certain ways. Perhaps the authors are trying to help the readers notice this about themselves.

JEROME FOUCAULTIAN (JF): I agree. Furthermore, OF, your ideas are shaped by the social and cultural ideologies of your time. Although I acknowledge that your group was the first leading advocate for people's telling their own stories, you then subjected these stories to the scientific metaphors and moralities of your era in order to give them the truth status of 19th-century science.

VB: Yes, admit it, old man. Your group advanced the field—maybe it even created the field—but you all blew the issue of sexual abuse badly. By creating a description of it as repressed fantasies, you inadvertently supported more years of oppression for women. I believe the authors may be asking the readers to imagine the effects of the descriptions and explanations they use. I wonder what the effects have been of other descriptions and explanations your group has created, OF—for example, the repression of instincts, defenses, and the interpretation of the unconscious as visible only to others. Now, the repression of sexuality . . .

JF: (*Interrupting*) That one really bothers me, OF. I'd like to comment on the effects of this from my point of view. Your society actually brought out in the open the issue of sexuality as something that could be commented on; it didn't suppress it. But your group subjected it to its <u>discourse</u> [social commentary that creates certain meanings][1] about what was normal and what was not, creating <u>marginalized</u> [those who don't fit the status quo] minorities, and thus supporting the culturally dominant ways of being. Sexuality wasn't repressed; it was <u>constituted</u> [created] along the lines the dominant culture of the times called for [inadvertently, consensus created deviance]. It's terribly frightening not to go along with <u>specifications</u> [what the culture says about how one should be].

OF: (*Smiling*) I wonder if these feelings you have for me are like the ones you have toward your father. You might consult *Totem and Taboo*.

MOD: Okay, okay. No need to get touchy with each other. We are here to talk about these cases, remember? What did you think about the way the problem was talked about in each?

OF: The first one is correct, although superficial. Intrapsychic conflicts must be explored in depth.

---

[1] Authors' note: To "translate" JF, we have <u>underlined</u> the words he uses in a particular way, and put our loose translation in brackets [ ] after each one.

VB: I like the second one.

JF: The point of view taken in the third one intrigues me.

MOD: I'd like to get each of you to bring forth your point of view here. (*To OF*) Why do you believe the first one is correct?

OF: Because the problem is in the conflicts of the mental apparatus of the person.

JF: Does it "hide" there (*chuckling*), like the "pods" in *Invasion of the Body Snatchers?*

OF: What do you mean?

MOD: He's just being obnoxious. JF, you of all people should appreciate that since ideas are subject to the limits of the cultural understanding of their time, none of you could think in any other ways. In fact, all of you represent points of view that were years ahead of your contemporaries. Anyway, why do you think about it this way?

OF: Well, our theories are well known; even though they have been softened, modified, or adapted in different forms over time, there have been some consistent themes. For example, work by one of our group members demonstrated that because of early experiences, a person's psyche develops in pathological ways.

MOD: Do I understand you are suggesting that individuals have relatively fixed personality structures and can have damage that limits them?

OF: Yes.

MOD: So the person's mental apparatus is the problem, and that causes all the bad things to happen?

OF: Yes.

MOD: Did you ever consider the effects of thinking about what you call "pathology" on clients?

OF: Unfortunately, the truth often hurts, but it is the road to health and it is necessary.

MOD: For example, therapy seems to have encouraged a more negative self-picture for Susan. She sees herself as hostile and rejecting.

OF: She is.

MOD: All the time?

OF: No, only when her ego falters.

MOD: But her ability not to be that way when . . .

OF: This does not matter, given the depths of the psyche.

MOD: Have you considered the effects on therapists of the way you think? For example, with Susan . . .

OF: Sure. The therapist realizes she needs long-term care; however, therapists must be very wary of her, as she will try to engage them in the repetition of earlier unsatisfying relationships.

MOD: But that's not Susan's experience—that she would try to do that, is it?

OF: Resistance and the unconscious.

MOD: And the therapist's ideas and experience?

OF: These should never enter in. If they do, the therapist needs additional analysis. My fantasies and ideas, of course, never affect my reactions. I'm completely objective.

MOD: One final question: As a woman, I'm apt to see this client as a person who is having trouble with relationships because assertiveness is not well received by men.

OF: This is your countertransference. She must learn to be more appropriately female. If she is not happy with this role, we must explore the unconscious basis in her early experience.

JF: I've had enough of this! This man not only is participating in what I consider subjugating cultural discourse [ideas in the culture that have the effect of reducing power for some], but is supporting systems of thought that allow his group to shape what is normal and what is not. Susan has been reduced to an object of study for him. He knows her only through his cracked lenses. This leads to a pathological reduction of her as a human being. The therapy she is in even has her trying to account for "deviances" that are actually being created by the descriptions he is using and by what the cultural norms demand. It was a lot quicker and cheaper for people during the era when all anyone had to do was say a few Hail Marys to be absolved of what the Catholic Church defined as sins. How can he not see that there has been a cultural assignment of identity to her as a woman, and that he is supporting it under the guise of a powerful, modern technology (which therapy has become), and is using it to brainwash her into buying into the culture, and . . .

MOD: Let's take a break!

The Authors Speak

Here is what we hope you will get out of this:

1. The cultural context of Freudian theory was modernism. This is seen in Freudians' attempt to tell us exactly how all things work. Coming from 19th-century metaphors, they believe that their

point of view is correct and not just a point of view. We see this in their emphasis on essences and absolutes, as well as in the description they came up with for their work—"analysis," the application of science (a scientific metaphor) to everything, including people.

2. Batesonian ideas represent a shift toward noticing the limitations of perspective.
3. Foucaultian ideas are radically different.
4. We hope you are wondering where you would place your ideas.

Part 2

VB: I'd like to discuss my preference for the second scenario and the way the problem is discussed there. Clearly this best fits my point of view, which *I* will own.

MOD: Go ahead.

VB: In the second story, I imagine the pattern is considered the problem. These patterns are part of relationships, and they include not only the family, but the therapist as well.

MOD: What do you mean?

VB: Well, for example, Betsy and her mom seem to be the ones involved with each other, while John is on the periphery. Does the therapist support the system pattern? I'm not sure from the story how this is going. Maybe the therapist is focusing on separating Betsy from her mother.

MOD: How do you understand the pattern's influence theoretically?

VB: Well, that's an interesting question, and observers might have different ideas about that, depending on what part of this theory they were attending to. For example, you could view the parents' behavior as causing Betsy's response and hers in turn as causing their response. This would be the notion of "circular causality." Or, as our later work has emphasized, you could see the pattern as a kind of feedback loop where one response affects but does not cause the other. We call this a "restraint." So, for example, in this case the parents are seeing and interpreting only a certain kind of response Betsy is making, and Betsy is seeing and interpreting only a certain kind of response her parents are making. The conclusion they inevitably come to is that no other response is possible or would make sense; this gives them the illusion of limited options. It doesn't make sense for them to respond differently, nor do they see the other as capable of doing so. This is the restraining effect of the loop.

MOD: Suppose they could notice other responses occurring?

VB: Then they would be as capable of behaving that way as anything or anyone else. The therapist must also believe that these possibilities are available to them. The difficulty is in getting them (the family and the therapist) to truly, and not trivially, notice these possibilities. In Betsy's family, this might mean noticing other ways they do communicate, other ways they can be or are with each other and/or with others in their outside lives. These alternatives must have meaning for them, or they will be rejected because of what the family members currently believe about each other and themselves. In contrast to what this family seems to have gotten from their therapist, I don't see the relationships as the problem, just the current pattern. I have trouble with some family therapies that suggest pathological motivations underlying the way people respond to each other and . . .

OF: What are you saying—that these people could be different without years of depth work? That if something else were pointed out, they would do it? This is difficult for me to understand.

VB: If you're thinking about what I said from your framework, I'm sure it is difficult. What I am saying and what I believe is that these relationship patterns are quite difficult to break. To truly notice other possibilities and other meanings requires hard work, but certainly not years.

OF: Patterns . . . why didn't I notice them?

VB: The restraints of your ideas are such that you weren't noticing other ideas. We are all affected by our ideas in a similar manner. I'm not even sure that in years you . . .

MOD: Can we get back to what you're saying? Have you thought about what effects this view of the problem has on persons and relationships?

VB: I'm not too happy with what has been done with these ideas by therapists who forget they are dealing with living persons and not machines. Our later work has emphasized that cybernetics is merely a point of view, like any other, that shapes what therapists see in the room. We have moved away from talking about causality in systems and begun to suggest that the problem doesn't reside inside relationships any more than it does in persons. Our work and the work of my esteemed colleague (*looks at* OF) and his group have been used to "hide," as my other colleague (*looks at* JF) jokingly suggested, the problem inside persons and relationships. This makes the problem bigger and more powerful, and it makes persons and relationships smaller and weaker and gives them pathological labels. The idea that families are fundamentally dysfunctional has negative effects. I see Betsy's family as completely capable of being another way.

JF: I'm really pleased to hear you say that. Families can be turned into objects of study from some "expert's" point of view just as individuals can, or as women can from a male's point of view.

MOD: We'll take a short break, and then we'll get to your point of view.

The Authors Speak

Our ideas here are these:

1. Batesonian work and family systems thinking can be seen as transitional (Zimmerman & Dickerson, 1994b). They opened the door, eventually, for family therapists to consider the influence of their point of view on what they experience in the room.
2. In a postmodern world, what we have are points of view and their effects. The question is not one of truth, but a question of which points of view are useful and which lead to *preferred* effects *for clients*. We worked in family systems models for years because we preferred the effects of this work over those of individual models. Now, because we don't like some of the effects on families of systems work, we work in narrative ways.
3. One effect of stories (a Batesonian metaphor would call them "restraints") on clients is that they do not notice things about themselves and others that would fit another story, one without a problem.

Warning: What follows next is a very tough section. We hope you see the importance of these ideas to our work. What you will notice is a radically different view of self, one that is created or shaped by discourse. You will also notice a radically different view of problems, also shaped by discourses or meaning systems.

Part 3

JF: I would like to comment on the relationship between views of problems and views of self in all three stories. I'm told that others will comment extensively on the third story later on.

MOD: Go ahead, then, but explain your "jargon" to us.

JF: In the era in which OF's thinking became dominant, a culturally created set of ideas (what I call "discourse"), was that all the meanings individuals created came from within themselves. These ideas about individuals led experts to believe that what persons wanted and how they behaved emanated from some "core." People's reactions were then subject to evaluation about whether they were acceptable to the majority and were "normal" or stood outside it, which meant they were "deviant," again for reasons that supposedly had to do with the nature of the individuals.

MOD: So what you are saying is that this—what you call "discourse" about individuals—actually shaped how experts thought about individuals and how individuals thought about themselves. This process must have rendered the effects of the culture invisible.

JF: Exactly, and it led to the theory that OF's group held about repression: that shaping comes from within the "nature" of the individual, instead of being created by cultural stories and experiences, which then encourage certain interpretations and certain actions. The "discourse" we have been focusing on is how the culture created a way of seeing the individual as the sole producer of meaning, rather than the culture as the creator of meaning. A word I find useful is "constituted." Persons or relationships are constituted [shaped] by the discourse or meanings that specify and influence them.

MOD: Could you refer to the cases? I'm getting lost.

JF: Yes. Susan has been recruited into a view of herself as deficient. This is not surprising, because her therapist is coming from a point of view that suggests to him that Susan *is* deficient. A microanalysis has been underway, with a resulting story evolving about her deficiencies and how they are created. How the story goes is that the problem is essential to Susan and that she lacks certain capacities to behave as other women do. The notion of "capacity" infers a contained self who is capable of some things but not others. From this point of view, it would, as OF suggests, take years to "fix."

VB: Can I interrupt here? The implication is that the view held by the therapist about what persons are and what problems are provide a relationship context that shapes the client's view. If this view is about lack of capacity and deficiency, then that invites the client to shape herself or himself in that way in the relationship.

JF: One further implication of the self's being determined by the effects of the influencing discourse is that we remain always capable of doing anything and being anyone. How we are at any time depends on what discourse is influencing us and in what context. From this point of view, we might be influenced by different discourses around different people. I believe we have all had that experience, haven't you?

MOD: I have. I guess I am influenced by a different set of ideas of how to be when I am here talking to you than I am by ones that influence me as a friend, a mother, and so on. It's all a matter of what experiences and ideas—what you call "discourses"—are shaping me in a particular situation. That gives me a number of possible versions of myself.

JF: I think you are getting it now. The next step would be to consider the effects of various cultural discourses on you. What are their invisible specifications? How do they affect you? And is the "you" they are creating one that fits your preferences? In our culture we have been taught to operate on ourselves to fit certain normalizing views.

MOD: You're losing me again!

JF: For example, Susan engages in comparison, a socially encouraged practice, and believes she falls short. She tortures herself because she is not docile, as the culture encourages women to be. She blames herself for what she experiences as a deficiency, because that is what she has been taught to do, and this makes her feel worse. She sees no difference between what the culture insists on and what she might want. She has been taught not to see this as even a distinction she can question.

MOD: I see. My point to OF about gender fits here.

JF: Yes. Also, it means acknowledging that ways women have traditionally been seen do not come from how they "are," but are the effects of cultural discourse. On a family/relationship level, Betsy and her family do the same thing. They submit to the expert description of them, which allows them to be known to the therapist and to themselves only in certain ways. They operate on themselves in ways that encourage being a family to fit certain cultural specifications. These specifications, aided by expert assertions, have, for example, determined a certain amount and kind of closeness, specific ways to communicate, certain kinds of involvement between generations, and so on. When they are not that way, they come up with pathological explanations to justify their deviance.

MOD: I can see why you prefer the view of the problem in the third story. If the problem is *self-doubt* and not the person or the relationship, this suggests that it lies in some discourse or meaning affecting the person. Separating the person from this meaning could allow the person to see other possibilities, as VB said. And since persons can and do continually create themselves, persons could seize upon these possibilities and shape themselves along more preferred lines. They could choose from whatever discourse is having the effects they want. *Lack of entitlement* brings in the level of cultural discourse and its effects, in this case for women. Would I prefer to feel greater entitlement? You bet! I could create myself this way in my relationships. This would support a new version of myself.

VB: Well said. You know, he (*looks at JF*) talks more than I do and is equally incomprehensible. You (*looks at Mod*) did very well to get that.

OF: What I'd really like to do is put him (*looking at JF*) on the couch. Not!

JF: You haven't heard anything yet . . .

The Authors Speak

Here, first, we want to ask our readers: How is this going? Are you still with us? If these ideas are hard (we find they are for us), stay with it. Maybe it will make more sense as we go.

Second, we want to respond to a colleague who read this chapter and asked, "Say again why you've decided to write this way." We really want people to *experience*, even in our writing, the effects of what we believe is a different view. We also hope it will help us better illustrate some critical differences inherent in our approach. These include a different view of problems, of self, and of points of view. We believe our thinking in these areas is radically different from traditionally held views. Our experience is that unless people understand these differences, they will have difficulty doing the work coherently, or they will do it in a way that is simply an attempt to apply technique—an attempt that we find is often likely to fail.

Our intent in presenting questions to you, our readers, and in creating the panel discussion is to demonstrate "deconstruction"— that is, to bring out the different points of view affecting the therapists in the three client stories, as well as the different effects of holding these views. These different ideas about persons, problems, and viewpoints, if understood, can also be seen to be behind what is producing our responses in the therapy room (as you will see later in this book). By using conversational forms, we are inviting you to bring your own experience to an understanding of the process. If you find yourselves more engaged than you usually do in theoretical discussions, then we have been successful. We believe that engaging your experience is critical, just as engaging the client's experience is critical to the work we do. Were you able to become part of the panel? What were you saying in response? What was behind your ideas? What experiences have you had that shaped these responses? Would you rather read straight theory?

Our preferred point of view is illustrated by the third story, because it fits with our values more closely than the others do. We both have had personal experiences in our lives that have led us to this particular point of view, that make it fit for us. For both of us, it meant a type of political resistance or a challenging of what was assumed to be true. For me (JLZ), it was in the late 1960s that along with many in that generation, I realized the truth we were being given wasn't by any reach of the imagination "true"—it was just the point of view of our government. For me (VCD), I was encouraged early in my life to have my own ideas and to express my thoughts; this encouragement came from my father, which in itself is counter to cultural discourse—a father actually inviting his daughter to have a mind of her own. This encouragement affected my later educational choices as I moved from a career as a scientist (objective truth) to one as a teacher and therapist, and continued to be interested in learning. These types of experiences have taken both of us away from therapy approaches that specify the truth of how people and families should be, or should be thought about, to those that leave the defining up to the individuals involved. In our own lives, we try to question cultural specifications by looking at their effects on us. We want clients to define their own experience in their own way and not be recruited into systems of therapeutic knowledge to understand themselves. We would like to invite our clients to question the culture's specifications by examining its effects on them. Are these leading in the directions they would prefer in their lives? Are there other, perhaps submerged, possibilities that could influence them and lead in directions they would like better?

We also have the experience of multiple selves and of creating ourselves along more preferred lines in the different relationship systems we are part of. In other words, we both live multifaceted lives in which we experience ourselves variously (as partners, parents, business associates, baseball fans, Deadheads, friends, etc.), and in which we are continually negotiating preferences within relationship contexts. So our belief in multiple selves is grounded in our own experience, and leads us also to believe in this possibility for others.

The Problem Speaks

I couldn't resist sneaking in and saying "hello" before we close. I will be out in full force shortly. Did you recognize me? It was me in all three cases. Yes, it was! I was able to hide in those first two cases in the many trees those kinds of views provide. I like it when people work that way, because I can be powerful and nobody knows it:

> *I was there, but no one named me*
> *Instead, you found some ways to blame ye.*

I can even write obnoxious poems! I really like those "self-contained" views of "ye." It helps my work when people believe they've created me themselves (or that their families have), or that once they are formed they are who they are forever. It's like I'm there for good. It has certainly been easy for me the last 100 years or so. It's harder for me to invade cultures where people live in connection with others, where their definition of themselves is embedded directly in their different relationships. With the way individuals have been isolated from others, and yet evaluated by an invisible culture, it is easy for me to work my way in. Since people in this culture believe there is one self that creates everything around them, making them feel deficient has been easy. I've even developed my powers so that I can trick people into believing their relationships are deficient. I have been greatly aided, of course, by concepts that classify and patholo-gize relationships and families (I love "enmeshed"). These concepts only follow one certain culture's norms. If you are from a different culture, then I can compare you to the dominant one and make you feel inadequate. And if you're from the dominant one, it's who you are!

Those problem fighters unmasked me in the third story, though. They named me instead of letting me hide in persons or relation-ships. They've also tried to unmask how I get therapists to play inadvertently into my hands by using systems of ideas that patholo-gize persons and relationships, making the persons even more vul-nerable to my self-doubts. Maybe I got back at the authors a little, though; they didn't admit that I was there, the same in all three stories, in order to make all three seem different. They just changed the name of the person in each case. How does knowing that affect you?

Anyway, I'll be around, and so will many of my close friends, associates, and work companions. Here I come!

CHAPTER 2

If Problems Talked

The Problem Speaks

I'm back! . . . and I've got some stories for you.

The Authors Speak

We'd like to interrupt the problem briefly because we don't want him to have a bad effect on you, the reader. He can be unsettling. We don't want you to be unsettled, but we do want to unsettle the commonly held notions of what a problem is—at least the usual notions that have evolved over the last 100 years or so. Given that we have all been recruited into these notions by the general culture as well as by the culture of psychotherapy, we want to do something dramatic to begin to shift your point of view in a different direction, similar to how ours has shifted.

   We are also a bit afraid (no—terrified) that you will see what we do as "technique" (some of you might read Chapters 3 to 5 that way), and we want to give you an experience of seeing the problem as separate from the person. We see the problem this way, not only because we have found that this is useful and has good effects, but because our theory views the problem as existing in the meaning systems that influence people. Our theory also suggests that this meaning is largely shaped by our culture. Therefore, you will notice that the problem tells you about various cultural "discourses," or meaning systems, that seem to support problems. These problems influence us, our colleagues, and our clients; at least the names and descriptions we use seem to fit for the people we talk with in our lives. By presenting definitions of these problem names as they might appear in a "postmodern dictionary" (in which problems define themselves!), we are indicating that we think of them as points of view that are socially constructed and that give meaning to our experience. They are not meant as truths.

We also bring in comments from clients so you can see the effects of the problem on their experience. (You will meet these clients again later in this book. They are clients we actually saw in therapy, but their identities have been disguised. The versions of their experiences and comments we give in this chapter are fictional.) They have felt like victims because . . .

The Problem Speaks

Truth. Victims. I like that. Can I talk now?

VICTIM 1: CINDY

The Problem Speaks

I found it really easy to pick on Cindy. She came from a family where everyone had such strong wills. If I can get hold of this strength and make it support me, what pain I can create! What made Cindy even more vulnerable was that her family lived in a land where expectations run rampant, where there were many specifications for how to be acceptable. I make use of these oppressive expectations to tyrannize people further because of their failure to live up to these expectations. Of course, if there are expectations, there must be *evaluation.*

Evaluation: I am powerful indeed. You know me, don't you! You experience my judgments, my torment, my pain. I have grown very powerful lately because there has been more space made for me in everyone's life. When people are encouraged to live their lives according to a lot expectations and specifications, they experience me through these.[1]

I imagine some of you must be familiar with this demon. When *evaluation* has this kind of family strength to work with, look out!

[1]Authors' note: This and all the other definitions in this chapter come from our imaginary *New Postmodern, Social Constructionist, Narrative Dictionary of Meaning.*

Among other things, **evaluation** loves to encourage **self-doubt.** These are two of my favorite forms, and I made sure Cindy experienced them.

How about you? Don't you feel me, too? When things don't work out well in a session, can't I get a hold on you? After all, you're the expert—what went wrong? Can you feel me take one of your strengths (such as determination) and use it to make you feel more **doubt**? I make you experience **doubt** and **evaluation,** with a really determined effort to make you feel bad.

The Authors Speak

Can we get back to Cindy? And stop bothering the readers.

The Problem Speaks

No! I'm having too much fun! . . . Anyway, I first got a hold on Cindy when she was a teenager. My most noticeable effect on her was to make her believe that to be worthwhile, she had to get boys to like her. This encouraged her to follow their direction in most matters. As you might guess, this did not please her parents. Of course, this allowed me to put great strain on their relationship.

Now, getting Cindy to operate this way was easy because she is a woman. I just bring in another version of myself, **lack of entitlement.**

Lack of entitlement: You women know me—yes, you do.
I take all your choices from you.
Put husbands, children, others first.
Otherwise **guilt** will make you feel worse.
Give up yourselves to them, I say.
Or be condemned to suffer each day.
After all, you matter less.
Be good girls and pass the test.

With **evaluation** and **lack of entitlement** squeezing Cindy, and with all that strong will to work with, it was easy for me to have **self-doubt** come in and take over her life. I do have to admit that we had help, but I'm sure that will come up later. Anyway, given what we got her to focus on in her life (boys and not performing at school), given the trouble we started between her and her parents, and given the increasing amount of discomfort we got her to experience, it was, as I said, easy to begin to direct her life more fully after high school. At this point, we had erased a good deal of her own sense of authority, and encouraged her parents to take authority and give direction. In fact, we left them no choice; they were loving parents who cared about their daughter and wanted to help.

We thus created a direction of steps that weren't Cindy's, along with the inevitable failures that followed. We bombarded her with *evaluation* through comparison. Comparison is my favorite tool! Through this kind of torture, people experience failure even though they haven't even considered whether these general specifications fit for them. Because Cindy was not living up to specifications around her, *self-doubt* became so overwhelming that all she experienced was despair and pressure. She and her family had no chance! What choice did she have? She went to therapy.

Cindy Speaks

It's very interesting. Very interesting. What I remember from when I was a teenager was doing things I didn't feel good about. I just did them. They seemed like the things to do. I don't know. . . . Pretty soon I was doing things out of school I shouldn't do and wasn't doing things in school I should do, and this became how my life was. I guess there were things I was supposed to want, but they began to seem impossible for me. I never did the right thing. I never handled anything very well. I tried to do what my boyfriends wanted, but I just began feeling worse and worse. I tried to do what my parents wanted, but I always failed. I began to realize I was incapable. Otherwise, things would be different. Just because something was wrong with me, though, this didn't take away the *pressure* that began to overwhelm me as a young adult to do things normal people did. I began to have a harder and harder time making decisions. I didn't know what I wanted. Every possible choice seemed wrong, or I would feel I couldn't handle it anyway. I felt worse and worse and couldn't take any steps that would help me be like others—in school, or at work, or with friends or dates. I supposed that if I was normal, I could do it—I could figure out what the steps would be. I began to wonder if life was worth it. There was so much *pain* and *pressure.* During this time I got sent to therapy.

The Problem Speaks

What I did to her was get her to know herself only through me. She can't manage her own life. She's helpless now.

Cindy's Mom Speaks

My God, I tried to help. Look what happened to my daughter. She wasn't always like this. I felt responsible. I tried and tried to get her to do things that would be good for her. She wouldn't do them without our pushing. But it was so draining. She would carry on and on, and I'd feel helpless and responsible. I was so afraid. Maybe she wasn't normal. Maybe she didn't want to try. Maybe she couldn't. I'm so tired.

The Problem Speaks

Look what I did to her and to their relationship! Listen to them:

CINDY'S DAD: We just wanted her to be normal.

CINDY'S MOM: We sent her to therapy.

CINDY: It was obvious to me my parents thought I wasn't normal. Why else would they do what they did? I wanted to be more independent, but I couldn't. That's why I leaned on them.

The Authors Speak

We hope you are getting a feel for seeing the problem as cultural discourse and for talking with clients from their experience. This is clearly different from filtering client descriptions through various personality, developmental, or therapy theories. What you hear is different when you privilege the client's experience and understand it as an effect of the problem. And, no, this is not Kansas.

HOW ABOUT SOME "NORMAL" WRITING FOR A CHANGE?[2]

Normal: Follows cultural specifications. Fits into dominant majority. Usually done without thinking. May or may not be appreciated, or enjoyable, or helpful, or anything else.

We are providing examples that make this point: Every story influencing a therapist about what a problem is, what a person is, and what therapy is has real effects on what is said, what is noticed, or what is done in the room. You have seen that these stories have real effects on how therapists experience themselves, on how they experience their clients, and ultimately, on how the clients experience themselves. Stories form the background against which everything is seen and interpreted, whether

---

[2]In later chapters, "normal writing" will be a regular feature. We won't mark it. After all, it's "normal," and so only other things need to be marked. (It's like "white privilege.")

these are personal stories for individuals, therapy stories for therapists, or cultural stories for all of us.

As people in the culture, either we are complying with the way the culture tells us to act, or we are forced to justify our differences. Often this justification involves that we notice what the culture calls "deficiencies" in ourselves or in those around us. Rarely do we justify how we do things through stating our own personal preferences. If we did, we'd act the way we want to or the way we think is right, regardless of the circumstances. Instead, we make up stories, influenced by our cultural store of stories and also by psychology, to help us organize this justification. Here are some examples:

1. "I'm a failure because of my [(a) terrible childhood, (b) overinvolved mother, (c) deficient behaviors, (d) whatever]. That is why I can't [(a) be cool, (b) work a standard job, (c) go to school more, (d) whatever]." We don't say, "I'm choosing to do these things because I want to [i.e., I don't want to act in traditional ways] or because the culture makes it difficult for me [i.e., I'm not cut from an average-person mold]."

2. "We can't help but act this way, because our daughter is unable to function. Maybe we were overprotective [or whatever]. We know we should give her space [or whatever]. We'd like to do [something], but we are doing [something else] instead. We can't help it." (See example later in this chapter.)

3. "I'd like to act kindly toward my partner, but she is acting aggressively. I know what she is doing is wrong, and I know I would *like* to act right, so she must have bad intentions. Therefore, I must protect myself and can't act right, or act the way I want." (Here "right" and "wrong" are determined by expectations about gender, such as "A woman shouldn't be aggressive." A story might be made up about the woman's family of origin to explain her problem.)

As Michael White (1991) has pointed out, stories affect what we notice (e.g., instances of failure) or how we interpret what we notice (e.g., "She's not normal" or "She's aggressive"). Jerome Bruner (1990) has commented that stories are often used by persons to explain the difference between what the culture expects and what persons are doing instead. In this way, people can justify what they are doing—by saying they are restrained by mitigating circumstances (e.g., a problem) and pointing to the imagined intentionality of others as limiting factors. This is equally true for therapists, whose stories may have them listening to the clients' stories more from the standpoint of their (the therapists') interpretations, understandings, and emphases than from the clients'. After all, clients need help, so the therapists must find out what's "wrong." If clients didn't need help, they wouldn't act this way. So therapists must do _____.

Do narrative therapists just ignore these "things" that other therapists see? No, what exists for narrative therapists is completely different, given that they have a different story. What exist for them are the experience and meaning of their clients (see the problem's comments and Cindy's story, above). How do narrative therapists justify this departure from the normative processes of pathologizing persons or families instead of problems? They prefer to support a story that casts problems in a bad light and addresses the issue of cultural effects instead. As you will see in later chapters, this is accomplished in many ways. Here we are addressing our refusal to participate in the usual therapy practices that we all have been encouraged to see as "truths."

Are you with us? Or is some problem interfering?

Problem: A meaning system that interferes with one's preferred direction. Located in the culture. Some-thing unpleasant. Any-thing that affects one in undesirable ways.

If a problem is interfering, what would you call it? Do you like serious or funny names? One reader has suggested *feelings of ignorance*—you know, the thing that gets you when you read about new ideas. This problem has certainly interfered with us from time to time. Or perhaps it's *tension.* We would understand this *tension* as an effect of normative ideas in the mental health culture—ideas that also affect how we experience ourselves as therapists and the work that we do. If *tension* between our different views is beginning to affect you, it could have you creating stories about us and why we do what we do that isn't "normal." It could create a process in which the more you read, the more you construct your meanings as different from ours, with the story that justifies your position becoming thicker and thicker. If we were to get feedback more directly from you, we could just as easily be swept up in this process. This happens with people and with families as well. As problems get bigger, meaning is less and less coproduced or shared.

Now, back to our other ways of writing . . .

INTERVIEW WITH THE PROBLEM (SORT OF LIKE INTERVIEW WITH THE VAMPIRE)

The Authors Speak

Why a vampire? Are problems mean? Are they evil? We had this debate with some colleagues. We originally wrote the problem as even more obnoxious than you might experience it now (if you can believe that). Some readers felt uncomfortable, so we toned him down. Yet, in many cases, our experience and that of our colleagues is that the problem is actually worse than we have presented him here, or at least usually pretty bad. Our colleague Stephen Madigan, told us he tried playing *anorexia,* and the feedback he got from the Anti-Anorexia League of Vancouver was that *anorexia* was much meaner and crueler and more evil than any of us can imagine. Yet we've also had the experience with other problems that they spoke to us in more subtle ways. How would you characterize the way a problem affects you? As a devil? Or a trickster? Or perhaps a questioner?

AUTHORS: You've reviewed in general how you managed to take over Cindy and interfere with her relationships, and she has shared her experience of losing herself to you. What we want to know is this: How did you become, in such a coherent way, something that defined who she was as a person?

PROBLEM: Well, it's the stories you tell about yourself that define who you are, right?

AUTHORS: Explain to our readers what you mean by "stories."

PROBLEM: Why should I explain it to them? They won't get it.

AUTHORS: Are you afraid they'll use these ideas against you?

PROBLEM: Against me?! Ha, ha.

AUTHORS: Then go ahead.

PROBLEM: Well, okay. I'm too powerful to stop. Take Cindy. When she had some bad experiences as a teenager, it was easier to connect them to other events in her life to form a "plot," like *failure* or *inadequacy* or *self-doubt.* These events, selected to fit the current situation, got strung together in a sequence, which led to the ultimate meaning Cindy gave to this evolving plot line—*self-doubt.* Well, anyone could see what it "meant"—that she wasn't normal. Because I am powerful, because I am supported by practices encouraged by people like yourselves, I can create this backward search that leads to an organization of a theme, which then takes over a person's life. I continue to move through time, adding more events from the past, creating new events in the future, dominating and directing a person so that all that is done, all that is noticed, is through me.

AUTHORS: (*Aside—muttering*)

PROBLEM: What did you say?

AUTHORS: I said, you seem to really enjoy "dominating and directing" a person's life so that how the person experiences things is organized by you, interpreted by you, given meaning by you.

PROBLEM: Yes, I do!

AUTHORS: This story idea . . . you didn't invent it.

PROBLEM: I didn't have to. People have been organizing their experience in story form since the beginning of time.

AUTHORS: Let's go back to Cindy. You've told us how you co-opted various actions in a way that began to mean something about her, to her. You then brought up other events and organized them into a sequence that gave her experience even more meaning. In other words, you created an action plot line in this story (a "landscape of action"), which in turn created a way Cindy began to think about herself—a description of herself that she began to think of *as* herself.

PROBLEM: Yes! Yes! Yes!

AUTHORS: But aren't people guided by more than this, by bigger things they think about, like their goals in life, their intentions (a "landscape of consciousness")? Like why they do what they do? What about a level of consciousness in their personal stories?

PROBLEM: Well, for example, it was quite easy to convince Cindy that any goals she had weren't realistic. Maybe they weren't hers, but only other people's goals for her. Maybe she had no goals. Maybe she was confused. And, if she made any effort, usually in response to another's encouragement, I would attack and make her feel bad, or put pressure on her, or make her not know how to handle it. As for intentions, just by having her not try, or try and fail, she had to begin to assume her intentions were not positive. Maybe she didn't want to succeed. Maybe she was afraid to go forward and so she didn't or wouldn't or couldn't. Maybe she didn't want to grow up. Maybe her parents . . .

AUTHORS: We get the picture. Could the same process be used against you—helping people notice other events, string them together to form new meaning, new versions of the self, noticing other intentions—you know, something like reauthoring . . .

PROBLEM: Reauthoring! Ha! Just try it.

AUTHORS: We want to ask Cindy and her parents some questions.

CINDY, HER PARENTS, AND THE PROBLEM

MOM: You know, listening to this makes me so mad. For so long I thought the problem was Cindy. I thought I had failed. Look what that problem did to us!

CINDY: I felt so bad. I knew what I was supposed to want to do, but because I thought I was incapable, I couldn't do it. I didn't even really know what I wanted anyway.

MOM: We knew how we wanted to treat her. We also knew we should trust her, but we couldn't, because of the problem.

AUTHORS: (*Aside, to readers*) We hope this is a good example of the justification process discussed earlier in the chapter—how this process leads people to do things that inadvertently support the problem.

PROBLEM: (*Aside*) Right on!

MOM: As a mother, I've been told I am responsible for my kids. How could I have done anything but try to make something different happen? Eventually I decided I must be incapable, and maybe a therapist could take over.

AUTHORS: (*To Mom*) Tell us about therapy.

MOM: We didn't know much about the first therapist. In seven years he wouldn't talk to us. The next one talked to us, but we felt blamed. Then I really felt responsible.

CINDY: I went in and talked. He didn't say a lot. I felt scrutinized. I felt evaluated. Occasionally he would say something that related to why I did things. By that time I knew I wasn't normal, and so what he said helped me understand *why* I wasn't normal. It gave me so much more to think about, considering myself in this way. Meanwhile, I got further behind in life, and felt worse and worse. My next therapist gave me lots of suggestions, which I needed because I was incapable. I followed some of his suggestions, but the pain was still there. I could really see how I needed another person to direct me. But what I did never seemed to work out. At 31 years of age, I felt things were hopeless.

PROBLEM: This works for me.

AUTHOR: Please be quiet.

CINDY: Who are you talking to?

AUTHORS: Never mind.

The Authors Speak

We hope, through the way we have written, that you, the reader, have a sense of our story—a meaning system about how to think in therapy that we have found quite useful. This way of thinking has affected our work and our personal lives. Later we share some possibilities about how to do some things to fight problems, along lines that are consistent with the way we understand problems and people, and that reflects our point of view. You may wonder about our use of the problem talking. We see it as reflecting our view of problems existing in meaning systems that affect people. We wonder how that is working for you. Does it help you understand this viewpoint better? Does it . . . ?

PROBLEM: I'm not done yet.

AUTHORS: What do you mean?

PROBLEM: I have more examples I'd like to give.

AUTHORS: You mean more stories about the ways you have linked together aspects of people's experience to create stories about people, about relationships, and about families that have unpleasant effects? And more demonstrations of the use of practices of therapy (done by caring therapists, no less) to help support you?

PROBLEM: Why blame me for that last point? I didn't make up the idea that there are things wrong with people, with families. Many therapies involve making up stories to account for why I am around. Such therapies are done by experts with more power than me; they are very engaging.

AUTHORS: But those therapies are well meant and have good effects. You don't.

PROBLEM: Well, I want to tell you some more about my efforts.

AUTHORS: Go ahead, but we're going after you with stories of our own—stories about helping people notice other possible, more preferred stories in their lives.

VICTIMS 2 AND 3: BRENDA AND EDDIE

The Problem Speaks

I could tell lots of stories about picking on couples. I do this countless times daily. After all, no two people agree on everything, and most people don't agree about the big things (you know, money, sex, relatives). And once they don't agree, I can get a problem pattern going just by employing the typical ways men and women have been encouraged to respond, such as men wanting to withdraw under stress and women wanting to affiliate more. Each does the one thing that maddens the other the most. Then, because this gender stuff is invisible, each begins to make up reasons why the other is doing what she or he is doing, and they aren't nice reasons. Throw in the power differential that men have been used to, and—pow!—I start to get bigger every day. It's not very different in same-sex couples, because there are always habitual reactions I can use to get each partner to make up stories about the other. And who says they're not also influenced by the gender stuff? Plus, with them, there are all those effects of being marginalized to help keep the pressure on.

Let me tell you, then, a story about a couple I've bothered for over 20 years. Now that's an accomplishment! How does the song go? "Brenda and Eddie met in high school. . . ." Anyway, you know the script. Brenda got pregnant, Eddie did the "right thing," and they lived unhappily every after. Brenda tried desperately to please Eddie and make the relationship and the family work—after all, it was "her job." (**Lack of entitlement** in action!) Eddie did what he knew how to do—work hard at his business. He also went out drinking with the boys and played a lot of basketball. (My colleague, *lack of responsibility*!)

Lack of responsibility: I'm good at getting you not to think about others. What I want counts, and I make you think only what you want counts. I get you to refuse to acknowledge the needs or experience of others. I get you married to your work instead of to your wife and family. I make you addicted to "rightness"—only mine and yours.

Over the years, as we (**lack of entitlement** and **lack of responsibility**) got more and more between Brenda and Eddie, they spent less and less time together. Brenda was overwhelmed by despair and negative self-evaluation. After all, she was supposed to make this relationship work and she hadn't done so.

Eddie took his drinking lifestyle more seriously. After all, what else was a guy to do? Now here were two very nice, caring people overrun by distance and getting into self-destructive feelings and habits. Affairs began to make sense. Brenda tried individual therapy; this turned out to be great for Brenda's affirmation but bad for the relationship. At the moment, I'm about to end the family life of two people who care about each other, as well as ruin things for their three kids. Could I be—*Satan*?!

Brenda Speaks

I tried so hard. For years I tried, blaming myself for not being good enough. If only I was this enough or that enough, he would be more involved. If I could be a better wife, then I wouldn't have to push so hard to get his attention. But I thought I was unable to be what he needed. Then I gave up. I'd had it with his partying and his lack of responsibility. I stopped seeing myself as the problem and started seeing him as the problem. If he cared for me, about me, about the kids, he would be more present, more talkative. So I began to believe he must not care. I began to do things separately, even though I preferred relationship. I had an affair. He didn't care, right?

The Problem Speaks

See what I mean? I was invisible, whether I influenced her view of herself or her view of Eddie's intentions, or whether I employed gender-trained responses.

Eddie Speaks

It's funny to call this "Eddie Speaks." For many years I didn't speak. I didn't even know I had anything to say. I loved Brenda. I was so young. I took care of her and the kids financially. That's what I was supposed to do. With the guys . . . we'd play ball and then have some beers. I was comfortable. Today I would say I felt a sense of connection. With Brenda . . . I tried to be in the relationship the way I thought she wanted. Eventually, I believed it was my problem— drinking and not doing what she wanted. But at first I just wished she'd stop bugging me, that she would be less needy. I never for one moment thought to wonder what I wanted from the relationship. Guys don't think about those things, do they?

The Problem Speaks

I did it to him, too!

VICTIMS 4, 5, 6, AND 7: JOHNNY AND HIS FAMILY

The Problem Speaks

> *Kids, let me tell you what's wrong with kids today.*
> *Kids, they're labeled **ADHD**, and it won't go away.*

You know what I love about **ADHD**? I can exploit what exists in "expert" descriptions and use it to make kids feel bad and parents feel hopeless. Sure, kids experience **hyperness.** Sure, people's brain wiring is different, leading some to greater expansiveness and/or fewer focusing abilities. But I didn't set up schools to privilege rote learning and detail work. Sure, I exploit the situation. These kids think *they're* inadequate because they don't function. I make sure they notice their "dysfunction" and not notice the advantages their open minds give them. Throw in a dose of **expectations,** especially with middle- or upper-middle-class parents, and they're down on the kid in a New York minute.

By age 10, Johnny's life was dominated by me. He had been inspected, rejected, and dejected for years. His older brother was just the kind of child his parents wanted; he did well at school, had conversations with them about serious matters, and had similar habits (whether about food, independence, leisure, or whatever). His parents were successful, affluent, and caring people. It wasn't very hard to take Johnny's inclinations and make them seem offensive, especially when combined with his failure to function in a manner **expectations** told the parents he ought to. His mother had to fight to hold on to liking him, because when **hyperness** was around it got her on the run. **Resentments** took care of the older brother, because of the time the parents had to devote to his brother, because of the demands his brother put on him, and because he didn't have the kind of relationship he wanted with his brother. His father was bugged by the **hyperness,** but mostly at night, and only when he was home. There went the family life they all wanted. Listen to them.

JOHNNY: I don't know; I just get hyper. I don't mean to annoy people. I just can't help it. It's a strong urge I can't control. I can't imagine what I want or how things in my life will be. I wish my brother would play with me more.

JOHNNY'S DAD: I care about Johnny and play with him, but I wish this insane behavior would stop. It's our responsibility to make him a functional person, isn't it? But he's not normal.

JOHNNY'S BROTHER: I sometimes feel Johnny does this on purpose, to annoy me. I'm afraid to do anything with him, because he might be hyper and I can't handle it. I wanted a brother I could do things with.

JOHNNY'S MOM: I pray for freedom. I can't help but react to the annoying things he does—sounds, gestures, around-the-clock demands on me. His refusal to go where we want or do what we want holds us all hostage. I feel too guilty to get a sitter so we can do things. I can't seem to set limits on him. Nothing works. It's like he wants to sabotage our whole family. I'm so very angry.

The Problem Speaks

Despite Johnny's having some deficiencies, I can still make the others think he's out to ruin things. And despite his having some interesting special abilities, I can get them focused on his deficiencies.

VICTIMS 8, 9, AND 10:
SHARON AND HER PARENTS

The Problem Speaks

I'm on a roll now. Let me tell you how I get to families when kids get to be teenagers. I fill kids' heads with how they're supposed to rebel, to be jerks to their parents, to start hanging out with other kids their parents don't like (and they're not even sure *they* like!), and to question the values and beliefs they have grown up with (even though they think they're not really such bad ideas). But I get in there and take on the role of *sneakiness* and try to create *distance* between parents and kids. After all, it needs to happen. It's just the first step in *separation,* and we all know that's a cultural necessity for teenagers and parents.

Separation: A necessary "developmental" task. Considered the "rule" for adolescence. Works hand in hand with "identity formation." Ignorant of cross-cultural information. Creates one "truth" despite widespread lack of interest in it. (See also *normal.*)

The next thing I do is drench the parents with a heavy dose of *fear* and *worry,* knowing that the slightest thing their kids do that's "off course" (read "not normal") will make them vulnerable to my power. Notice how I keep changing what's "normal" and what's "not normal." I trick parents into seeing whatever their kids do as "wrong," and then I tell them that's just what happens when kids get to be teenagers.

So, I create a strain or a *rift* in the relationship. By then it's all over. The kids are gone. The parents think they have done a bad job. They only hope that someone else can save their kids—a therapist, a teacher, college (not a boyfriend or girlfriend). I totally disempower them. Then I use *guilt* to really get them to obsess about their decisions. They end up making life miserable for their kids and for themselves. I get them to disconnect. Listen to Sharon and her parents:

SHARON: They don't know. I'm doing my thing. I'm making new friends, trying things out. Who cares about grades, anyway? Besides, I like this guy, even if he does make me a little scared. I don't much like having to sneak around, though. I mean, sometimes I wonder if my parents aren't right. I wonder if I don't agree with them. How could that be? I really need to move out. Then they'll know I can make it on my own.

MOM: I don't want to have to monitor her every action, but she has changed so much since she went to high school. We don't know her any more. Have we lost her? Is it my fault?

DAD: I know this stuff happens. I have grown kids from my first marriage. They just do their own thing, and, unfortunately, it's mostly disappointing. I had hoped it would be different with her. But it's not. I guess that's just the way it is. Maybe she'll learn when she's on her own.

SHARON: I feel so alone.

The Problem Speaks

I am getting between them. I have convinced them that this process is inevitable. So I can be present and bring them pain, but they think they can do nothing about it.

The Authors Speak

Well, he's had his say, but after all, *we* are writing this book, and we and our clients will tell the ends of these stories. In the chapters that follow, we discuss some ways of talking with each other to get him on the run. And we continue to try to make it interesting for you. Are you still there?

CHAPTER 3

Finding the Enemy
and It's Not Us

THE PROBLEM BY ANY OTHER NAME

When the problem came into their lives, they were all sleeping. But it came nonetheless. Gary, at least, knew it must have. Too much had changed. Their world was topsy-turvey, even though everything still looked much the same. At any rate, it made him feel like his house was full of strangers. Whatever connection they had seemed completely gone. He carefully watched his wife, Judy. Although she did the same things daily—got up and went to work, cooked dinner in the evening—he was wary. He couldn't quite put his finger on what was wrong, but there were crease lines in her forehead that hadn't seemed to be there before. And she was very curt, short with him where she had been pleasant in the past. They had difficulties in their relationship like anyone else, he supposed, but it was such a treat to be with her. They seemed to be able to talk about their problems, as Gary and his first wife had not been. And in general, he knew she respected him—and vice versa. What was wrong now? It wasn't quite that the respect was gone, but something seemed to have moved in and taken over. Whatever it was, it had taken away their closeness, their ability to talk things out; she wasn't even admitting anything was wrong. But he knew things weren't right.

Mostly the havoc the problem had wrought was noticeable with Sharon, their daughter. Gary hardly ever saw her any more. She would come home from school and go to her room. At least that's what Judy said, because by the time he came home she had disappeared. She would only eat with them if they made her;

she either said she wasn't hungry, or picked up something else or ate a snack as soon as she got home. When she did deign to show up at the family dinner table, she scowled, sulked, answered any queries with monosyllables, and usually left the table early and went back to her room. Gary suspected she was on the phone a lot, because he could hear her talking in a low voice.

What scared Gary the most was that this devastation seemed to be invisible, but it also felt to him like it had happened before, maybe in just this way—a sudden disaster that left wreckage in its path, but that was silent, invisible, and unstoppable. A similar problem had hit his family in his first marriage; it had destroyed his relationship with his wife and taken away his children. But he couldn't quite put his finger on how it had happened. How could something so devastating sneak up on him this way? However it did, the problem took away relationships, connection, and closeness. It left only itself, a huge cavernous rift, behind.

One afternoon when he was at work, trying very hard to keep the fear that had settled into his very being from infecting his work life, the phone rang with a call from his wife. "Meet me at the hospital," Judy said. "Sharon has been in a car accident."

Gary's heart leapt into his throat and lodged there. "Is she all right?"

"I don't know, but I think so. I knew something awful was going to happen."

How did she know something awful was going to happen, he thought, as he raced toward the hospital. What did she know? Why hadn't she talked to him? How had their lives gotten so rattled? Was that why those worry lines had appeared on her forehead?

When he arrived at the emergency room, he found that Sharon was fine, at least physically. She seemed a little shaken up, but she still had that scowl on her face. "What happened?" he asked.

"Nothing, really."

"How can that be? Your mother said you were in an accident."

"She exaggerates."

Judy interrupted. "The school called. She took off in a car with one of the boys in the group she has been hanging out with. They think he was on something."

Sharon's scowl deepened. "They're so nosy. He was perfectly normal."

Suddenly the problem was in the room. It was only because they were in a hospital waiting area that their voices did not become shouts and angry invectives. Gary struggled with how to escape this powerful force. Where was this problem taking them? How had it become this huge rift between them, ruining their lives?

A week later, they were all in a pleasant-looking therapy room with a woman who was calmly asking questions. Where was the problem? Had it followed them, preceded them? And what kind of therapist was this person? She was talking about **worry** and *fear* and **sneakiness** as if these were real entities.

The crease lines that Gary had seen on Judy's face, her taciturn behavior, her shortness, were talked about as effects of *worry.* Gary's own distress, nervousness, and feeling like walking on eggs were seen as by-products of *fear.* And Susan was even agreeing that *sneakiness* had gotten her to shut herself up in her room, not talk to her parents, and act uninterested and sulky. This therapist talked about these things as enemies to their well-being; she noticed how they had stolen away their closeness as family members, and had led to an even bigger culprit, which she called a *rift.* What was she getting at?

What interesting questions she was asking. Gary commented that he really didn't like thinking that he had lost Sharon forever, although the idea that a *rift* had gotten between them all made him think so. He actually would rather think of Sharon as continuing to have a close relationship with him—one in which they could talk about her plans, her ideas, and he could share his thinking with her. He heard Judy say that she was so upset by *worry* that she had decided to put the clamps on Sharon's plans and question all her requests. Gary wondered why he and Judy hadn't talked about it more. Then he thought that perhaps it was because of the *rift.*

Sharon said she didn't much like the *sneakiness;* it was "stupid." It took her away from a sense of mutual trust with her parents. It kept her from being able to share things with them, and she missed that. Gary wondered if she experienced the *rift,* too. Then she said that once she had been out with friends and had wanted to go somewhere else with them; they said, "Just come along. Don't call your folks. They'll say 'no.' " And, in spite of their pleadings, she decided to call. Gary was astounded. How did she do that?

He thought about a car ride he and Sharon had had recently. They had talked about her thoughts, her plans. He had refrained from giving advice, just listening and enjoying their time together, and she had shared her ideas with him. That was counter to the *rift,* wasn't it? How had that happened?

Judy told about what she was thinking on the occasion when Sharon called. *Fear* and *worry* had made things so difficult. For a while at least, she'd decided to "lighten up." "After all," she said, "I really had to trust that Sharon would make good decisions in the long run. If I never let her make decisions for herself, how could she ever learn what would be better decisions for her and what not?"

They weren't too sure how they reconnected. The *rift* had tricked them into thinking they were completely destroyed. But somehow they were beginning to reclaim what they wanted for themselves. Gary knew there was still work to be done, but in the room they had started to explore how the problem had tried to take over their lives. They were beginning to pay attention to what they really wanted, for themselves, for their relationships. When they returned home, Gary heard Sharon and Judy both giving sighs of relief (mirroring his own) and Sharon saying, "There's no place like home!" But he thought, "This place we're in isn't Kansas, either!"

THE FAMILY AND THE PROBLEM

The problem preceded the family as they came into the therapy room. There was an evident strain between the parents and their daughter. It showed up as anger in both parents' voices, **worry** and *fear* in Judy, and *fear* and *frustration* in Gary. It manifested itself in Sharon by her looking down and away, refusing to talk, and finally saying, "They're worried about nothing; it's no big deal." This strain, which then began to be discussed as a *rift* in the relationship, was telling Judy that she was losing her daughter and that she no longer had any control over her, now that she was a freshman in high school. The *rift* told her that Sharon was more interested in her peers—friends who were not of her mother's choosing—and was more influenced by them than she was by her mother's ideas. It also told her that she would have to clamp down more, refuse to let her daughter go out, monitor her actions, screen her phone calls, and check out her choice of friends. It had gotten her to think that perhaps she should begin to pay closer attention to Sharon's education—make sure she did her homework, check her assignments, and find out whether she was attending all her classes. In short, the *rift* got her to worry increasingly. For Gary, the *rift* told him that his daughter couldn't be trusted. (After all, he had experience with teenagers; having adult children from another marriage, he knew that they strayed easily from the path.) The *rift* was influencing him to make sure Sharon knew the rules and obeyed them—rules about curfew, where she was, who she was with; rules about homework and chores; rules about the use of alcohol and drugs. The *rift* got him to be angry at Sharon and frustrated when it seemed she wouldn't listen.

The *rift* influenced Sharon differently. It got her to become more secretive, to tell her parents little, to scowl, to look away, to not show up, to hide in her room. It got her to sneak around, to lie about where she was going and who she was with. It got her to tell them not to worry about her schoolwork, even when she herself was worried about her falling grades. It tricked her into thinking they didn't really care about her, so it got her to confide more in friends. It even sometimes got her to hang out with people she wasn't sure she liked, because the *rift* told her that her parents didn't really care much anyway.

The Authors Speak

As we continue to describe the work we do with the persons who consult with us, we will also comment on our thinking about the process. We want to make transparent our thinking about our thinking, and to do this by situating our ideas in our experience. We plan to stress what we have found to be important in this work. We hope, then, that "The Authors Speak" will be another opportunity for you to access your own experience about what is important as you read about the work.

As far as *rifts* go, this is what the *rift* seemed to be up to, and how we—the family and I (VCD), the therapist in this case—ended up talking about it. The *rift* came to represent the meaning system affecting the family.

The Problem Speaks

I am very powerful. I don't know, though, what I think about being called *rift.*

MORE "NORMAL" WRITING[1]

How did everyone come to construct the problem in the therapy room as a *rift*? What did each parent say? What did the daughter say? What was the therapist thinking? How did the therapist respond? We have talked about how we view the problem as a meaning system embedded in the cultural (sociopolitical) context. However, what was the meaning system, or the narrative, of influence on this family? How do we decide to respond to a relationship problem, such as the one we have described as the focus in this case, and when do we focus instead on a specific behavior or attitude—for example, in a family, what the parents might describe as something their son or daughter is doing (or not doing) or thinking? Why not focus on the pattern, such as the one that became noticeable in this family (that of *controlling* on the part of the parents and *sneakiness* on the part of the daughter)? Finally, how does the therapy go? What are the steps?

This chapter illustrates the clinical process, beginning with the first phone call and the decision about who should come to the initial session. It shows what kind of thinking occurs in the therapy room and how we co-construct problems and their effects. We comment on what gets "externalized" (i.e., behaviors, patterns, and/or cultural or personal narratives) and when. We hope that a map for therapy, including a step-by-step description of the work, will emerge, with an emphasis on the "unmasking" of cultural "truths." We and others who are enthusiastic about these ideas see such "unmasking" as crucial to this work.

---

[1]This is our last reference to "normal." We're confident that you'll be able to tell when the writing is "normal" and when it isn't!

The Authors Speak

What we hope to stress here, again, is that our map is influenced by our theoretical position regarding problems and persons. Therefore, we give our attention to the *clients'* description of their experience.

STARTING OUT

The Problem Speaks

I put looks of concern and worry on the faces of the parents, and a scowl on the young person's face. Often I have a teenager refusing to come into the room—staying in the car or yelling, "I won't go in there!" from the waiting room. Sometimes I can even jump over phone lines, putting anger in the parent's voice, or tears and frustration.

Our introduction to the problem usually comes through the first phone call. When the *rift* took over this family, the mother, Judy, called. The *rift* became noticeable when their daughter, Sharon, was in a car accident in which she was lucky to be alive; she had been a passenger in the car with a friend from school, who was stoned. She was 15 years old and a freshman in high school. The parents were scared. To them, this was a very frightening indication of the bad direction their daughter had started to go in, including a dropoff in grades, a certain secretiveness, and hanging out with what they considered less than desirable friends.

Often parents ask us to see their teenagers, with the idea being to "set them straight" or "turn them around" or "fix them." When the *rift* took over this family, it gave the parents the idea that their daughter needed "fixing." In many cases, a useful response could be something like the following: "When problems come into people's lives, they tend to affect several people. Who do you think is affected by this problem, besides your daughter?" Usually the caller answers, "Oh, we all are!" We then ask whether it would be possible for everyone who is affected by the problem to come in together, at least for the first meeting.

What we are interested in is how the "problem" is affecting not only the young person, but also the others in her or his life. In families with adolescents and younger children, we believe that the problem must most certainly be affecting others in the household. For example, *rifts* encourage parents into certain explanations of their children's behavior; these explanations in turn encourage parents to respond in ways that are often counter to the ways they might prefer for the growing up of their children. As the examples in Chapter 2 demonstrate, these ways of responding can inadvertently support the problem. As we discuss later on, the prevailing metaphor of separation in families with adolescents—a metaphor that supports the creation of *rifts*—has an effect on everyone.

The Problem Speaks

They think they can get me this way, but I outwit them by masking my effects and getting therapists and clients alike to think that I only have one or two people under my control—certainly not the whole family. I can get each person in the family to develop stories about the others that make them "bad." Then I can make a case for separating and isolating, rather than for the family members' working together. Besides, we all know parents and adolescents are supposed to fight . . .

We have found that it is easier and more efficient to start with more persons in the room, rather than less. Working this way, we can notice the effects on the larger group and perhaps pull the whole group together to fight the problem. It also becomes easier to separate the one person from the problem, and then the more people there are who refuse to cooperate with the problem, the weaker the problem gets.

In this case, if the parents had originated their concern with "She is lying and is not to be trusted," and we had seen only the daughter, then we would only have had access to her description of the problem, which would probably have been some negative response to her parents' concern. It would have been more difficult to construct the *rift*. The same situation occurs in couples. If a woman were to complain, "I can't trust him any more," and come in for herself about what to do, we might end up discussing the effects of the lack of trust on her (among which might be anxiety, fear, anger, or depression); we would thus lose direct access to the experience of the effects of the problem on both people and also on the relationship. We also lose the possibility of helping both persons stand up to the problem in the ways that it is getting them to respond—ways that do not fit their preferred picture.

If we bring a family in only after first seeing an individual, our experience is that these sessions can privilege the original client's experience, that person's relationship with the therapist, and his or her efforts to escape the problem. As can be readily seen, this puts the therapist in a position in which new persons in the room may experience him or her as attending to the first person's experience and efforts more than to theirs. This has the effect on them of diminishing their experience, and they become increasingly vulnerable to listening to what the problem is saying about the first person. A possible exception to starting with more rather than less is when an individual calls for herself or himself. In very rare cases, this can even be when the individual is an adolescent, as in the case of abuse or extreme fear of the parents' response. However, we are careful to check the intentionality of the caller. For example, is the call inspired by a parent thinking the young person "needs someone to talk to"? Is an individual adult wanting to come in by himself or herself because the thought is that the other person "doesn't want to"?

The Authors Speak

We find that the question "Who else is affected by this problem?" continues to be a meaningful one to ask. Indeed, we find that mapping out all the effects of the problem is often where we start this work.

IN THE ROOM, PART 1: JOINING

The Problem Speaks

I like to get clients to start their complaints immediately. After all, they are there to talk about me. It undoes me when therapists try to get clients to talk about themselves separately from me.

We find it helpful to spend some time at the beginning of the first session finding out about people's lives, so we ask them to fill us in briefly on how they spend their time. This question allows for a short description from clients about how they see themselves, without getting into a lengthy (and at this point unnecessary) history. There are several beneficial aspects to this initial practice. First, it sets a stage for openness and empathy in regard to a low-risk topic. (We have found that even teenagers are willing to respond to this question.) Second, it initiates a structure for communication that we continue throughout, in which we talk to each person separately. In this way, we can try to understand and appreciate each person's perspective, as distinct from whatever story another might have for them. The third reason, and perhaps the most important, is that it allows us to get to know people as persons separate from the problem and to appreciate their areas of competence. Having done this, we are aware that we have collected a great deal of information about how people see themselves, to which in the future, as the problem story unfolds, we might be better able to return as we search for contradictions to the problem story.

For example, in the family experiencing a *rift,* if we had started with the problem and learned that the mother was acting in ways that seemed overcontrolling and perhaps dictatorial, even though we knew that this behavior was the effect of *fear* and *worry,* we might have missed that in another area of her life Judy was well respected as the director of a nonprofit agency dedicated to women's resilience. Or if we had begun with the parents' description of their daughter's *sneakiness,* which got her to sneak around and end up doing risky things, we would not have heard that Sharon was a star athlete and a bright student, or that she had a history of enjoying doing things with her parents. In many cases, what gets co-constructed as the problem is affected by this initial practice of joining as much as by further discussion about each person's perception of the problem. Certainly, a *rift* as a problem construction has meaning in a context in which doing things together has been valued. Also, during this initial "joining," we ask clients whether they have any questions to ask us—perhaps similar to ones we have asked them—or anything they might be curious about. Often clients seem stunned or bewildered by this question, and usually end up asking about our professional degrees or experience. Sometimes they want to know whether we're married or have kids or have dealt with similar problems before.

The Authors Speak

The intent here is to establish a context of collaboration, rather than one in which we might be thought of as "experts" subject to very different rules from those for "clients." We want to be transparent about our position as different from "set-off, high-up" therapists. This also sets a direction in which clients can question us about what we might be thinking or why we ask the questions we ask.

During this time, we usually inform our clients that we take notes during the session. Although it is obvious that we do so, we want to let them know that the notes are specifically about what they say, and we often tell them what we are writing down as we do it. They are not interpretations or hypotheses. We also invite the clients to review our notes, or offer them copies, or comment that they can take their own notes if they want.

CONSTRUCTING THE PROBLEM

The problem is most often described as something "in" the other person, or something the other is doing *because* of something "in" him or her (a characterological flaw) or "not in" him or her (a deficit).

The Problem Speaks

As I've said earlier, I love this way of thinking, confusing me with the person. It lets me hide and be powerful.

The Authors Speak

We are taking it somewhat for granted that you are understanding our talking about the problem in an "externalized" way. We find when we work with clients that using externalizing language from the beginning is extremely useful. Without explaining what we are doing, but simply using a language that locates the problem in a meaning system rather than in persons or relationships, we are creating a context in which the client begins to experience herself or himself as separate from the problem. This way of speaking that talks about the problem as an object and thus gives it a "life" is what we are discussing here.

What's in a Name?

The next step in an initial session is to inquire about the problem. Usually we try to be very specific: "What I would like to hear next is how you might describe the problem that brought you here. Who would like to start?" From the outset, the problem is seen as separate (it has brought them there), and each person is asked about his or her own perspective. As stated above, most often with families and couples, the problem described is something that one person sees the other person as doing wrong, brought on by some flaw or deficit in the other. Sometimes, however, the problem is expressed as an experience *between* them, such as the **rift** in the family described here. Other possibilities might be **conflict, hostility, trouble, misunderstanding, mutual despair,** and the like. Externalizing language is used from the beginning, and some formulation of the problem is attempted that will capture as wide a range of experience as possible.

Several choice points become immediately available. Does the therapist begin by externalizing the "problem behavior" or "problem attitude," such as **stubbornness, slipping, defiance, sneakiness** (or perhaps, if present, more complex problems such as **ADHD** or **anorexia**)? A first answer to this question is that as the therapist listens to each client's description, he or she responds with externalizing language. An immediate decision about what to call the problem becomes less important than talking about it in an objectified way and in a way that fits the client's experience. For example, in this case, as the parents described the problem as one of continued lack of trust in their daughter because of her increasing distance from them and presumed sneakiness, a possible response could have been, "How does *sneakiness* affect you?" From the beginning, problems are seen as separate from persons and are talked about in this way. The parents might then have answered that Sharon's *sneakiness* led not only to a *lack of trust* but also to increased *worry* and *frustration,* which in turn directed them, particularly Judy, to *control* more. Several possibilities for problem construction/externalization would immediately have become available: (1) *sneakiness* as the problem seen by the parents and also experienced by Sharon; (2) a pattern of *sneakiness* on the part of Sharon inviting *controlling* on the part of the parents, and vice versa (*controlling* inviting *sneakiness*); (3) a *rift,* which was both the effect of this pattern and the problem that continued to encourage the pattern and that the pattern supported.

The choice of whether to externalize a single behavior or attitude problem, or the problem pattern, or some relationship variable, depends greatly on (1) how the problem gets discussed by the family or couple; (2) what the effects of the problem are and how strong a hold it has on the family or couple or individuals in the family/couple; and (3) whether or not other institutionalized ways of thinking (e.g., therapies, schools, churches, etc.) have previously influenced the clients. Addressing a problem like *anorexia* directly, while paying attention to its effects on all, is quite useful. Likewise, *depression,* which other therapies and/or cultural understandings might create (as opposed to people's own experience of sadness), may be more helpful to externalize separately. These problems end up with such a hold on persons that they shape their identity, and so must be challenged.

The Authors Speak

Are you following this? We believe that this part of the work is extremely important, but we are also aware that writing and talking about it is difficult. We are worried that you will find this somewhat dense. If we could engage you in an exercise here, we would do so, since we have found this to be a very helpful way to teach problem construction. Instead, what we are trying to do here is give enough examples to make the point. How is it going?

Externalizing a Single Behavior/Attitude Problem

When families (or individuals) come in with a story about a particular member (or about oneself) that is experienced as a very powerful influence on all their reactions, externalizing this problem separately is most useful. For example, I (JLZ) saw a family in which the parents and the older son reported that the younger son, Johnny, had made all their lives miserable for years (see Chapter 2). On the basis of Johnny's experience, we talked about *hyperness* as the problem that affected him by inviting anger, frustration, and impatience. This problem then affected his parents' and his brother's reactions to him, as well as their relationship with him. Although the pattern and relationship effects could easily be seen (given that *hyperness* invited silence and led to a lack of closeness in this family), since the story started with the Johnny, *hyperness* "became" the problem. Shifting away from *hyperness* started a direction of noticing new things about this boy, as well as new possibilities for the family's relationships.

Externalizing a Problem Pattern

With families and couples, we often find it useful to pay particular attention to pattern. This is not to say that we believe any specific pattern "exists" in families and couples, but that various patterns can be constructed by the therapist in a way that helps those "caught" in them to notice them. The ideas about pattern are well established in Batesonian theory and in most systems theory thinking and writing. What we bring to these ideas is a different theoretical understanding, based on social constructionism and narrative: We are interested in how one person's behavior may affect the other in a way that he or she creates meaning about it.

In the example of Sharon and her family, the parents noticed what they experienced as *sneakiness,* and they used this experience to justify making responses that their daughter experienced as *controlling.* They would probably rather not have reacted this way, but they saw no other choice, given the *sneakiness* and given the culture's demands on them to take responsibility for their daughter's growing up (and to do so quickly). The meaning attributed to the other's behavior is influenced by cultural, and sometimes personal, stories. When we focus on pattern with couples or families, it is usually because one or more persons' meaning making about another's behavior has influenced each person in a way that his or her response is perceived as the only one possible. If we externalize the problem pattern, we externalize each end of the pattern, looking at the effects that the problem has on each person. We do this when there are reciprocal accusations and minimal talk about the relationship. Separating people from these problem patterns can be a helpful first step, particularly as this process helps them to notice other possibilities with regard to how each person might respond, as well as what to expect from the other. Also, noticing the influence of cultural narratives on these patterns helps people externalize the demands on them to act in certain ways.

Externalizing a Relationship Variable

How in this case did I (VCD) decide to externalize a relationship problem instead? From the beginning, the parents experienced and articulated the problem of *sneakiness* and *controlling* as a strain or a *rift* in the relationship—something about which they were particularly concerned. This came up in the first session when I asked the parents how the difficulties they were experiencing with their daughter were affecting them. Gary responded first with "It has created a huge strain in our relationship," and Judy chimed in with, "We have always been so close; this is really hard." I then turned to Sharon, asking her a similar question: "How are these difficulties affecting your relationship with your parents?" She answered, "We don't talk to each other as much as we used to." What I became interested in was how that was a concern, and what I learned was that this family had a history of closeness. The parents' relationship with their daughter was highly valued by all three of them. They had all become increasingly distressed by the distance that began to occur with the onset of the difficulties they were experiencing.

In this case, no one in the family wanted the *rift* in the relationship. They were particularly invested in keeping the closeness and connection they had all had. So exposing the problem as the *rift* became at the outset a problem that they could all join forces against. In this context, then, *sneakiness* could be seen both as an effect of and as something that contributed to the *rift* or disconnection; *controlling* was also seen as both an effect of and as contributing to the *rift*.

The Problem Speaks

I did my best to trick this family. I even got the parents to think that *controlling* was a way to alleviate their concerns and get rid of me. Of course, it only made me stronger. And I gave Sharon ideas of *sneakiness* and got her friends to support her in this endeavor by getting them to say, "Don't call, don't let them know what you are doing. They won't let you do what you want. They don't understand you." One of my ploys is to tell members of families that the others don't understand!

The Authors Speak

Again, we believe it can be very helpful for couples and families, no matter what kind of problem is identified (one affecting a person, a pattern, or a relationship), to team up as a family (or couple) to fight against the problem.

From the outset, we are also thinking about what might be the cultural (sociopolitical) narratives of influence on clients. With the family described above, I (VCD) was attending to the parents' description of *worry* or *fear,* and was wondering how *fear* not only might be a response to their experience of their daughter's seemingly irresponsible behavior, but also might be influenced by a larger cultural narrative about parents' responsibility to bring up their children to be independent, worthwhile adults. We believe that the cultural discourse about adolescents' needing to separate from their parents and find their own identity influences parents to take on the task of making sure their children do this in highly prescribed ways. Situations are set up in which parents and adolescents become competitors for the "right" way, rather than allies in a process of adolescents' beginning to narrate their own stories. (See Chapters 9 and 10.) A focus on the influence of these larger cultural narratives is what makes this work dramatically different from other forms of therapy, which psychologize about what is inside persons and relationships. These cultural narratives form the backdrop against which family and personal stories are created.

Often we hear the question: "How can you think about what question to ask, since it seems you have so much going on in your heads?" Our answer would be that we all have a lot going on in our heads. What we try to do is remember that from our postmodern perspective there are many viewpoints, so we try to understand each client's meaning. Specifically, we want to know what the narratives of influence are on this person. This is a position of respect and curiosity; however, it is *not* a position of neutrality. In other words, once we can get to the meaning system affecting the client's constructions, we then take a position *against* cultural narratives inevitably influencing these constructions and having effects the client does not prefer. For example, in this case, what did Gary and Judy think about feeling so responsible that they had to put pressure on Sharon in unhelpful ways?

More about the Problem and Looking at Its Effects

Recently a woman in her mid-40s came in with a story of illness, anxiety, and guilt. During the initial joining, she said that she had decided to make this appointment as a birthday gift to herself. She was married, had a 10-year-old son, and spent her time primarily as a housewife and mother—roles she enjoyed along with several other interests, the chief of which was sculpting. She had previous experience as an accountant, but decided not to continue that work when her son was born. Her story included her father's death following a heart attack two years previously, surgery for her husband a year before, and her own continuing difficulties with allergies. This constellation of the experience of family illness had brought forth a burden of guilt, which told her that she was not success-fully undertaking her job as a mother or as a wife. This burden of guilt came out in the following way: As I (VCD) asked her what was troubling her, she responded tearfully, "I just feel so *bad* all the time. I get angry and begin raging at my son, and my husband and I can't talk without fighting." When I responded with what that "feeling bad" was all about, she said, "I'm not doing it right; I feel so *guilty*." Thus, the initial discussion focused around the experience of **guilt** and how it affected her.

Often in a first session, the client's description of her or his experi-ence is unfocused and rich in detail; it becomes important to respond to the story with questions about a possible "candidate" for externalization, phrased in consistently externalizing language. Also, when clients first begin talking about a problem, they usually include in their description others in their experience who also have some relationship with the problem. In this case, for example, the client specifically included her mother and her husband as those who had greatly contributed to the experience of **guilt** in her life. A consistent way of thinking that is helpful to us in these cases is to think of the "others" contextually. That is, we think of them as participating in the client's experience—both as persons who may have inadvertently cooperated with the creation of a problem story, and as audience to first the problem story, and later a preferred story. Questions that continue to speak of the **guilt** in externalizing language, but that also acknowledge the client's inclusion of others in her descrip-tion, might include the following: "Since you had an experience of being trained in **guilt** in your growing up, what do you think some of its training techniques were?" This question locates the **guilt** training in history, but also thinks of it as something that developed in a context. We do not think of it as something "caused" by someone else, but as something that arose in a particular cultural meaning system.

A helpful way to arrive at an appreciation of the problem's influence is to ask "effects" questions—for example, "How did the **guilt** affect you?" If the response includes something like "It made me feel like I wasn't taking care of things the way I should," then we might follow with "What other effects did that have?" until eventually **guilt**'s field of influence is mapped out as extensively as possible. It is useful to ask about the effects on how a person views herself or himself, or others, or her or his relationships with others. Another way of asking this question that we have found helpful is "What does the **guilt** tell you?"

What also often happens is that when "effects" questions are asked, other candidates for externalization become available; one of the effects may then become a better choice in terms of capturing the client's experience. In this case, what became apparent was that **guilt** had become a *burden of responsibility.* This eventually became externalized as *expectations.* By co-constructing *expectations* as the problem, the client could specifically list all the *expectations* that were influencing her. In future sessions, other ways of talking about the problem could be located in *expectations*—for example, "How does this fit your experience of *expectations* making demands on you?" This particular construction could also open space for alternative possibilities centering around the notion of "resigning" from the job of meeting *expectations'* demands.

"Effects" questions are asked in every case as tools for understanding the extent of the problem's influence. In the example of Sharon and her parents, in which a *rift* had opened up between them, "effects" questions brought forth Judy's experience of feeling guilty, of doing something wrong, of feeling isolated; they also included the experience of *fear.* The *rift* told Gary that he needed to take action, that he had to "correct" the problem. For Sharon, the effects were those of increasing isolation and more *sneakiness.* It is through the asking of "effects" questions, as well as the use of externalizing language, that separation from the problem begins to occur.

The Authors Speak

We cannot stress enough how much we believe in constructing problems in their cultural context. Cultural discourse becomes the problem, not people or families. For example, *expectations* as a name for the problem of the woman trained in *guilt* better reflects the cultural meaning system. It calls upon the discourse that requires certain things from women as wives and mothers.

By carefully mapping the influence of the problem on people's lives and relationships, the therapist and each client can notice how much of the client's experience has been affected by the problem (and the cultural narrative that supports it), and perhaps how little is left for what might be considered preferred aspects of her or his experience, which have been marginalized. Often clients include the effects of the problem in their description of what is "wrong." In these cases, it is useful to respond to them with externalizing language—again with the intent of separating them from the problem, and also to slow down the process and allow them to notice the negative effects the problem has had and is continuing to have on them. So, for example, with the family, if Judy had included her experience of *fear* in her discussion, one response could have been "So this *rift* has had the effect of *fear* on you; what other effects has it had on your life?" To Gary, a possible response could have been, "Since the *rift* has gotten you to want to take action in your daughter's life, how has that further affected you?" The idea here is not only that the problem has affected people, but that the effects have further effects. For some clients, beginning to really notice the effects of a problem in their lives is critical to their deciding to work to take their lives back from the problem and begin to move in a new direction.

The Problem Speaks

I hate these questions. When clients begin to see my effects, they start to really stand up against me.

Intentionality

A very useful area of exploration is intentionality. When problems occur in relationships, they influence one person to make meaning of the other's intentions. To extend the effects of the problem to the interpretation of intentionality, a helpful question is "What did the *rift* tell you about [your mom, your dad, your daughter]?" or "What did the *rift* tell you about their intentions?" In the case of Sharon and her family, the *rift* told her that her parents did not care about her, and vice versa. Again, the advantage here was that the problem was the culprit; the problem told Sharon that her parents didn't care. Questions about the problem's intentions would begin to challenge the inevitable direction in which her thinking was taking her: that her parents truly did not care about her. With the individual woman, the question might be "What did *expectations* tell you your son thought [or your husband wanted from you]?" Her response might be that *expectations* told her that her husband wanted her to get over her allergies faster so that she could take care of him. They also told her that her son thought she was always only angry, that she shouldn't ever be angry, and that he (her son) was suffering unduly. The *expectations* had clouded her experience of herself as a parent who could get upset sometimes—an upset that would not necessarily have a negative effect on her son (or her husband).

Advantages for Clients

This extension of the field of influence of the problem has a twofold effect on a client. Clearly, the therapist's intent is to understand the client's experience of the problem's oppression. The effect this has on the client is one of a profound experience of empathic appreciation. When the therapist continues to ask clients about their relationship with the problem, and to respond with externalizing language, clients begin to notice not only how much the therapist is interested in and is trying to appreciate their experience, but also how they are not the problem. Clients report the resulting experience of empathy in terms such as "having a relationship with a therapist who cares about me," "feeling like we were taking a stand together against the problem," and "feeling that she was on my side." (These phrases are taken directly from clients' statements.)

The Authors Speak

One of the common misconceptions about narrative therapy is that it is located primarily in the cognitive domain. Certainly, since the work in the room is language-based and is a searching for meaning, this misconception is understandable. However, we see narrative as located in experience, and this includes not only affect and cognition but the physical expression of the experience as well.

The second effect on the client is the opening of awareness of what may lie on the periphery of the problem field and may *not* be affected by the problem. These may include behaviors, attitudes, knowledges, or times with others that seem to go differently—that is, anything counter to what the problem would predict would be the case. As the therapist continues to ask questions that extend the field of influence of the problem through "effects" questions, these previously unnoticed experiences often slide into view and are available to be considered by both client and therapist. For example, they can consider what the *rift* might have affected, but, as becomes obvious to the client and the therapist, hasn't. Sometimes, as in the case of the family with the *rift,* the clients' very presence in the therapy room is something that can be seen as counter to the influence of the *rift.* They want to be there.

Unique Outcomes

These contradictions to the problem are called "unique outcomes" and are aspects of a client's experience that would not be predicted by a reading/telling of the dominant story. However, these possibilities are always present in the client's experience; they have been lost, not attended to, not stored in memory, not "storied." Often these unique outcomes (contradictions) "pop out" in the course of conversation about the problem. This can happen without the therapist's needing to ask direct questions to bring forth these events. It is usually important to take note of these contradictions, to punctuate them or call attention to their existence—for example, "Oh, so that's different; that doesn't fit with how the problem has taken over your life." However, it is never safe to assume that what we as therapists notice as unique and outside the influence of the problem is preferred by our clients.

In our teaching, we have noticed that the enthusiasm of those beginning to work this way encourages them to go on and on or be "impressed" by what they think of as unique outcomes; they may perhaps jump too quickly or too strongly to these events. We wonder whether this is the influence of some idea that we are "looking for positives." Unique outcomes are determined by what the problem is and not what the therapist decides is "good." When our clients offer, or we notice, some unique outcome, we have found that a much better tack is simply to note the unique outcome and to be curious—perhaps asking, "What do you think about this? Do you think it was a good or a bad thing? Is it more or less helpful?" We have generally found that it is not a good idea to begin to explore the "history" of unique outcomes too soon, especially if unique outcomes are noticed in the course of mapping out the influence of the problem.

Our experience is that there is a danger of going too fast—of not fully understanding and appreciating the extent of the problem's oppression. Occasionally, we have found that if we jump too soon to an appreciation of unique outcomes, then our clients feel misunderstood or feel pressured to move more quickly than is comfortable. We often tell students that it is preferable to err in the direction of going too slowly; the clients will let us know whether they are ready to move on. Often an attention to unique outcomes does occur in the first session. If, in noticing these develop-ments, we have moved too fast, our experience is that clients are less apt to slow us down directly; after all, they too are influenced by the dominant narrative telling them that therapists are experts. However, we have found that they find some way to let us know—by shifts in conversation, by action, or by disconnection.

The Authors Speak

What we want you to notice here is the importance of keeping pace with the client.

In the case of the family with the *rift,* what became apparent in the course of the first session was how important it was to all the family members to keep their closeness and connection. They referred often to how close they had been to each other as the daughter was growing up. By focusing on the relationship variable, the parents began to notice the peripheral experiences of closeness and of shared and open communica-tion that were continuing to occur but had gotten lost in the problem story. I (VCD) noted and commented on these experiences in the first session, but did not extend or expand upon them in any detail. They became information for future reference—entry points to another, more preferred story.

With the woman for whom *expectations* became the influencing problem story, I paid attention to times in which she might have not given in to the demands of those *expectations,* times that she resisted or had considered resigning; these emerged through our conversations about the effects of the problem. With this client, her statement that she had made the appointment as a birthday gift to herself could be seen and commented on as an opening to a new story. She, indeed, indicated that this was a sign of resistance to her experience of *expectations.*

We are always interested in identifying at least one unique outcome in a first session—again, not to extend it in any way or to make something of it in a way that could appear to discount the client's perceptions, but more simply to open up the possibility of some experience that is counter to the problem narrative.

The Problem Speaks

I must redouble my efforts! If they begin to notice other possibilities, it will weaken my influence.

The Authors Speak

We think it is important to remember that the therapy process is a back-and-forth one. We are paying attention to the influence of cultural narratives on each client, while simultaneously attending to other possibilities, contradictions to the problem story. How do we decide when to focus on the influence of the problem and when to shift focus to other, perhaps more preferred, possibilities? Mostly what we try to remember is that our clients give us the clues. Michael White has suggested that it is most helpful for therapists to stay just behind their clients, to follow them.

IN THE ROOM, PART 2:
STARTING A NEW STORY

When a *rift* was talked about as the problem in Sharon's family, it said to me (VCD) that a connection would be preferred. So I began to pay attention to instances, either brought up in conversation or implied, when connection and shared communication had occurred. I asked questions about these instances: "How did these become possible?"

"What did you think about them?" "What did you all do to create those possibilities in your lives?" I listened with both ears, each attuned to different stories—one to the problem narrative, the other to a counter-narrative. When I noticed a contradiction, I asked about it. By the second session with the family, I could readily pay attention to a counternarrative, to preferred directions.

What makes alternative stories possible? For the family we have been discussing, the experience of connection was a powerful one and had not been completely subsumed by the *rift*. Most often, in subsequent sessions, we begin by asking about preferred developments (e.g., "How have things gone more in the way you would like?" or "Catch me up on developments"). In this case, the family members gave responses indicating that they were able to focus on their successes and move rapidly in a new direction. The therapy was completed after six sessions over a total of three months; their relationship was thus reclaimed from the *rift* in a rapid, straightforward manner. In a family where the problem may have a longer history and is more influential, other work to deconstruct the problem needs to be done (see the next section), and more time must be spent in slowly reauthoring a counternarrative.

A longer, more back-and-forth process occurred with the individual woman. *Expectations* had an entrenched history, fed by family and cultural narratives. Although unique outcomes were noticed and explored from the first session onward, each session included a discussion of the influence of the problem and of victories over the problem. Her experience was one of increasingly noticing resistance to *expectations* and fighting against them, and the session time became more filled with accounts of her successes. At the same time, the influence of the problem was still noticeable, in particular since it also seemed to affect her physically, contributing to her allergies. Because the pace of therapy was geared to her account of her experience, it became a pace that she, rather than I, set.

The Authors Speak

We believe that clients have the experiences already that are problem-defeating.

Before pursuing how the therapist and client co-construct more preferred versions of their self-narratives, it is important to notice another aspect of the back-and-forth process of therapy. As the influence of the problem on the life of the person is mapped, and as unique outcomes are noticed and brought forth, it also becomes more apparent how larger cultural discourses are influencing people. These larger cultural discourses take the form of "taken-for-granted realities." So, as part of the back-and-forth process, we discuss those practices next.

DECONSTRUCTIVE PRACTICES, OR "UNMASKING" CULTURAL DISCOURSES

Recently, taking a walk and thinking about how to formulate what to write next, I (VCD) saw a neighbor doing some work in his yard. It was a beautiful Sunday morning, so I jokingly said to him, "You shouldn't be working so hard!" His response was "I *don't know* why." We laughed together and I went on my way. I started thinking: I hadn't asked him *why* he was working so hard; my comment reflected some meaning system that was influencing *me*. His response, and in particular the intonation, indicated that it was an unreflected activity; he was just doing it for whatever meaning that was influencing him. *I* was the one questioning it.

What we want to discuss next is this: how we do take certain things for granted, how we do respond unthinkingly in our lives, without examining how it fits. Often it is not necessary to attend *explicitly* to the larger discourse of influence; rather, it may be more important to think about it in the way we have discussed—that is, by including it in the way we construct the problem. At other times, it is very important to specifically deconstruct these grander narratives in the interest of a client's progress.

The Authors Speak

It is our experience that problems like to take advantage of situations in which what we are doing doesn't actually fit what we prefer.

We return to our previous examples. Sharon's parents believed that the *rift* was happening now because their daughter was a teenager. It had happened with Gary's children from a previous marriage when they were teenagers. Certainly, other parents talked about it this way: "They all go through this; it's just part of what happens." Sharon had a similar reaction: "My friends told me not to call; they said my parents wouldn't understand, that they wouldn't let me do what I wanted to do." Drinking and drugs, fast cars, irresponsible friends, bad judgment, and "risky business" are all part of the growing-up process. Doesn't the culture tell us so?

For the individual woman, weren't **expectations** part of her job as a mother and a wife? Her mother said it would be this way, and her husband wondered when she would get it right. There are just certain things that women do; they are responsible for their kids' welfare, for their making good decisions, for their having friends or not, for their happiness. They need to protect their children. And they need to take care of their husbands—to give them good meals, clean the house, attend to domestic details, and listen to their woes. After all, husbands deserve it. They are doing their jobs; they are the breadwinners; they put the food on the table. It's all a "given."

Do these ideas seem familiar? Do you find you are somehow influenced by them? Are they in any way offensive? They may seem more offensive when they are spelled out so blatantly, but rarely do they come spelled out in our lives. Usually they are more subtle, less obvious, and more insidious; they hold us hostage and make us think we should like it.

These are the "truths" of our lives; they influence the way we think about ourselves, the decisions we make, and the actions we take on our own behalf. And they are rarely challenged. When clients talk about them, they are "givens," "the standard definition of," "what's 'normal,' " "the way it is," or "what I was taught." These truths are so "settled" in our lives that we are apt to think we agree with them. How many people talk about the stress we all feel as if it were simply the status quo, something to be expected—something we hope we will outgrow or retire from? Where did we get this idea that stress is to be expected, that we should put up with it? This question, along with any question we might ask about "truths" or other "taken-for-granted realities," could stop us and allow us to think about whether or not we want such experiences as part of our lives. In some cases, a response might be to justify putting up with it because of needs—to work and make money, for example. In other words, the "truth" of one's experience is created by the effects of these "realities." Several different aspects of this discourse could be challenged. For example, we could look at stress-increasing ideas, habits, and lifestyles, or we could look at the needs themselves.

The Problem Speaks

You see how insidious I am. I can so easily convince people that things just "are"—immutable, unchangeable "truths"—especially if I have been around a long time and have a well-established history in people's lives.

These "truths" are the effects of the influence of some cultural discourse. A "discourse" can be considered as a set of ideas that have evolved over time, contributed to by all of us and shaping us in a way that we come to take for granted, "as if" it was always there. (See Kathy Weingarten, 1991, and Rachel Hare-Mustin, 1994, for some extended definitions and helpful analyses.) We continue to use the term "discourses" throughout, because we believe that this term embodies, more clearly than any other, the ideas that we are discussing. We may alternately use such terms as "cultural beliefs and ideas," "grand narratives," or "larger stories"; however, none of these quite capture the meaning that we think "discourses" does. We use this term, in spite of the notion that it may be thought of as "jargon."

Discourses are created at different historical points, and so are influenced by the prevailing practices of the culture. Discourses support the power of some persons or groups (e.g., men's rights over women's); indeed, those who help create the dominant discourses seem to benefit from this position. They only fall when other discourses challenge their influence and take their place. More recently, the work of Michel Foucault (1979, 1980, 1984a, 1984b) and others who situate themselves in the realm of social and cultural psychology, anthropology, and various critiques of history and philosophy have drawn attention to discourses that have subjugating effects on persons. It is in this context that a stance of deconstructionism takes place.

"Deconstruction" is a term that has been borrowed from literary theory. In the tradition of Jacques Derrida (1981, 1991), it would have the effect of *erasure*—of directing our attention to what is and of what is not in whatever is stated or indicated. As narrative therapists, following the thinking of Michael White (1991), we would think of deconstruction as a practice of questioning or challenging what is considered "given" or "taken for granted" or viewed as a "settled certainty" by looking at the factors producing these givens. In this way, externalizing conversation is a deconstructive practice, for it challenges the "truth" of problems as existing in persons. The practice of externalizing is predicated on an understanding that sees the problem in the discourse or the meaning system. It is therefore a practice that objectifies subjugating "truths" or discourses rather than objectifying persons. (See Stephen Madigan, 1996, for a more extended discussion of these ideas.) What is deconstructed here is the way views of problems are produced (i.e., a discourse about problems). These views are not truths, but can be traced directly to certain assumptions created by discourse. Bringing forth these assumptions, challenging these assumptions, or cleverly operating with different assumptions—these are the practices of deconstruction.

The Authors Speak

Often, in our work, a discourse as such is not directly questioned. We may address behavior patterns, relationship variables, or personal feelings and attitudes, in such a way that the discourse is not directly brought into the foreground; it is, however, always in the background, always there. As we describe the clinical work, we give examples of how a discourse is always in the room, is attended to by the therapist, and is always addressed either directly or indirectly.

IN THE ROOM, PART 3:
QUESTIONING CULTURAL DISCOURSES

In the example of the family experiencing a *rift,* I (VCD) could have attended to the "normalizing" view of adolescents—that is, the necessity of separation to achieve "identity." From this normative discourse for adolescent development, a *rift* is to be expected and predicted; an adolescent or family may even be considered abnormal if it does not occur. If we were to accept this metaphor as "the way things are," then a *rift* would not necessarily be seen as a problem; more likely, the problem would have been constructed around some so-called "deviant" behavior on the part of the adolescent, such as sneaking around or lying or falling grades, or perhaps lack of trust on the part of the parents. As it turned out, partly because we do not subscribe to the dominant discourse that requires separation as a sine qua non, I instead attended to what was problematic for the family: the *rift* in their previously experienced, and still desired, connection.

The Authors Speak

This is an example of a deconstructive practice in our thinking.

By externalizing *rift* as the problem, I brought back into view a marginalized discourse, one of connection as a possibility for families; this allowed the family to focus on a preferred counternarrative. In other cases with families with adolescents, problems are often talked about as somehow "symptoms" of what "we all go through when our kids become teenagers." Unless those ideas are questioned, examined, challenged, and/or subverted, we will all continue to replicate a cultural oppression of people through these "taken-for-granted realities."

When we keep our ears attuned for meanings that the family members are attributing to the problematic behavior or attitude that they experience, we begin to notice the influence of these cultural beliefs. Because they are taken for granted, their influence is often not noticed, even though the power of the discourse is far from subtle; it is, in fact, pervasive. With this particular family, it was easier to notice the cultural influence, because a *rift* was clearly *not* what they preferred. However, more often it is considered normal. For example, in one family in which an 18-year-old male, a recent high school graduate, was struggling with his parents about taking charge of his own life, the problem was presented as a "quickness to anger," and the solution presented by the family was that he just "needed to get out of the house, to be on his own." The mother constructed a scenario in which this young man could gain a sense of responsibility and independence by experiencing the structure and safety of college, where he could make his own mistakes and learn from them. This conclusion can be seen as an effect of the separation discourse, which suggests that a college experience may provide this context better than the home environment. Both mother and son were attending to this conclusion, despite their both talking about how important being close was to them (and also understanding that a college environment does not always, or necessarily, provide structure and safety). The son said he wanted to solve some of these "anger" problems before he left for college, so he would know he could come home and share things with his mom. For the mother the experience of anger and arguing clearly had painful effects, and she wished for an easier time between them. When I (VCD) invited them to consider how to escape the influence of **anger** and to notice their own and each other's efforts, they reverted to the cultural "truth" of the necessity of leaving home. Their comments were "It's 'normal,' " and "He has to find out on his own." Such ideas seem to have a blinding effect, preventing people from noticing other possibilities. They also are isolating, cutting people off from each other, leaving them adrift, with an overall effect of disconnection and disempowerment.

Likewise, for the woman experiencing the burden of **expectations,** the influence of cultural and familial discourses was apparent. How do women get to be responsible for home, kids, husbands, and households? What did **expectations** tell this particular woman she should do, and where did **expectations** get their power? How did they get passed down and inadvertently supported by her mother and by her husband? These **expectations** had constituted this wife and mother in this way (i.e., good mothers are *always* responsible to and for others); their effects included depression and guilt, as well as stress, which weakened her to ongoing allergies. Some physical illness may be one subjugating effect of discourse. (In another deadly example to be explicated later, anorexia can be seen as an effect of this subjugation.)

It was clear from the first session that this woman was experiencing the oppression of a dominant discourse. Usually, when we think in terms of the influence of discourse, we notice early what may be affecting our clients. It is most helpful to attend to each client's description, using her or his language and construction of the problem as a starting place. For this client, the initial description of the problem contained expressions of guilt, of overwhelming responsibility, of illness, of anger, and of depression. I initially externalized these as possible candidates for continued discussion of the problem. At the end of the first session, the client left with an appreciation of what a heavy **burden** responsibility had been in her life, and we considered the other experiences (guilt, anger, depression, illness) as "effects" of this problem.

Although I (VCD) might have noticed other societal and/or familial expectations (cultural discourse) that contributed to this **burden** and were possibly present for this client, I did not question or bring them into the room explicitly. Rather, I addressed them more through the use of a problem construction that could capture the influence of discourse, as well as through a set of questions that could reflect both this understanding and a sociopolitical stance.

The Authors Speak

To explore further how deconstruction occurs, we now look at some possible questions that can be asked. What questions might you, the reader, ask, or about what in these narratives would you be curious?

Types of Questions

When clients first present with a problem, the therapist can ask, often even prior to "naming" the problem: "How does this problem affect you?" and "What conclusions about yourself and others has the problem led you to?" Besides questions that address ideas and beliefs, it is also important to ask questions that address behaviors and activities flowing from these unexamined beliefs. One way to think about this, from a deconstructive viewpoint, is to consider these behaviors and activities as "strategies" or "techniques" that people have been "coached into" by the problem. It is evident that this way of formulating questions continues to refer to the problem as separate and as having some power over people. This way of talking about the problem is also more compelling than the usual ordinary rhetoric of therapy conversation, which has been popularized, made more familiar, and perhaps trivialized by the mass media and by a proliferation of self-help books. Here are some examples of questions that could have been asked of the individual woman:

- What do **expectations** tell you about yourself as a wife, as a mother?
- How do **expectations** team up with **guilt** to affect your responses to your husband and son?
- What tricks or lies do **expectations** use to get you to do what it wants?
- What purpose do **expectations** have in getting you to do what it wants?

And of Sharon's parents:

- How has this *rift* affected the way you think about yourselves as parents?
- What activities does the *rift* direct you into?
- How does this experience of a *rift* get you to respond to your daughter?
- Does it make you more wary and suspicious, or help you to be more understanding and supportive?

And of Sharon herself:

- How does the *rift* get you to think about your parents, yourself, and your relationship with them?
- What strategies does this *rift* coach you into in terms of responding to your parents?
- Does it get you to be more honest and forthcoming, or trick you into dishonesty and sneakiness?

So a set of questions can focus on how the problem affects the way people think about themselves, about others, and about their relationships, and also on how it directs their actions. When problems are seen as "tricking" people, or "coaching" them to perform certain actions, or "training" them in specific lifestyles, then clients tend to perk up and notice effects of problems that they may not prefer. These questions, then, have the effect of opening space for clients to become aware of other possible ways of being in their lives.

Another set of questions can look at how past experience may have recruited clients into the problem. In other words, what about their personal history has contributed to the evolution of this problem? Often this history has an inevitability about it, given certain meanings that people have attributed to events over time. These meanings have a family settledness about them. As one mother said about her 11-year-old daughter, who seemed particularly "resistant" to parental directives, "She has the 'Smith family stubbornness,' " The mother then proceeded to list all the attributes portrayed by members of her extended family that seemed not unlike the "resistance" or "stubbornness" her daughter was displaying. This had taken on the flavor of a "family trait." Questions can be asked in this area, although we find it more useful to put the majority of the focus on the cultural foundations for problems.

The Authors Speak

In general, we find beginning with cultural discourse and then moving to the influence of family/personal stories to be a helpful progression. The latter may not be necessary or helpful, given the "psychologizing" that people typically engage in on their own.

The following questions could have been posed to the individual woman:

- Where do you think *expectations* come from?
- What individual or group might be most likely to voice these *expectations?*
- Do you think others might suffer from similar *expectations* in their lives?
- Do you know anyone, yourself included, who really likes these *expectations?*
- What about your past experience helped recruit you into a lifestyle of *expectations* (as a woman, as a family member)?
- What training in *expectations* do you think you received in your life?
- Do you think others in our society receive a similar training?
- Whom do they serve the most?

And to Sharon's family:

- Do you know other families that share your experience of discomfort about a possible disconnection or a *rift* in the family?
- Do you think disconnections or *rifts* just happen, or do some cultural or family ideas support them?
- Why do you think that is?
- Does it fit for you?
- What did this past experience tell you that may have made you more vulnerable to a *rift* at this time in your lives?

The Problem Speaks

These therapists are using my preferred language—a tricky thing to do. I try to play the final trick by making myself invisible. Now they've tried to unmask that—but I have lots of power, because everyone knows what I have to say is true.

Making the Invisible Visible

How do we notice what is taken for granted? How can we question what we have previously not questioned? It becomes a dilemma when we consider that we are all always influenced by whatever cultural and familial beliefs we have encountered. However, paying attention to the notion of cultural influence can itself alert us to the subtle indicators of the "givens" in our lives, and to the effects of these "givens." So, in general, what we listen for are words and phrases that are clues to these influences. When clients say, "It's a given," or "It's normal," or "That's the way it is," or something similar, we perk up our ears. Our intention is to explore the ideas that influence people, not to destroy them; to question them, not to leave persons without an anchor or without some sense of constancy in their lives. Our experience is that discourse can take us away from our experience, or get us to make sense of our experience only against some standard or norm. We believe that by questioning the discourses of influence, we allow people to consider their preferences more clearly, and to decide whether or not the ideas that influence them "fit" for them.

We also pay attention to certain discourses to which we have become so attuned that they have been rendered invisible. These can have particularly subjugating effects on persons. For example, we are watchful for the influences of gender constructions on couples—the effects of these on the partners' ideas about themselves and each other, as well as the effects on their relationship. We also notice how gender constructions affect the ideas parents have about their male and female children, or ideas about how men should be husbands and fathers and women should be wives and mothers. We look for the influence of developmental discourse on beliefs about what is "normal" for adolescents and children of different ages, as well as the effects of this discourse on what parents and kids think about education and work. We notice the effects of psychiatric/psychological diagnoses on people. We pay attention to discourses about sexuality, including the construction of sexual preference, as well as ideas about sexual intimacy. We are attuned to how socioeconomic discourse has influenced the development of class and the effects of poverty on persons. We are sensitive to the particularly oppressive practices of racism and the invisibility of white privilege. To show how some of these influencing discourses make themselves apparent in the therapy room, we include a few examples.

IN THE ROOM, PART 4: EXAMPLES

Example 1

Recently, a husband and wife who had decided to separate presented with a problem of intense antagonism and hostility that had gotten between them. (In the first session the husband indicated that the problem was his wife's hostility, while she indicated that the problems were her husband's single-minded interest in sex and his cluelessness.) By constructing the problem as *antagonism* (mutual) early on, the couple could consider this as a focal point against which both partners wanted to move. Since these two clients indicated only a 1% possibility of their getting back together (even though they were interested in therapy together), a starting point of helping them to notice a problem that affected them similarly and pervasively seemed more helpful than addressing the problem in a pattern, or in a small thing they might see as affecting their relationship, or directly in cultural discourse. As is most often the case, the influence of any discourse can be seen first as background to whatever problem is presented; it becomes foreground as questions are developed to tease out the history of the problem.

In this case, the gender stories were not brought into the fore until after several sessions; sufficient space between the partners and the power of the *antagonism* had to be created first. When the larger cultural influences that supported the problem were attended to, it became apparent that the gender story affecting the female member of the couple was *self-sacrifice*—an idea she had grown up with, which told her that after many years of sacrificing her own needs and wants in the service of being a good wife and mother, she would in time be appreciated. For the male member of the couple, the gender story influencing him was *entitlement*—a belief that he knew best what would in the long run serve his family. Along with this was the *male sexual drive* discourse (Hare-Mustin, 1994), which told him he was *entitled* to having his sexual needs met by his wife on demand. It is not difficult to see the intersection of these gender stories (discourses) as a ripe breeding ground for the development of *antagonism.* For these clients, although some progress was made early against the influence of *antagonism,* the shift in their willingness to reconsider relationship as a possibility came when therapy began to address (deconstruct) the gender stories. (This was not a privileging of recommitment to relationship over separation, but a privileging of what evolved as the preference of each member of the couple.) In this case, the clients wished to have some kind of relationship, and that is what the therapy continued to focus on.

Example 2

In another example—one influenced by both gender and developmental discourses—a mother came in with her 15-year-old daughter and complaints about the daughter's *anger.* They had been to several therapists with no apparent respite or reduction in the *anger;* the whole family had been seen, the parents only, the daughter only, and the mother only. Since this was a situation in which the problem seemed clear and agreed-upon, and several therapists and therapies had been tried, what was immediately addressed was the influence of discourse. In this case, the mother (in fact, both parents) believed that girls should not be angry or show anger; on the other hand, might not this *anger* be a sign of moodiness, a beginning of the "necessary" separation that adolescents "must" undergo? The mother had developed the idea (an influence of developmental discourse) that her daughter would only "come back" to her after she had grown up and moved away. It was only when the *anger* was deconstructed as perhaps the only way the young girl could see as available for "having a voice" (Brown & Gilligan, 1992; Gilligan, 1990) that possibilities for conversation and mutual understanding were opened up. Again, awareness on the part of the therapist of the possible kinds of discourse that might be influencing families allows for a noticing of what is not being said. These influences must, however, be approached with caution, without the belief that "This is the answer." Respectfully questioning persons about their experience, and their understanding of their experience, opens the door to what the narratives of influence might be; these are not assumed.

Example 3

In the third example, the intersection of the influence of developmental discourse with the effects of thinking from a perspective of psychiatric/psychological diagnoses becomes evident. In this blended family, the stepmother was a therapist and the father had been diagnosed for most of his adult life as having a bipolar disorder (and, more recently, adult ADHD). The daughter was brought in because of her difficulties in school and her general uncooperativeness at home. The father attributed the daughter's difficulties to a possible psychiatric/psychological problem; if this were diagnosed properly, he thought, either medication or an appropriate treatment protocol would result in "cooperation" on her part. The stepmother was open to the therapy process (she preferred that someone else do the work, rather than her having to take on the role of resident therapist at home), but she tended to attribute the daughter's difficulty to both a "normal" adolescent rebelliousness and a reaction to the father's "disorder." The daughter said that of course she was rebellious, because that's what 15-year-olds were. She added, "Nothing's really wrong—it's just Dad's manic–depression that's a problem." When she was asked where she got the idea that 15-year-olds were rebellious, she responded, "Everyone knows that." She was then further asked whether that was okay with her, whether she liked that picture of herself; she said, "No, I don't really like it."

Questions could then have been asked about what the daughter did prefer and how she might be interested in developing a different picture. In this case, however, there were also overlapping diagnostic labels to be considered. Because the daughter attributed the problem to her father's diagnoses, she saw her reaction of anger as the only possible response to what she perceived as her father's inconsistencies, anxiety, and overcontrolling behaviors. This perception called for further deconstruction of the diagnostic labeling. The father was thus questioned about what the effects of bipolar disorder and adult ADHD were on him. He talked about a "constant noise" in his head and a pervasive experience of anxiety. When he and the stepmother were asked about what that might look like to his daughter, they responded, "A tremendous amount of worry." With continued questioning, they acknowledged that it led to behaviors of "needing to control." Often the influence of discourse is so powerful that it continues to stand up to examination, so that even though clients may not like the effects of the discourse, they still can see no other option. With this particular family, an ongoing questioning of the *anger* (rebelliousness) and of the *anxiety* (worry) became a thematic strain throughout the therapy process. This work continues to remind us to follow the clients, to be willing to pay attention to detail, to realize the powerful influence of the problem, and to deconstruct the dominating discourse patiently.

Example 4

Recently, an experience with a training group brought up another possibility, which called into question whether it is always helpful to bring forth the influence of discourse directly. In this scenario, a member of the group had asked to be interviewed by one of the supervisors about what she believed was a particularly difficult situation for her as a therapist-in-training. The rest of the group observed from behind the mirror, after which a reflecting team, exchanging places with both the interviewer and interviewee, went into the room to ask some questions about the interview. It became apparent (at least to the supervisors) that the trainee was being affected not only by a discourse about how to be a good therapist, but also by a gender discourse about self-worth. However, the reflecting team did not address "discourse" at all, but rather asked reauthoring questions about preferred possibilities, as well as some successes in the life and the therapy experiences of the trainee. Afterwards, the trainee responded positively to these questions and seemed empowered by them. At the end, when one supervisor asked the other supervisor (the interviewer) why he had asked the questions he asked (a common practice in our training groups), the possible influences of discourse were brought into the fore. Although all members of the training group, including the interviewee, agreed that these influences were present, none of them thought it was necessary to address them. In fact, the direction the interview had gone and the aspects of it that the reflecting team focused on seemed very fitting to the trainee's needs.

What this example calls into question is how and when to make the influence of discourse explicit. Does deconstruction primarily serve its purpose in the subtle though powerful process of externalization, a practice that puts the problem squarely in the discourse, without calling specific attention to whatever is the discourse of influence? Does it do this by constructing a problem that somehow incorporates the influence of culture, as well as by focusing on the negative effects of the problem on the clients? Our experience is that this is often the case.

Example 5

In another example a lesbian couple presented with extreme difficulties of mutual blaming. The problem was constructed as **blame** of self and of others, but the work went very slowly and with little success in separating the couple from the problem and its effects. Our supposition was that there was some cultural discourse affecting them, perhaps a lesbian discourse about how partners are to respond to or be with each other. This discourse can lead to certain mutual *expectations,* which, when unfulfilled, can engender a response of **blame.** Little movement was made, even with some deconstructive questioning about what couple messages might be influencing them. Eventually, we consulted a colleague, a therapist who was "out" as a lesbian. The couple had agreed to be videotaped, because they, too, were stymied about why this problem had such a hold on them. The consultant watched a videotape of one session with the purpose of trying to unravel what might be the discourse of influence. Her comments addressed a specific expectation that she noticed might be operating on this couple. She said that often a woman in a lesbian relationship expects her female partner to be there to meet all her needs and, thus, becomes extremely disappointed—perhaps even blames the partner—when this is not her experience. This *expectation* does not seem to operate in the same way for women in heterosexual relationships, because a heterosexual woman, although she might want such taking care of from her male partner is not encouraged by the same *expectation,* given the gender training that affects both of them in their male and female roles.

The Authors Speak

It is important to say here that in cases where we might not have the knowledges of certain cultural influences, we have found it very useful to consult someone who can help us understand how a specific cultural discourse might be affecting our clients. We find this especially helpful when the race, ethnicity, class, age, or sexuality of the client and the therapist are different.

Example 6

In this sixth example, a therapist from a training program was seeing a black man in his mid-30s who had come in because of a pervasive experience of *depression.* He reported that he had been "wrestling with this demon" since he was a teenager and that it "spoke to him of his identity." The supervising therapist had some idea that the *depression* might well have been an effect of the oppressive practices of *racism,* so when she went into the therapy room at a prearranged break to consult with the therapist, she raised some questions about how the therapist might talk with the man about the effects of *racism.* She wondered aloud whether *depression* might be a tool of *racism* or a ploy that it uses to keep persons who are not of the dominant white majority down, or to make them think something is wrong with them. When she left the room and went back behind the one-way mirror, the man's first remark was, "You mean *depression* might *not* be about my identity?" He went on to say that previously he had no hope, but now he could see hope in his future.

Although *racism* is certainly not invisible in our culture, it is often invisible in its effects. In this example, by not assuming that the problem was "simply" a psychological one (one that those of us in Western, white culture have defined), and by bringing into the room the very real probability that this man had experienced *racism,* the client could for the first time feel free from the experience of *depression* as his identity. By continuing to focus on the discourse of influence (white privilege leading to *racism*), the therapist and the client could move to a new level of self-confidence and freedom of action. By separating from *depression,* the client (and the therapist) could protest the effects of *racism.*

Example 7

A brief example of work with a family involves a conversation with the father, in which he talked about how he had been working on escaping habits of *evaluation,* which had negative effects on his wife and children. In a discussion about his anti-*evaluation* voice, he attributed his love of nature, his spiritual self, and something he called a "tribal sense" to his family-of-origin experience. However, much of this also fed *evaluation,* because he believed the involvement and closeness he had with his family had to do with the fact that they were "lower class." He was embarrassed by this background (he was now a professor) and said *evaluation* used this to tyrannize him and to place too much emphasis on money and success.

He preferred an anti-*evaluation* direction because it emphasized involvement in relationship, play, and acceptance. He was questioned about the "lower class" definition (i.e., What made his family lower class? Who decided that upper and lower has to be based on money? What effect did having less access to resources have on his view of himself? If he had a rating scale, where would he put "upper" and "lower"? Based on his scale, where would he rate his family? What effect did that have on *evaluation?*).

He looked relieved and said he never realized before how his family had been so defined by the culture. He later said this conversation really helped shift his view of himself and supported a new story for him.

The Authors Speak

We are not interested in replacing one "truth" with another, "better truth," but rather in simply questioning how we accept certain conditions, situations, and events as "realities" in our lives. Our intent is to "unmask" these "realities" so that we develop a clearer sense of what are the discourses (narratives) of influence. From this perspective, then, we approach clients from a position of respect and curiosity, wanting to understand their meanings and how they are affected by what is influencing them. This is very different from an intention of wanting to replace people's ideas and beliefs with something we might think is better, or intending to "break down" or "destroy" people's meaning systems. We are interested in challenging certain "taken-for-granted" ideas and realities, in that we believe that discourses can have subjugating effects on people, and that the problems that develop in people's lives are oppressive. We do not wish to replicate certain oppressive positions that have developed in society—for example, the occurrence of misogyny, racial prejudice, class bias, heterosexual dominance, and other subjugating influences. For these reasons, we are always interested in reflecting on our own position, deconstructing the narratives that influence us—in fact, deconstructing narrative therapy—as a means of questioning our intentions, with the purpose of continuing to operate from an ethical stance of openness and respect for our clients and a political stance of protesting discourse that has subjugating effects on persons.

The Problem Speaks

You must know I want to have the last word. I continue to affect people—even you—in ways you do not suspect. All this nonsense about "discourse" and "deconstruction"! I hope you realize this is just another bit of jargon invented by theorists to make them seem smart. I outwit them all, but I do it in everyday language and in the dailiness of people's lives. That is how I am often experienced as impenetrable, indestructible, and immortal.

AUTHOR: Remember what the caterpillar asked?

PROBLEM: What—and why does it matter?

AUTHOR: "Who are *you?*"

PROBLEM: So?

AUTHOR: The answer: "I hardly know . . . at least I know who I *was* when I got up this morning, but I think I must have been changed several times since then."

PROBLEM: I think I must be missing something.

AUTHOR: We think so, too. See what's up next.

CHAPTER 4

I Knew Who I Was When I Woke Up This Morning

The Authors Speak

What we have found is that once persons begin to experience themselves as separate from the problem, and, even more, to understand the problem as existing in a meaning system, they seem to notice other possibilities spontaneously. They begin to appreciate other self-narratives. In fact, they begin to experience themselves differently as persons. It is this experience of other versions of self that we want them to notice, and that we also want you, the reader, to notice here.

OTHER VERSIONS

The following questions were what I (VCD) asked in response to statements from Gary, Judy, and Sharon in the next-to-last session with this father, mother, and daughter, who were experiencing a *rift* in their relationship (Chapter 3).

To Gary: "What has happened in the direction of taking the *rift* out of the relationship?" "Was this a surprise to you?" "How do you suppose the situation invited that conversation?" "Do you think that perhaps she thought you would be able to refrain from giving advice?" "It seems this is important to both of you [taking the *rift* out of your relationship]."

To Sharon: "How did you decide you could put *sneakiness* behind you and give your mom a call instead?" "When did you realize that the *sneaking* was 'stupid,' as you put it, and that it was contributing to the *rift*"

To Judy: "Tell me more about this 'direct connection' that you made, that 'lightening up' invites a 'more relaxed' relationship with your daughter and that 'not monitoring' her behavior invites 'more sharing' on her part." "In the past, *fear* told you that if you didn't monitor your daughter's behavior, something bad would happen; how did you put the *fear* behind you?" "What does this tell you about you as a parent, that you could embrace *trust* as something you wanted more than *fear* in your relationship with your daughter?"

In the process of extending the field of influence of the problem on this family, the parents first, and then the daughter, had begun to remember times of shared communication—times when Judy and Sharon had a special closeness, and when Gary and Sharon had had helpful conversations. What also became evident was that these times were in the not-too-distant past; they could easily be brought into memory. As mentioned in Chapter 3, we call these other possibilities or contradictions to the problem story "unique outcomes," and consider them to be "entry points" to an alternative story. Michael White (1988) has used the term "unique outcomes" instead of "positives" or even "exceptions," because they are outcomes that would not be predicted by a reading of the problem story. They are interesting in that they have meaning *in relation to* the problem story. Clients may experience these events as positive; more importantly, clients experience them as preferred, and therefore they can be helpful in creating a different story.

When working with families with adolescents, we find it useful to imagine the ways they are influenced by the culture. As we have discussed previously, a familiar cultural story for parents is that adolescent sons and daughters will "naturally" begin to drift away; they will no longer wish to talk to their parents, will prefer the company of friends, and will stop sharing their thoughts and ideas. We believe that teenagers are also influenced by this story, in that they begin to see no other alternative than to withdraw from their parents, particularly if the parents show more *fear* and *worry* than they have shown previously. Inevitably, parents are apt to express *fear* and *worry* in more noticeable ways, given the dangers they know their youngsters will confront. It is our belief (Dickerson, Zimmerman, & Berndt, 1994) that this is how problems centered around separating and drifting away may develop. "Separation" is a constructed cultural story. It is a process vulnerable to problems because of the erosion of connection between family members. Separation of teenagers and parents becomes the goal rather than a process of evolution. We believe that this separation discourse encourages teenagers to keep their ideas to themselves and not share what they are thinking and doing with their parents.

With this family, it would not have been a surprise to me if the parents had shown interest in continued communication and the daughter had indicated *no* interest, given how pervasive the separation metaphor is and how peer relationships can inadvertently feed the idea that teenagers need to separate from their parents. However, Sharon clearly was also experiencing the loss of closeness with her parents, and was able to articulate that she "wanted it back." When she was asked about how she was able to put *sneakiness* (an effect of the *rift*) behind her, she said it was just "stupid." It contributed to the *rift.*

PROBLEM: If I had convinced the family and the therapist that I was *sneakiness* instead of *rift* I would have had a better hold on them.

AUTHORS: Is this because *rift* reflects the culture in a way that *sneakiness* doesn't?

PROBLEM: Well, that's a "duh"!

TURNING IT AROUND

For this family, the turnaround toward increased communication and closeness did not happen immediately. Although we attempt to find at least one unique outcome in a first session, this is not always done easily, and sometimes only a glimpse of something counter to the problem can be found. Because we are always on the lookout for contradictions, sometimes they "pop up" in the process of asking questions about how the problem affects people; then we can show interest in and curiosity about these unique outcomes. At other times they become noticeable in the "gaps," the things not said, the experiences not storied. Sometimes we find that it is helpful to ask specific questions to elicit something from the clients' experience that does not fit their telling of the dominant, problem-saturated story. The oppressiveness of problems tends to subsume people's experience and blind them to events or intentions counter to the problem. Another way to say this is that the problem "marginalizes" what could be seen as preferred developments in people's lives.

The Authors Speak

We really hope that what we say here won't be marginalized.

When we attend to unique outcomes, we also think about how to ask questions that will allow the clients (and us) to notice whether these events are preferred. Sometimes the problem tricks people into not knowing what they think or what they want. That is why it is imperative to work with them to create sufficient separation from the problem. Only then can they begin to notice other possibilities. Thus, as we continue to ask questions about whether these events are good or bad, helpful or not helpful, interesting or not interesting, fitting for them or not fitting, clients can begin to make their own distinctions and decisions about these events and whether or not they might be preferred. We believe that unique outcomes have a history; our interest is in situating them in a narrative that can then move forward into a present and a future that fit more what clients might want in their lives, not what the culture might tell them.

Unique Outcomes: Recent and Distant Past

We often begin by asking questions that will indicate how clients may have had some influence over the problem—for example, "Were there any times in the recent or not-too-distant past in which this problem may have tried to get the better of you, and you didn't let it or you pushed it away?" With Sharon and her family, such a question might have been "Are there times you can recall when you might have experienced a strain or a *rift* in your relationship, but you were able to fend it off and not let it develop?" Often clients, without much reflection, will respond with an emphatic "No!"

The Authors Speak

We believe that this response is an effect of the oppressive power of the problem.

Our timing in asking such questions then becomes of great importance. We are most apt to pose one when some opening for alternative possibilities or some gap in a client's experience has already been noticed. In that way, we can then locate an example or a unit of experience in the client's more immediate past. If this does not seem possible, we search for unique outcomes in the distant past.

For example, with the couple experiencing **antagonism** (see Example 1 at the end of Chapter 3), it was helpful to recall earlier days in the marriage when the spouses had worked together as a couple, in which there were no signs of hostility or **antagonism.** Going in this direction can usually assist people in marking the beginning of the development of a problem in their lives; going back *before* the problem may help them focus on a lifestyle and a history they prefer. It also assists people in noticing how problems insert themselves in their lives and take over in ways they do not like. This process increases their experience of separation from the problem. With this particular husband and wife, over the course of therapy the pre-*antagonism* history even began to color their more recent past, and they frequently referred to their "history of closeness." This continued to be the case even when their decision to divorce became firm. Separation from the problem had been sufficiently maintained that the "closeness" spoke of their interest in having an ongoing, friendly relationship.

The Problem Speaks

I try to blind people to any times they may have gotten the best of me. I don't like it when therapists wedge these unique outcomes between me and the clients—I have to work harder to blind them.

When the Problem Is a Lifestyle

At other times, even distant history has been tainted by the problem story. This is usually the case when the problem has the increased weight of a "lifestyle" or a "career," as often occurs if there has been a psychiatric history (one that includes hospitalization or ongoing medication); examples are schizophrenia, bipolar disorder, or a pervasive experience of depression or generalized anxiety. Sometimes parents will say of their children, "They were born that way," or "They have always been difficult." Our experience is that these histories often become even weightier if they include traditional psychiatric/psychological interventions; such interventions, by objectifying persons, tend inadvertently to support the development of the problem. (See Gremillion, 1992, and Gaines, 1992.)

We have had success with "lifestyle" problems, because we find we are able to notice some contradictions to the problem story even in these cases. However, the work is slow and the progress occurs in small steps. One example is the case of a middle-aged professional, an orthopedic surgeon, who decided to come to therapy because of an increasing experience of **hostility, anger,** and **guilt.** In weekly therapy over a year's period, a story unfolded in which he discussed his early childhood experience of emotional abuse—an experience that led to various hostile, angry, and guilty feelings; a sense of "never getting it right"; fear of possession by the devil; obsessive thinking and compulsive behaviors; and hostile fantasies of hurting children. This experience affected his practice as a surgeon, getting him to overdo workups on patients and constantly question his decisions. It affected his relationship with his wife, whom he saw as someone to "mother" him. It affected his behavior toward his grown children, whom he treated with criticism; it got him to plot revenge against his parents. It led to hostile fantasies toward his grand-child. It led to patterns of overindulging with food and alcohol. One of the most telling moments (and a turning point in the work with this client) was when, in a discussion about his success as a professional, this question was asked: "Who in your past would be least surprised to know about the caring and concern you show your patients?" He quickly responded, "My grandfather." What then transpired was a touching history of his relationships with all his grandparents, but in particular his connection with his paternal grandfather. This connection was a unique outcome with which the problem history could be contrasted, and from the standpoint of which he could reconsider his past and rewrite his history. From this close and loving relationship, he could develop an alternative story that included the preferred qualities of a gentle, caring man rather than those of an angry, obsessive one. The question that opened these possibilities was a question that located an experience in a relationship—one that could help him see himself from another's eyes. The unique outcome was from the distant past; it reflected his current experience of success as a physician, but also brought a past meaningful relationship into the present. This is an example, then, of noticing contradictions in the present and assisting clients in developing a history that supports these contradictions.

The Authors Speak

We discuss the importance of a community of support, as well as the reflexivity of this experience, later. Also, it is important to emphasize that these unique outcomes are *experiences*, not cognitions.

Unique Outcomes: The Present

Another way of bringing forth unique outcomes in the present is to notice directly, with clients, a current behavior that is counter to what the problem might indicate. As stated previously, this is often our first line of questioning. A clear example is the presence of clients in therapy. This can be brought forth by asking about the clients' intention in seeking therapy for the problem. What does this tell clients about themselves as persons? Does this fit more their ideas about themselves or how the problem might be directing them? How was it that the client just described—the surgeon experiencing **hostility, anger,** and **guilt,**—was interested in coming to therapy? What did this tell him about his own preferences? What about the family members experiencing a **rift**? Wasn't their being in therapy itself counter to the problem? In families, it is more often the parents who decide that therapy is indicated; we often tell young people that we want them to show up, that they don't have to talk, but that we suspect they will want to tell their side of the story. Even spouses or partners who seem intent on blaming each other can respond that they are interested in bettering the relationship or in increased communication or in cooperative parenting.

The Authors Speak

In a family or couple where mutual blaming is taking place, this does not tell us as therapists that we should "fix" one person or the other; rather, it tells us that each member of the couple or family has some idea that their relationship could be better. Our interest is in asking them, "What gave you that idea?" and "How did you mutually decide that therapy was something you wanted to pursue?" We want to help people access what might be in their own best interests, and then notice their intentionality in that regard.

Sometimes unique outcomes occur in the present in quite unexpected ways, and it is helpful to be on the lookout for them. For example, in a recent therapy session, the husband in a couple was working on overcoming the *anger* in his life; this *anger* was intimidating to his wife, was scary for his grown daughters, got between him and his friends and coworkers, and took over when he was behind the wheel of a car. I (VCD) was talking to him about how he might have managed to stay in the driver's seat, rather than let *anger* take over, when a door-to-door vendor came to the therapy room and walked in uninvited. My response was one of quick anger: I stood up, said firmly, "This is not okay. You need to leave," and followed the vendor to the front door. I then quickly came back to the therapy room, apologized for the interruption, and visibly cooled down. The husband remarked, "That's just how it happens for me; the *anger* happens so quickly. When I saw that you got control over it, I realized that I sometimes do, too." It became a turning point for him to notice his own attempts to be in charge, rather than the *anger*'s being in charge. In subsequent sessions, not only he but his wife noticed how much calmer he was behind the wheel, and how this being in charge was generalizing to other areas in his life.

Often we first notice unique outcomes in the "plot line" of the story; that is, they appear as events or behaviors within a particular time frame. From the perspective of narrative theory, we refer to these as occurring within a "landscape of action" (Bruner, 1990). However, some unique outcomes in the present occur in the area of personal characteristics, preferences, goals, values, philosophies, and intentions. We refer to these as occurring within a "landscape of consciousness." As mentioned above, people's intentionality in terms of coming to therapy is a clear example. However, at other times—even in an opening session, in the midst of relating the oppressive effects of the problem—a client may voluntarily say, "We really do love each other," or "I'm not depressed all the time," or "We haven't given up on our son." We believe that most people's story of therapy is that it is a time for talking about problems; why would people go to a therapist and say how well they are doing? However, our interest is in taking clients in the direction of noticing how they might be doing well, or have been doing well in the past, or are interested in doing well in the future. So when clients volunteer these contradictions to the problem story (unique outcomes) early in therapy, we at least comment on them—for example, "I would be interested in hearing more about the history of that love. Could we come back to that in a few minutes?"

The Authors Speak

Our experience is that by attending to the client's experience, we can maintain the balance between extending the field of influence of the problem and noticing unique outcomes on the one hand, and not jumping to these outcomes too quickly on the other. When unique outcomes do pop up, we often emphasize them or punctuate the sequence, so that we can return to them for further expansion of meaning as the therapy continues.

Unique Outcomes: The Future

By focusing on the "landscape of consciousness," we can also question clients about their future hopes, goals, and desires. This set of questions becomes increasingly important at two junctures in the process. The first is when unique outcomes seem particularly difficult to locate in the past or the present; we then ask clients to imagine a future time when things might look the way they would like. Often the problem has brought such hopelessness and despair into clients' lives that future possibilities seem hard to imagine. However, even asking a question about the future may invite some hope back into their perspective. An example that occurs frequently is in families with adolescents, where parents might say, "I know that sometime in the future, after they have left home and experienced the world a bit, they will come back to us." One question that might follow this remark (and would also attend to the influence of cultural discourse) could take this form: "What is it that you know about yourselves, your son/daughter, and the connection between you, that tells you there will be a future time of closeness?" or "If you could make that time sooner rather than later, what is it that you know about your relationship now that you might want to capitalize on?" We think it is important not only to notice clients' preferences, but also to begin to draw attention to what is already present in their sense of themselves and their relationships (counter to any subjugating effects of the discourse) that can help them begin to appreciate themselves differently.

In another example, the surgeon described earlier, who was beginning to notice and perform a more preferred story of anti*hostility* and pro*caring,* related an incident in which his father had his 80th birthday and no one was there to help him celebrate. I (VCD) asked him what he envisioned for his own 80th birthday (at the time, he was 56). He responded, "I would like my wife and children and friends to share it with me." I then asked, "As you continue to live this life of attention to caring and love for the people in your life, can you imagine how rich that celebration might be?" His eyes welled with tears, and he responded with gratitude that he was taking this new direction in life. This speaks to the second juncture in the therapy process when focusing on future possibilities is helpful—when we "thicken" the alternative, more preferred story.

The Authors Speak

Our theory suggests that contradictions to the problem story (unique outcomes) already exist in each client's experience, but that these contradictions have been marginalized and thus not noticed or attended to, and have therefore gone unstoried. We also believe that this position is very different from one in which we need to give ideas or suggestions to the client. Our experience is . . .

The Problem Speaks

Excuse me, but part of my power is my ability to see in exquisite detail a past in which only those events that support me are noticed. I make these events into small stories that make up the larger, dominant story that has me as all-powerful.

The Authors Speak

That is quite a trick, for you to push aside some experiences in favor of others that support you. You might muster a history; however, we also think that there are other histories, made up of events that support preferred stories, and that you have overshadowed them. When we search with a client for unique outcomes, we do so with the intention of shedding light on these events, bringing them out of the margins, making them not trivial. We then work with the client to notice a string of events that support unique outcomes. Thus, we begin to bring forth a different history—one without you. Because we see unique outcomes as entry points to alternative stories, we use these outcomes to help clients construct a new narrative. These outcomes *mean* something other than you. There are other possibilities, other discourses available, besides the ones that support you. When clients indicate a present attitude or behavior that is clearly preferred, we try to help them locate that attitude or behavior in some part of their past, which you have blinded them to or misinterpreted for them.

To return to the story of the surgeon burdened with **hostility** and **guilt,** we see that he also had a current experience of being a caring physician. The **hostility** and **guilt** had a noticeable history, located in an emotionally abusive growing-up experience. What was the alternative history, one that supported a story of **caring**? It had its origins in a past relationship with a grandfather. The questions asked in therapy shed a light on that relationship experience in such a way that this client's personal history could be rewritten, revised to fit his more preferred account of himself. How we work with clients to develop these alternative stories is the stuff of which much of this work is made. In these sessions, the problem is talked about less and less, and becomes less and less predominant.

The Problem Speaks

Who . . . me?

IN THE ROOM, PART 5: THE ONGOING WORK

When clients come in to a second session, as well as to subsequent ones, we generally begin with the question "How are things going in the direction you prefer?" or a variation, "What has been happening since last time that is more the way you want?" Sometimes we begin with a review of the summary with which we ended the previous session—a summary that includes the problem's effects, as well as each person's experiences that are separate from the problem. Often, especially early in therapy, clients will want to recount the problem or present another variation of it and its power; this makes it difficult even to notice, let alone to describe, alternatives. Sometimes we comment, "When problems take over people's lives, they become very good problem watchers. What did you notice that was outside the influence of the problem?" Or, "I find it useful to start with developments away from the problem. Would that be okay?" Often, at the end of the first session, we suggest that people notice how the problem affects them *and* the times they were more apt to escape its influence or fight back. If the problem is particularly oppressive, we may simply suggest that they "spy on it," notice its influence, direction, and strategies, and compare this to what they want. A second session can easily begin with a question about both the problem and any alternatives that have occurred.

It is not unusual for clients (at least very early) to respond to the question of how things might be going in a preferred direction with a comment such as "They're not." Or, if they are asked what has changed or what is new, they may answer, "Nothing." In such a case, we find it most helpful to respond first by following the client, particularly if the problem has been chronic and very oppressive. How is the problem encouraging, demanding, convincing the client in a way that it is continuing to take him or her away from the preferred direction? This response continues to privilege the client's experience; it is respectfully curious about what they are noticing in their lives and how the problem is affecting them. We also believe that since problems blind people to what possibilities might be present or to what contradictions may have occurred, a second response might be something like this: "When the problem occurred in the past two weeks, were you more apt to find yourself affected by it in the old way, or did you also (1) notice any slightly new responses, (2) imagine what you could do differently, (3) notice that you noticed that 'the problem was getting a hold on you'?" These questions gently remind the client that noticing the problem in a new way is already a turn in a new direction. We also remind ourselves that perhaps we need to do more work with some clients in mapping the influence of the problem, or that perhaps we have not sufficiently understood the problem and could find another way to construct it and externalize it.

A few years ago, in working with a family whose high-school-aged son was falling behind in his grades, we discussed the problem as one of **stubbornness.** As the family left the therapy room, the mother turned to me (VCD) and said, "It's not **stubbornness** at all; he's just lazy!" My response was, "Oh! Well, that's what we should talk about, then." In the next session the problem became redefined, with the son's concurrence, as **lack of effort.** This appreciation of the family's understanding of the problem allowed restorying to occur much more rapidly than if I had insisted on my construction of the problem.

The Problem Speaks

She missed me here. She forgot to think about how I'm in the culture. What she didn't see was the discourse about first-born sons needing to succeed, and how this was specifying of the parents' pursuing and the son's difficulties. You see, this family came back five years later with the son continuing to suffer from academic failure. The therapist paid attention to my cultural partners the second time around, but I won't let you in on what she did . . .

The Authors Speak

(*Aside, whispering*) I'll tell you later. See Chapter 9.

Further Externalizing

Depending on the power that the problem is exerting on a client, couple, or family, subsequent sessions are illustrative of the back-and-forth process of further eliciting the effects of the problem, perhaps further externalizing other narratives of influence, continuing to bring forth other, more preferred possibilities, and enriching or "thickening" an alternative story. As indicated previously, an initial presentation of the problem may suggest that the therapy focus on behaviors or attitudes, and when this problem is externalized and sufficient space is created between the client and the problem, then other narratives of influence become apparent. The work becomes a further externalizing and deconstructing of whatever problem stories arise in the course of therapy. Each session is an iterative or unfolding process of externalizing, deconstructing, extending the field of influence of the problem, searching for unique outcomes, finding a history of the contradictions, and continuing to develop and maintain whatever alternative story evolves.

As is always the case when working with clients in therapy, we focus first on the problem presented in the beginning session(s). Sometimes therapy proceeds quickly toward developing an alternative story, particularly if the problem has a short history or seems situational; in these cases, the therapy is often completed in a few sessions. This was the case with Sharon and her parents, as described earlier. In other instances, given the pervasive influence of subjugating cultural narratives and oppressive personal stories, further externalization and deconstruction are indicated. We have discussed this previously (Dickerson & Zimmerman, 1992, 1993; Zimmerman & Dickerson, 1993a, 1993b, 1994b), where we describe our work with couples and families. (We also address this again more specifically in Chapter 6.)

We do believe, however, that all problem stories have been informed and shaped by larger cultural discourses. Thus, whether we address such a discourse directly as the major narrative of influence or not, we always attend to its shaping effect; by intention, it is in our thinking and often in our language in our externalizing conversations. As we have been suggesting all along, we try to choose a name with the sociopolitical implications that the larger discourse has dictated. For example, instead of *self-doubt* (for women), we might suggest *evaluation* as the problem; or rather than *overresponsibility* (again for women), we would mention *expectations.* As a possibility for men, the problem of *overentitlement* can capture the cultural influence. This problem can have effects on men of *withdrawal* or even *fixing;* when we explore these effects with them, they say that they are not helpful either personally or to the relationship. With women, a counterstory of *self-confidence* or *entitlement* or *believing in self* might be helpful, whereas with men a counterstory of *being present* or *responsibility* often seems to fit. In those many instances when we name a problem in a way that seems to fit a person's experience better (e.g., *doubt*), we still *think* about it in a way that reflects the culture's influence.

The Authors Speak

Would it be redundant to say again that cultural discourses are what this work is about?

Clients provide clues that further attention to the shaping effects of discourse would be useful. When there is very little movement away from the problem, or when clients show an interest in continuing to explore what are experienced as troubling ideas and beliefs, we see these instances as times when further deconstruction can be helpful. The examples discussed at the end of Chapter 3 illustrate this process:

1. The spouses who experienced *antagonism* as the problem between them (Example 1) began to notice the influence of gender constructions on their perceived roles as wife/mother and husband/father in ways that had fed the *antagonism.*

2. The mother–daughter dyad in which the daughter's *anger* was the presenting problem (Example 2) began to experience some relationship change only after the influence of gender stories for young girls was deconstructed in a way that allowed the daughter and the mother to have conversations rather than arguing matches.

3. The family members struggling with *anxiety/overcontrolling* and *anger/rebelliousness* (Examples 3) were able to move toward greater

mutual understanding once the influences of diagnoses and developmental discourse were brought into the room.

4. In the examples of sexuality, race, and class, once the problem was seen as having been encouraged by sociopolitical contexts (i.e., *blame* from a lesbian cultural message of mutual *expectations*, *depression* as a ploy of *racism*, and *evaluation* as fed by an experience of coming from a "lower class" background), the clients experienced a degree of freedom from the problem that then allowed a reauthoring to more readily occur.

Bringing In Our Own Experience

Since cultural discourses, our own personal narratives, and our experiences as therapists also influence us in the therapy room, we often find ourselves thinking about how we have heard a similar story from another client or how we have had a similar experience. Sometimes clients are interested in our giving them advice, making suggestions about what they should do, or telling them what we think about something. Certainly a therapist who has spent many years working with individual clients, couples, and families may have some exposure to a variety of ways of doing things, and may also have some ideas about what works well. We are cautious about how our own ideas may or may not be helpful to these particular clients, so we ask questions about the clients' experience, believing that they have some ideas already available about what works better or fits best for them. This is not to say that we do not share our experience; however, we do so within the context of "situating" our questions. For example, we might say, "In my time of working with families, I have heard [such and such]; would you be interested in some of those ideas?" At another time we might say, "I could tell you what I think, but I would also be interested in hearing how you think my ideas would fit for you." It is in these ways that we continue to privilege each client's experience.

Naming the Counterplots
and "Thickening" Preferred Narratives

The direction of therapy is to continue to assist in developing a more preferred narrative, one that is counter to the problem story. When further externalization occurs, then the process of attending to unique outcomes, asking whether or not these contradictions are preferred, and beginning to develop an alternative story continues in much the same way as before.

With Sharon and her parents, the opening question in the session mentioned above was this: "What has happened in the direction of taking the **rift** out of the relationship?" Another way of addressing this changing direction is to "name" the counterplot—for example, "What has been happening to strengthen **closeness** in relationships in this family?" In much the same way as we work with clients to "name" the problem, finding a problem construction (externalization) that captures their experience, we also work with them to "name" what is counter to the problem. When the problem name is an attitude or behavior, such as **defiance** a countername might be an attitude of **determination.** This naming became helpful as a counterplot in work with a 12-year-old boy; once **determination** was named, an amazing story of goals, ideas, and plans in this young man's life could unfold. In another example we have given—that of the woman burdened by **expectations** (see Chapter 3)— we could describe a story of personal qualities as a text of **self-acceptance** and **competence,** which would further along the woman's resigning from **expectations** (a problem reflecting the influence of cultural discourse). Often it is useful to find a name for the alternative story early in the process, as it becomes an anchor or a seed for the development of this more preferred story; at other times, naming a contradiction to the problem story is premature until the story becomes "thickened" through continued questioning that promotes the client's authorship and agency. At all times we attempt to employ the client's own (and our own) creativity, using examples from imagination, experience, the mass media, film, literature, and so on.

When a client experiences the narrative flow of the work early, we find it is helpful to name the sessions, as if they were chapters in a book that the client is writing. For example, in one time-limited therapy process (in a training setting), the client was asked at the end of the first session whether she would be interested in giving a name to what had occurred. She and the therapist (along with a supervisor) decided to name the experience "Escaping the Problem's Influence." The subsequent sessions were called "Taking Steps in My Own Behalf," "Preferred Developments," "My New Story, Part I," and "My New Story, 33⅓." We have also used the practice of naming events in training/teaching settings. (In Chapter 11, we will discuss how our training is isomorphic to the therapy process.) Restorying is a process that readily occurs in the teaching context, so we often create exercises in order to help students attend to their performance of a preferred story. They will name their experience as "Meeting the Challenge," "Taking Off," "Noticing Choices," "Challenging Discourse," "Stepping Up," or the like.

We have often found it helpful to name the problem story with a problem designation, but to give the counterstory the client's own name. With one young adult woman whose experience in her family was one of failure and not measuring up to what she saw as parental expectations, the problem story was called "The Black Sheep Story," whereas what she preferred was called "Laura's Story." (See also Chapter 6.) The over-arching advantage is that externalizing and locating the problem in its sociopolitical context becomes the vehicle for protest, for challenge, for resistance against any and all of the subjugating practices of cultural discourses.

The Authors Speak

In this sense, therapy becomes a political act, countering the nega-tive effects of the culture.

The advantages of naming the problem story and the counterstory are many. First, it allows a noticeable separation between the problem and what people want for themselves. Second, it tends to focus the process by providing a framework within which the alternative story can be mapped. Third, naming assists clients in experiencing their own personal power in creating more of what is preferred or in choosing what influence they want to respond to. Fourth, and perhaps most important, it tends to create (even while it is forming) the new description, shaping people's ongoing experience and affecting what they do and how they think about what they do.

Whether we name individual chapters or name the overall new story or both, it is through continuing to notice events that contribute to the new story, and asking questions to help a client develop a history of preferred developments *and* extend the meaning of each event, that the story becomes not just a blip in experience, but a rich and well-developed narrative. In every case, it calls forth the experience of persons' being agents in their own lives and authoring their own stories, always in the context of a community of meaning and as a preferred response to what clients have previously experienced as the negative effects of some cultural discourse. This brings us to the therapist's role in asking questions to elicit this elusive activity or quality, called "agency."

The Problem Speaks

What do they mean by "agency"? If they think of me as existing in meaning systems or in dominant cultural specifications that influ-ence people, isn't it inconsistent to think that people can make their own choices, separate from these meaning systems? How can they talk about "agency" if all meaning is always negotiated in a context? And why am I talking this way?

The Authors Speak

The question of "agency in a person" disconnected from contexts of meaning and relationship makes little sense to us. The question that fits better for us is this: What marginalized experiences speak of an alternative truth? So, of the multitude of discourses that we are always living within, which, and what about which, do we want to have influence us? In this sense, "agency" means that each of us can play a part in choosing what to let guide us and in what contexts, based on a consideration of *all* of our experiences. We are therefore less interested in why some things seem to stick and not others, why certain aspects of our experience get attended to and not others. We are more interested in whether or not what sticks or gets attended to is what fits for us. Is it helpful, useful, pleasing, desired, preferred?

The problem occurs when we are subjugated by the culture's normative specifications as well as by some of our personal experiences in ways that keep us from distinguishing between what some or most of our experiences and preferences are telling us to believe or value and what the problem is telling us.

The Problem Speaks

Now they're acting like I'm not here. But I make it very hard for people to pick what *they* want.

AGENCY, AUTHORING, AND AGENTIVE GAPS

Restorying or reauthoring occurs as clients begin not only to notice but also to recount those events, actions, and behaviors, that fit better for them than those the problem story has recruited them into. It also occurs in the process of developing a history—extending and expanding events over time, or what we might describe as developing a plot line. The new story becomes richer as characters other than the protagonist are included, those who are part of the client's reauthoring context. Earlier in this chapter, we have given some examples of questions that helped facilitate this process. We have referred to this as bringing forth a "landscape of action"—events that occur in a sequence over time, with both a distant and a recent history, with an imagined and preferred future, and with persons and their actions as parts of that historical development. We have also referred to a "landscape of consciousness" or "landscape of identity"—a person's experience of meaning in a narrative. This includes personal characteristics; desires and preferences; goals, purposes, and intentions; philosophies, values, and beliefs; and a commitment to a way of life and ways of being. These two "landscapes" are seen as relevant to the development of narrative (Bruner, 1990) and as critical to a narrative approach to therapy (White, 1991).

Narrative requires a narrator and a protagonist, and in most instances of self-narrative, the narrator and the protagonist are one and the same. The exceptions occur when a problem story takes over a person's life, or when another's story becomes dominant (e.g., parents' stories for their children, one member of a couple's story for the other, or the culture's stories for all of us). In these cases, the problem can trick clients into thinking they are still authors of their own stories, when in fact the problem has taken over and has taken on the narrator's voice. The countertrick requires a wresting of authorship away from the problem. This process, as we have intimated, is one that calls for a great deal of attentiveness to a person's preferred narratives, as well as a vigilant opposition to the subtle influences of cultural discourse. In order to assist in that process, the therapist's task is to develop agency with and for the client, always attending to the client's world of meaning and experience, and continuing to call attention to agentive gaps. This means working with clients to notice previously unnoticed aspects of their experience, occurring in either the landscape of action or the landscape of consciousness, that reflect personal agency in a preferred direction.

If we believe that these events occur with intentionality, and we do, then our work with clients is to bring forth the small units of experience that surround the preferred activity in as much detail as possible. This requires first noticing what clients may not be noticing, and then asking questions to bring forth agency—such as "What happened before that?" and "How did you think to do that?" and "Where did this idea come from?" and "Could you relate the specifics of that incident?"—so that clients can appreciate their agency in these events. This process of question and response thus "thickens" the account of an activity and the meaning attributed to it into a narrative.

The Authors Speak

You might think about what questions in what domain will be most helpful to clients in this reauthoring process.

Questions Revisited/Landscape of Action

Often the turning points in people's lives are first noticed in a particular action or incident in which clients clearly *do* something different from what the problem story would suggest. In the family experiencing a *rift* each member noticed the change during a different event. For Gary, it occurred when he was on a drive in the car with Sharon, during which father and daughter were able to have an enjoyable conversation. For Sharon, it occurred when she made a decision to call her mom to ask about going out with friends, rather than just going out without asking, as *sneakiness* would suggest she do. And for Judy, it happened in a series of events in which she began to trust her daughter rather than assume she was making bad decisions. In fact, Judy recounted what, for her, was a key question in therapy: "When you back off from *fear* and *worry* and become okay with your daughter making decisions for herself, how can you keep the *fear* and *worry* from telling you the decisions have to be good ones?" By beginning to operate from *trust* (a counterplot), she could assume that many of her daughter's decisions would be "good," or that those she considered "bad" her daughter could perhaps manage. When a therapist and client are beginning to thicken an alternate story, it is often helpful to focus on one of these specific events and to ask questions about the event, using both landscape-of-action and landscape-of-consciousness questions. These questions are not asked in any particular order, nor does one start with one landscape and conclude with another; in all cases, questions are posed in response to clients' statements.

What we have found helpful is to switch landscapes if clients are having trouble with questions in one of them. For example, if clients can't say how they took such-and-such a step or even have trouble owning that they did (maybe it happened "because the moon was full"), we might ask questions such as these about the significance of the step: "Were you glad it happened?" "Do you prefer to respond this way?" "Why do you?" "Does it fit some goal?" In other words, we go from landscape-of-action to landscape-of-consciousness questions. After these sorts of questions, perhaps we return to the landscape of action, either present or past: "What did you do that fits that goal?" or to shift time, "In the past, what did you do that fit that goal?"

The Authors Speak

By listening carefully to the client and using our own instincts and intuition, we move between landscapes and across the dimension of time.

The questions put forth here are intended merely to illustrate these ideas. So, for example, with Sharon, I (VCD) asked first whether anything in particular had occurred that was more in the direction she hoped, away from the *rift* and toward more *closeness.* When she responded with the incident mentioned above, I could then have developed more of the narrative around action in the following ways:

1. Focusing on sequence, I might have asked, "What led up to this particular decision? For example, was there an incident that got you thinking more that calling would be a good thing to do?" Or I could have asked, "Was there anything in particular that led up to this decision or that prepared you for it? For example, did you have a memory of other times in your life when calling your parents about your plans led to an experience of mutual trust and understanding?" An infinite variety of questions could have been asked here. What seems to be helpful is to break down the sequence of events in a finely tuned and detailed way, to assist clients in seeing the actions they took, and thus to bring forth an experience of personal agency.

2. I could also have attended to the time variable of the narrative. I might have focused on the near past of the event with the following type of question: "Had any actions or events occurred recently that told you your parents might be responsive to your call in a way that would lead to more closeness?" Or the future could have been invoked: "Since this event reflected more what you might want to continue in your relationship with your parents, what events do you think might occur in the future in which you would find yourself wanting to do similar things?" "As you continue to act this way in your life, can you imagine what different ways *closeness* might look in your relationship with your parents at different life stages—for example, if and when you decide to go to college, get married, choose a career, have children, and so on?" Such questions as these are, of course, geared to specific clients and their histories and preferences.

Other possible types of a questions about the landscape of action— which can include aspects of or can be alternated with landscape-of-consciousness questions—include the following:

1. If the time variable is looked at as a rite of passage, we may ask questions that situate events in an in-between stage, clearly moving from a "before" to an "after" that is more how the client wants her or his life to be. (This type of question incorporates aspects of landscape-of-consciousness questions, because it refers to "wants.") The first question asked of the 56-year-old surgeon about what he would want to happen on his 80th birthday is an example, especially given his experience of transformation from being in the grips of anger and hostility to seeing himself as a caring and loving person. A possibility for Sharon and her family might have been this: "As you see yourselves moving away from

this time in which an experience of a *rift* dominated your lives to one in which *closeness* predominates, what other steps do you see each of you taking?" These kinds of questions also focus on the process as a stepwise one, not necessarily something that happens suddenly (even though a sudden shift is often people's experience).

2. "Future-looking-back" questions can be very helpful in the process of cementing a new story. These questions often take this form: "When you think about yourselves five years from now, when your daughter is 20, and you are sharing an intimate moment and/or relishing the closeness you all share, and you imagine that you are looking back to now. What steps do you see yourselves having taken to reach that time?" This question has many parts: It can be geared to address each person separately; it can focus on the particulars of the five-years-from-now time; it can break down the specifics of each step in terms of people, events, and time. And, again, any of these questions can be interspersed with landscape-of-consciousness questions, moving back and forth between actions and intentions, behaviors and desires, doing and wanting.

Landscape of Consciousness/Landscape of Identity

However restorying begins, we find it useful to help people bring forth counter narratives or alternative stories that are rich in both landscapes. Our belief is that even though the course of people's lives may begin to take them in a direction that supports a more preferred story, it is helpful for them to notice how this fits into their overall intentions. Without a restorying of intentions (e.g., "I was doing bad, but I'm now doing good"), they will be less apt to maintain the new direction. It is all too common that people again call to mind events that are painful or have brought difficulties into their lives, especially if these events still speak truths to them about who they are and why they do what they do. Types of landscape-of-consciousness questions that may be helpful in this regard include the following:

1. "When you think about this time in your daughter's life, and this experience of disconnection or of a *rift,* what do you wish were the case?" Or, "Looking ahead to how you want to continue your relationship with her, what ideas do you have about how your relationship will be?" And, back to a landscape-of-action question: "What specific events might you create that would lead to your future picture?" As we have suggested above, the landscape-of-consciousness and landscape of action questions interact within the context of therapist question and client response. So, as the questions above indicate, we either focus on wishes, desires, and

hopes and then try to locate them in events and behaviors, or vice versa (i.e., we focus on events and ask the client about intentionality).

2. We can also focus on values and beliefs: "When you think about what your daughter is choosing that you support and are pleased about, what about her choices tell you that perhaps she learned some of her values from you?" Or, to Sharon: "When you find yourself making decisions that lead to more *closeness* in your family, what values do you think you are holding?" And "Do you suppose you might come by those values 'naturally'? That is, might not these values be similar values to ones your parents hold?"

3. As the alternative story begins to become the dominant story for the client, we can bring forth meaning at the level of commitment—for example, "As you have renewed your commitment to connection and *closeness* in the family, do you have any ideas about how you might continue to call attention to that renewal?" With the woman experiencing *expectations* as the counterplot was thickened around *competencies* we could have asked, "Since you've resigned from *expectations,* what commitment have you made to a focus on *competencies* in your life?" Landscape-of-action questions can also be interspersed, as we ask about contracts, rituals, and both long-term and short-term goals.

The Authors Speak

Our experience is that it takes time for people learning this approach to think in terms of questions in the room.

The Problem Speaks

I keep trying to get them to listen mostly to me . . .

The Authors Speak

(*Aside*) What the problem hasn't quite gotten yet is that we are moving him further and further away. We have, in fact, created some "space" between him and our clients. We think you will find this space a helpful place in which change can occur. Maybe the problem will become less powerful. We shall see . . .

%

CHAPTER 5

Things Are Closer
Than They Seem

ON (NOT) DOING IT WITH MIRRORS

Several years ago, our favorite baseball team was in the National League Championship Series. This team, to the surprise of most of the baseball world, lost the series. Since the other team seemed clearly inferior in several aspects of the game, the explanation given was that they must have "done it with mirrors." The implication, of course, was that the winning team won in some magical way. Many therapies seem to have a magical component—an experience in which both the client and the therapist are unclear about how change happens. Explanations are given retrospectively in an effort to understand the therapeutic process. Instead, we see our work as having an intended direction and with specific desired effects. Our use of "mirrors" is intended to promote a reflexive position, which we believe can both create and enhance the restorying efforts of the client, instead of having the obscuring effect that smoke and mirrors and magic often connote.

The Problem Speaks

Going underground, becoming invisible—that is how I work *my* "magic." When therapies try to use *their* "magic" to trick me, I outsmart them. But when therapists use the mirror of reflexivity and transparency, they "unmask" me. Suddenly I become visible. But you are too "professional" to talk this way, so . . .

SPACE—THE FINAL FRONTIER

When we think of noticing something previously unnoticed, the metaphor that comes to mind is that of "space." For example, we often hear women comment that when they are in the company of men, the men "take up all the space." Women's words, ideas, and thoughts seem to carry less weight, less importance; there is little or no "space" for their thoughts to be expressed. Members of other groups that are marginalized and that are lower in status on the hierarchy of privilege often describe their experience as one of having no "space." This is the case for people of color when in the presence of European-Americans; for people who have been designated as lower-class in the presence of persons with class privilege; for gays and lesbians in a dominant heterosexual society; and for women with respect to men in a patriarchal society. Might it not also be the experience of people who are oppressed by a problem?

To continue this metaphor, we see that the dominant culture takes up most of the space and pushes to the edges those experiences that lie outside its normalized standards and values—so much so that even personal preferences are viewed in that space. If people notice that their wishes and desires are outside the dominant values and standards, they distrust them and, taking a more "normal" societal stance, quickly push them to one side. Is there ever space for people to examine how they have just gone along with the status quo, and whether doing so is even what they want? How, then, can people begin first to notice and then to voice· their marginalized, and perhaps preferred, experiences? For example, how does a woman pushed around by **expectations** access her experience of **competence** and **self-confidence?** We believe that this can be done through a creation or an opening of space—where discourse and its interpersonal context are pulled apart. In therapeutic interactions, we see that one way space can be opened for clients is by creating reflexive practices in the room. We think that it is most helpful for clients first to experience themselves in a reflexive position toward themselves and others.

The Authors Speak

We are raising the question "Could it be here, in some reflexive space, that change occurs?"

The Problem Speaks

I hate to admit that it is harder for me to hide when this space is created. I have nowhere to go, and it is indeed frustrating. However, I am still very slippery and very fast, even though these therapists think they are outsmarting me with their ideas of space and reflexivity.

The Authors Speak

One author to the other:

JEFF: Do you think their minds are on overload?

VICKI: Well, maybe this brief interlude will be a needed respite.

JEFF: Let's tell them, "Clear your minds, grasshoppers." I loved it when Master Po would tell Kane that in the TV show *Kung Fu*.

VICKI: You are weird.

The concept of "reflexivity" seems to capture this idea more precisely, for it is more than "reflecting." It is a process in which ideas can bounce off other ideas; aspects of experience can come to the fore, so that persons can begin to notice and examine previously held assumptions. It is an in-between place—between persons, between representations and persons (e.g., letters from others), between experience and persons (e.g., music). Reflexivity seems to occur in a space where the clients and the therapist can begin to generate new meanings and examine them for possible preference. Alternative knowledges or new stories become available for clients to begin to perform. There are numerous possibilities for helping clients assume a reflexive position. Here, we mention some of the ones we explore in our work.

BRINGING OTHERS INTO THE ROOM

"Who might be most apt to notice?" Notice what? Notice this new way of being, of performing—this new version of self. This is the question we ask any client who is beginning to perform a new, more preferred story. There are many other possible questions, all directed toward helping first the client and then others to notice a performance that reflects new meaning. Clearly, clients are the first to notice—often in subtle ways, but sometimes more dramatically. The latter happened with the orthopedic surgeon described in Chapter 4: "If someone had told me a year ago that I would feel really different, that I would think of myself and see myself in a new way, I wouldn't have believed them. I thought therapy meant just feeling better about some things and for a while. I didn't know I could actually experience myself as a different person." In other words, he no longer experienced himself as a man overcome by *anger* and *hostility;* he was living a life of caring and consideration for himself and for others. Thus, we want to explore those questions that not only will "thicken" the new story for the client, but will help it become the dominant one. We talk here about ways for clients to begin to reflexively notice their own preferred possibilities; these include ways that the therapist can construct the interview, as well as ways that the therapist can use himself or herself to create possibilities for opening space. First, we will explore some further ways of questioning, which can help a client find himself or herself in a reflexive position.

Experience-of-Experience Questions

- Who in your past would be least surprised about these developments?
- Would it surprise you to hear that I'm not surprised that you took this step?
- What would your son notice about the steps you have taken that he would be pleased about?

Questions such as these allow clients to notice themselves from the perspective of another—in these cases, a significant other person from the past, the therapist, or a family member, respectively. In a way, these questions allow other relationships into the room (not just a therapist and a client), and/or they put clients into a position where they see themselves the way the therapist and others see them. Bringing other relationships into the therapy can have the effect of others' carrying the burden of the work. Michael White (1995a), borrowing from Barbara Myerhoff (1982), has dubbed this process "re-membering." Persons can restory their lives in the context of their most significant relationships; therefore, work with the therapist does not have to count as much. These questions could be followed up by actually bringing people in; they would be a powerful audience for the development of an alternative story. Questions can be asked across time (past, present, future) and can be asked in either the landscape of action or the landscape of consciousness, as in these examples:

- What did that teacher notice you were doing that would have her conclude this about you?

- If I asked your friend Joe to tell me what it is about you that allows you to take on such a project, what would he say?

A variation of this type of question is a "future-looking-back" question, which involves the client consulting her or his own knowledge and experience—for example, "Five years from now, when you look back at the steps you have taken, will you see that you have many more steps to take or that you are near the end of your journey?" Such questions help the client think about what she, he, or the other is thinking. This is a reflexive process, which creates the space for noticing possibilities that have been outside the client's usual view.

The Authors Speak

It is our experience that these types of questions are generally evocative and are among the most useful we ask.

Asking Questions to the Ceiling

Even when questions are asked in an indirect way, as "experience-of-experience" questions are, clients are still being faced directly with questions and thus are in the position of respondents. Once the clients are in this position, there is an overwhelming pull to give some kind of answer or response. This inclination leaves little room for them to reflect or consider the possibilities available, or to explore the many experiences they may have had that could enrich their thinking and thus their responses. If, however, clients feel no need to respond—and one way to bring this about is not to ask questions directly—then they may find several more ways to think about their thinking and their lives.

In the past, for example, I (VCD) would suggest to students who were interested in working with adolescents that it is often helpful not to make eye contact with adolescent clients—to look at the floor, or at the ceiling, or out the window, while one is conversing with them. This takes the young persons "off the hook," as it were, and allows them to respond or not (something that doesn't usually happen when young people are "called to the office," which therapy often feels like to them). It subsequently became clear that this practice is useful for other clients, not just adolescents. So, for instance, if you had watched me work with the family with the *rift,* you might have seen me leaning back, looking at the ceiling, and musing out loud to Gary and Judy, "Let me think about this. I wonder what ways you may have given *fear* the slip in the past and focused more on the closeness and connection between you and Sharon?" Sometimes clients will spontaneously respond. At other times we may offer some examples that they have offered previously or that we have heard from others. Almost always, when we look at our clients, they are nodding or smiling or also looking at the ceiling (no doubt looking for answers!), and in some way indicating that they are operating from a reflexive position.

Two Talking, One Listening

Whenever there are more than two persons in the room, there is ample opportunity for people to find themselves in a reflexive position. Contrary to what many other therapies try to create, we are not so interested in attempting to get people to talk to each other (because usually the problem takes over the conversation).

The Problem Speaks

Who, me?

Rather, we talk to each person in the room individually about his or her experience of the problem and preferred directions. So, for example, when working with a couple, we may talk with one person for some time about the problem and the problem's effects on his or her life and relationships, while the other is listening to the discussion.

The Problem Speaks

I can keep people from hearing what the other is saying. I fill their heads with my thoughts so that they can't even pay attention to a different perspective.

Often, especially early in therapy, we realize that the problem is filling people's heads with its thoughts. What we try to do is help clients notice its influence. Constructing the problem and listing its effects seem to reduce its power. At first clients listen primarily to the problem, but over time our continued talking about it in the antiproblem ways that we do (externalizing) does open up space for clients to notice their own ideas.

The Authors Speak

Our experience is that others in the room who are listening to these conversations also notice new things—not only about the person to whom the therapist is talking, but also about themselves.

Over time, a person in the listening position begins to listen in new ways and begins to hear the other from a different perspective. In other words, the problem is no longer getting the listener to make meaning of the other's actions or to attribute some ill thinking to her or his intentions. This "listening in" or "eavesdropping" can also trigger new possibilities for listeners; it can allow them to call to mind unique outcomes in their own lives or in their relationships in which the problem was not able to trick them. So, for example, as I (VCD) talked to Sharon, who had triumphed over the *rift*'s attempt to get her to continue to participate in *sneakiness,* her mother was listening to her daughter's more preferred intentions and behavior while *at the same time* recalling her own efforts to beat *fear* and *worry* and to develop a more trusting attitude toward her daughter.

This also happens in cases where the problem has gotten a firm hold on people because of an outside influence that has disrupted a family or an individual. In one such instance, a 13-year-old boy had been molested by a male adult, who had seduced a group of young boys by offering them alcohol, cigarettes, and pornographic material. The effect on the young man was one that included *anger* but also *noncaring,* and the effect on the parents was one of *fear* and *confusion,* particularly about how to parent their son. As I (VCD) talked to the young boy about how he was continuing to act in caring ways in some aspects of his life, in spite of the influence of *noncaring,* the parents were able to notice their own efforts at escaping the influence of *fear* and *confusion* by taking more action in helping their son set limits for himself. The reverse also occurred; that is, the son could see that limit setting on the part of his parents was a helpful thing to him, because it set a context of safety in which he could recapture some of his preferred (more caring) ways of acting in his life.

In earlier sessions in therapy, the problem seems to have more of a hold. For instance, with the spouses experiencing *antagonism,* (see Chapter 3, Example 1), each was certain that the problem was the other who was antagonistic. When the problem was externalized between them, each was better able to hear the other speak. It was only in this way that the early history of closeness could even be acknowledged. Sometimes in the course of therapy, I (VCD) would also experience the effects of the problem—in this case, *antagonism*—and find it difficult to notice the couple's progress. Then one or the other member of the couple would remind me that they had indeed been communicating more openly or had worked together as parents to help one of their kids.

Taking a Break

Simply taking a break is a practice that may be underrated by therapists of any theoretical persuasion. The Milan team introduced it as an important step in their process, but their use of it was to enable the therapist to develop a hypothesis about what was happening for the client (Selvini-Palazzoli, Boscolo, Cecchin, & Prata, 1980). Since our work is antithetical to hypothesis construction and is geared more toward understanding the client's meaning (the client's own hypothesis), we think of taking a break as an opportunity for both therapist and client to engage in some processing of reflexivity. In other words, we leave the room and take a break when we think a problem has interfered with our own reflexivity. We find we can then think about the client and what we can ask that would be helpful to him or her without the problem's influence being as strong. We often suggest to interns/trainees that they take a break when they are stuck. We are finding now that we can usually take a break in the room by looking at the ceiling and saying out loud, "I wonder what I think about this," or "Let me ponder this," or "Give me a minute." This is a way we have of creating space. However, physically leaving the room is sometimes the best (if not only) option when a therapist truly needs to escape the problem's influence.

The Authors Speak

Our experience is that clients are undergoing a similar process: "What is happening? What am I thinking? Am I doing/saying what I want?"

Situating

"Situating" is a process that further allows clients to experience themselves in a reflexive position. It is a very specific kind of self-disclosure in which the therapist says what led to the content of a particular question— that is, what personal experience, or previously held theories, or newly concocted fantasies were in the therapist's thinking. Situating has the effect of removing us as therapists from the position of experts and prevents our comments from being accepted as "truth"; rather, it places our questions and our thoughts alongside those of our clients and of others as simply other perspectives, other views. In this way, it primarily offers information only, and allows clients to take whatever they want from the questions and the perspectives. The situating of our comments allows us to be "transparent" in a way that backlights our personal biases and viewpoints, as well as providing a social, cultural, historical, and political context to our questions and comments.

One of our ways of introducing situating into the therapy room is to ask clients at the end of the session what questions they may have about our questions. Generally, clients are so unused to this question and so caught up in the problem that such a question has little or no meaning for them. They occasionally offer a general comment on how the therapy is going, or ask what we think about how they are doing. One possible way to get the conversation going is to ask them about a particular question we have asked—for example, "Well, I wondered if you were curious about why I asked where you might have gotten the idea that your son would do better if he were away at college." In this way, we can do further deconstruction of our own thinking, thus inviting clients into reflexive positions that will (we hope) involve them in further thinking or perhaps questioning. In regard to the example just given, we might talk about "separation ideas" in the culture and ask clients to consider what fits for them.

We may also situate a comment in other clients' ideas. For example, we might say to one client, "Other clients who struggle with similar problems tell me [such and such]; I wonder what you might think about this." Such a statement/question often allows clients to ponder their own resources and notice other options.

Recently, upon taking an "emergency" call from our exchange, I (VCD) talked with a client who was seeing another therapist not currently available, and said to him: "My clients often tell me that when they are experiencing a crisis or a difficulty and they can't easily get hold of me, they have conversations with themselves about the problem." This started a process that was very different from one in which I might have been influenced by the idea that I had to fix things. The notion that other clients have found something useful, and that a client himself or herself may know best about how to handle the difficulties he or she is experiencing, can take hold much more readily when the information is coming from others who have experienced things in a similar manner.

What we have found useful and now tend to do more frequently is to situate some of our questions as we go. So we might say, "Tell me how you think your son's going away to college would be better for him than staying at home, and might be a solution to the *anger* that you both experience. I say this because my experience from talking with other parents is that they are influenced by some idea that *separation* is necessary for kids to grow up. I wonder what you think."

Another time, in a consultation group meeting, one of the participating therapists said, "Once you start to say, 'Let me tell you why I asked that question,' I go into an altered state. I immediately begin to think about what I'm thinking and all the possible ways I could respond to your question."

Yet another recent example is that of the young boy who was experiencing *noncaring* in his life. Situating the question about what habits *noncaring* may have gotten him into was done in the following manner:

"I'm asking you that question because in my experience with other young men your age, they tell me that *noncaring* and *nonthinking* often get them to do things they wouldn't do otherwise, like sneak drinks from their parents' liquor cabinet, or sneak a cigarette, or try smoking marijuana. I wondered if this problem had gotten you to do any of those things."

The Authors Speak

JEFF: Vicki, I would like to ask you how you thought that was helpful.

VICKI: I believe it was helpful in two ways. First of all, it gave him time to think about his own experience, separate from having to respond immediately; that is, it created "space." Second, it allowed him (and his parents) to notice that some choices kids make are effects of the problem and are likely not preferred by them.

JEFF: What I find is that this sort of conversation creates an opening for clients to reflect on their own experience; they then can compare their own experience to what the therapist says and notice more clearly whether it fits for them. Often this has the effect of helping them get clearer about the meaning they want to bring to their own lives.

End-of-Session Summary

A further practice for creating an experience of reflexivity is to construct an end-of-session summary with clients. The therapist composes this summary from the session notes (thus staying close to the clients' experience) and uses externalizing language. Usually it is helpful to make a distinction between the problem story, with its subjugating effects on clients, and the story they may prefer. Earlier in therapy, the summary may include only the beginnings of an alternate story, a unique outcome or two, and questions for noticing. In the middle of therapy, the summary may focus on antiproblem strategies and on possibilities for continued reauthoring. And near the end of therapy, the summary reflects a more "thickened" preferred story. These summaries allow clients to consider how therapy is going for them and whether they are proceeding in ways they like. Summaries also become anchors for the clients in their lives, as well as starting points for subsequent sessions.

For example, with the young boy experiencing *noncaring,* a summary might go as follows:

What seems to have happened here is an experience of *noncaring* as an effect of the *abuse. Noncaring* has gotten you (*to the boy*) not to pay attention at school, to fight with your brother, to get into hassles with your mom and dad, and not even to have fun with your friends. For you (*to the parents*), it has brought *fear* and *confusion* into your lives, getting you not to know whether you know how to be parents to your sons, and making you question your own ideas and intuitions. For you (*to the boy's brother*), it has brought up feelings of *unfairness* and gotten you to argue with your brother and with your parents. However, what I am also paying attention to is how *noncaring* has *not* taken away your ability (*to the boy*) to talk with your parents and to "know they will listen," as you told me; and for you (*to the brother*), it has not taken away your interest in sharing time and energy with your brother; and for you (*to the parents*) you have not strayed from your continued efforts to have discussions with your sons.

A summary may end with a suggestion that all members of the family notice what the problem is doing to them, and also notice how they are continuing to fight its influence. When summaries like this are offered, our experience is that family members often nod, give verbal agreement, sometimes add (or subtract) a word or two, and generally seem to be reflecting on how the summary fits their experience.

The Authors Speak

Clients often tell us how important the summary is to them, and they will remind us if we forget. They also remark on how helpful it is that we take notes, using *their* words. We also often begin each subsequent session with a brief recap of the preceding session's summary, thus reminding them of the direction they are going—remembering that this direction is set by the clients, not by us.

AUDIENCES

An Event with Meaning

I (VCD) have a memory from when I was a little girl, maybe nine years old, of the day when my father laid down stepping stones in our backyard. After having dug the holes and laid the stones, he proudly showed them off to my mother. My mother responded critically, saying that they were too far apart, and that neither she nor we (their two daughters) could easily walk the path—we'd have to leap! Why does that memory stick with me? One reason, I suspect, is that I was in a reflexive position; I overheard a conversation. Another reason is that it had some meaning for me. Why did it have meaning? Was it that my mother rarely contradicted my father, so that when she did, it was noticeable? Was there some gender importance involved (my father's assumption that his steps would fit us all, my mother's unwillingness to defer)? My father responded by adding more stones, making it more of a path, so that it would fit everybody's step size. What did I make of this? Was I learning the importance of respect for other's wishes, sensitivity, listening, saying what one wants? This event eventually became one of the small stories that made up a dominant personal narrative for me.

What we realize is that people seem to remember those events that have meaning for them, and that reflected-upon events are imbued with meaning. We also know that people live in a context of others, those who have noticed other performances (sometimes ones previously dictated by the problem). In our work we try to help clients perform new meaning and enter into new stories, and we are interested in helping them develop audiences to these new performances—ones that they, rather than the problem, direct.

Individuals as Audiences

To return to the example of the orthopedic surgeon, when he remarked (and he continued to do so) on the performance of his new story, it was helpful to ask repeatedly what his wife saw and how his sons and daughters were responding. No story is performed without an audience; all of us live in a context. We believe that for any new story to truly become a dominant influence, it needs to become public. It has to be noticed or announced. Recently, the surgeon shared a conversation he had with his wife and a grown son, in which he was discussing his own parents when his son said, "Well, they might be able to change. After all, you did!" He was quite pleased to be able to relate this incident. There had occurred a spontaneous noticing on his son's part. It was an answer to the question he was often asked: "When you are around your son, can you imagine being a way that your son wants you to be—in a way that you both prefer?"

When clients begin to perform a new meaning, not only are they the first ones to notice it; they often are the only ones to do so. This is why, with couples and families, we don't invite others to notice how someone else is doing until they spontaneously do so. The noticing of another's performance usually only occurs after one has noticed one's own steps. We catch up with each person's development individually, and only when it is clear that she or he is noticing new developments do we ask about the other. In the example given above, if the family had been in the room, one question to the son might have been "What did you see that let you know your father had changed?" However, this question would have made sense only after the son had made the spontaneous remark or had otherwise indicated that he noticed the developments.

Our experience is that early in therapy, the problem is often so powerful in its "blinding tactics" that it is almost impossible for people to notice anything but what the problem wants them to notice. In fact, we often talk to our clients about how the problem may have inducted them into its "Problem Watchers Club." This membership has a coercive effect, making it even harder for anyone to notice steps that people may be taking away from its influence.

The Authors Speak

This is all the more reason why we believe it is critical to assist clients in creating audiences for the performances they prefer.

Leagues as Audiences

What would a performance be without an audience? Problems are isolating. They make people feel alone, outside, not fitting. By helping clients create a community of persons who can support and notice their progress away from problem stories and toward alternative stories, we are challenging individualizing psychologies. Such psychologies support the notion of problems "in" people; they also support the problem's tactic of creating audiences and getting members of the family, and others in a supporting cast, to become "problem watchers." Creating counteraudiences is something that "leagues" can do. The first antiproblem league that we know of was the Anti-Anorexia/Anti-Bulimia League, started in New Zealand by David Epston (1994). He created archives, consisting first of letters written by him and to him from the clients with whom he was working who were suffering the effects of anorexia and/or bulimia; later, he added videotapes to the archive. The texts of the letters and tapes were stories of his clients' battles with these problems and their small steps toward beating the problems. Although the league members never met face to face, these archival documents became tools for the therapist and each client to use to work together and join with other clients in sharing ways they had found to fight the problem. We in California have used David Epston's archival material and have begun to develop our own archives to draw upon in our work with clients.

The Anti-Anorexia/Anti-Bulimia League in Vancouver, begun by Stephen Madigan (1994), has become a league whose members do meet together. The members are currently publishing a newsletter, selling

T-shirts, and acting as consultants on reflecting teams for work with others struggling with these problems. They provide a community of support and offer truly "expert" opinions. The idea of leagues is catching on for other problems, such as ADHD, for which an alternative body of knowledge (archives) may be necessary to offset the cultural "truths" that are circulating to support the problem. Both anorexia/bulimia and ADHD have a great deal of support in the culture (i.e., the encouragement of a certain body type for women, and the rampant specifying and diagnosis of children in schools). Leagues offer an alternative culture and an alternative body of knowledge to support clients. In addition to support for other versions of self, the possibilities for developing anti-problem strategies, all from material generated by clients themselves, are enormous.

The Authors Speak

We find that reading a letter or showing a videotape from another client with a similar problem not only allows the client present in the room to be in a reflexive position, but also allows us to question the client about how her or his experience relates to what the client from the archive is suggesting. We provide a specific example of this in the next chapter, where we talk with a client about *bulimia.*

Other Ways of Circulating Preferred Stories

A colleague who works with parents in a workshop format shared the following story. She usually ends her first meeting with parents by asking them to notice something they might do with their kids that fits their preferred ways of acting, rather than the problematic ways that concern them; then she starts the second meeting by asking for examples of these kinds of experiences. A recently divorced father told of his weekend with his son. Previously on weekends he had struggled with disciplining his son, constantly telling him not to do things. This particular time, however, he picked up his son and asked him what he would like to do. The boy, a seven-year-old, said, "Nothing." It was raining outside, and the father suspected the boy was not looking forward to spending a long, boring weekend with his uptight father. The father took him to his house, then spontaneously said, "Let's put on our old clothes and go out and play in the rain." The boy was delighted, and the father reported that he hadn't had so much fun with his son in ages. In fact, he said that people who were driving by honked and waved. The colleague said that the rest of the parents applauded and that many of those present (including herself) had tears in their eyes. What happened here? Not only did the father begin to implement elements of a new, more preferred story, but he was in a situation where he had a ready-made audience (which the workshop leader had helped create).

Once a new story has become more noticeable to oneself, then circulating that story to a larger audience seems crucial to one's continuing experience of oneself as narrator and protagonist in the newly authored story. As stated above, the creation of leagues can be very helpful to this process. The very existence of a league adds a structured experience of a community of like-minded others; this experience is especially powerful, since this community and its knowledges have been marginalized by the dominant culture. There are other possibilities— perhaps less structured, but equally viable—for circulating preferred stories. For example, we often ask, "Since you have had some successes over this particular problem, would you be willing to share that information with others—that is, what things you specifically did or thought that might be helpful to someone else?" The effect is an empowering one for clients, because it allows them to see themselves in the position of having knowledge about the problem and about ways to deal with it successfully.

One way in which preferred stories can be circulated is for the therapist to hook clients up together. Sometimes, while working with a client, we notice that he or she is struggling with a problem similar to one that a former client (or another therapist's client) has struggled with and developed some expertise about. Since we typically ask clients whether they would be willing to share their expertise with others, we find it fairly straightforward to call former clients and ask them to act as consultants. This hookup has a circulating/reflexive effect in both directions: The former client is pleased to share her or his victory, and the current client is happy to have some support for his or her struggle. We have done these hookups by phone predominantly, sometimes by letters, and even occasionally by having clients meet together, with the therapist facilitating the exchange. This process seems to create an interesting space in which clients and problems meet in a new way, with the therapist taking a back seat.

I (JLZ) have had a number of recent experiences in which facilitating a connection between clients was, according to their feedback, extremely helpful. A woman experiencing **hopelessness** in a marriage heard from another woman about her experience of a new direction in her marriage as well as new efforts from her husband, despite repeated warnings from **hopelessness** that "It will never happen." A woman feeling overwhelmed by **obsessions** was connected to a client who had pushed **obsessions** out of his life; he offered hope to her. Another woman spoke to a former client who had been going with what she herself wanted, instead of submitting to *specifications* that privileged what others thought best. This provided support for moving in a direction away from what the dominant culture requires of women.

Documentation

A great deal has already been written about the power of documentation by the person who has made it a fine art, David Epston (White & Epston, 1990). David's consistent and continual use of letter writing as a part of his therapeutic practice has had immense positive effects on his clients, and also on those of us who have learned of the power of this practice from him. What we address here is the reflexive position that this practice creates for the client. Imagine having met with a therapist and returning home (dare we say "reflecting" on one's experience?), and within 24 hours receiving in the mail a letter that summarizes the session (including one's own words). Perhaps this raises a further question: What kind of different space occurs when one is reading a letter about one's experience?

Clients have reported that the experience of reading letters allows them to separate themselves more clearly from the problem and its effects; thus, it provides some space for them to notice other possibilities. In addition, therapists who are new to narrative therapy and social constructionist thinking have said that letter writing is an excellent way for them to fine-tune their thinking about what happened in the session, to review their notes, and to think more clearly about how to construct a problem that captures the client's experience.

We have used other kinds of documentation as well, also suggested by White and Epston (1990). Some years ago, when working with adolescents in a group setting, I (VCD) would end a time-limited group by asking that the group participants construct graduation diplomas or certificates or awards for one another. So, for example, a certificate might read "Courage to Stand Up for Oneself" for a group member who had overcome some timidity or what looked to others (teachers, parents) like sadness or depression. Another certificate might read "Respect for Others" for a young person who had been marked as defiant and rebellious. The group members would then discuss where they might display these certificates so that parents would see them. Some members would suggest that they hide them somewhere in their rooms, where parents would inevitably search them out. Others would suggest taking them home and immediately attaching them to the refrigerator. The outcome would most frequently be a conversation in which parents would ask what the certificate meant, and the young person would have a chance to talk about her or his new story. Many parents commented on how powerful these certificates were for them to see and appreciate, and how important it was for their children to know that they were being seen and appreciated.

REFLECTING TEAMS: REFLEXIVITY CUBED

As we have been saying, a reflexive position can occur when people find they have some space to consider, think over, examine, and explore their own thinking in relation to something else. In particular, it allows them to wonder about multiple possibilities for understanding their experience. We have utilized, and have described here, several ways to create a reflexive position in the therapy context:

1. The therapist speaks to one person in the room at a time while others listen.
2. The therapist wonders out loud about what might be occurring in the room.
3. The therapist takes a break, so that both therapist and client can have some thinking time.
4. The therapist constructs an end-of-session summary.
5. The therapist makes specific suggestions to clients, asking them to pay attention to or notice some preferred ideas, intentions, or activities.
6. Audiences are generated (through the use of individuals in or out of the room; leagues; other means of circulation; and documentation).

However, what we are currently finding most helpful is the structured creation of a reflecting team. In our use of a reflecting team, the members interview one another, raising questions about things that have popped up in the interview as possible preferred outcomes.

Listening to others (two or more) raising questions, without having to respond immediately, may put the client in even more of a reflexive position—one that allows possibilities for pondering while at the same time keeping them in relationship. When this occurs, a space is created in which clients can call to memory past incidents, make new associations, attend to some (but not all) questions, and generally wonder about what is being asked. When therapists on a team are purposefully raising questions about previously marginalized but possibly preferred experience, then this reflexive space is created. When, in addition, they offer their own experience as a basis for the origin of their questions (i.e., they situate their questions), then clients also have the space to compare their own experience to that of the team members. Whether there is a fit or a difference between the clients' experience and the team members', clients consistently report that this is the most helpful aspect of the process. This suggests that an experience of being in a reflexive position may offer a great deal more to clients than the usual listen-and-respond mode that characterizes most therapies.

The Set-Up

Reflecting teams are most easily utilized in training settings or in group consultation work, where several therapists or trainees are already present. The following structure is how we ordinarily structure the reflecting process. It starts with the therapist's meeting with the client and the team's observing behind a one-way mirror. After a short interview (perhaps 40 minutes), the team and the therapist and client change places. The team members then raise questions about what they heard for a short period of time (10–15 minutes). After this team interview, the two groups change places again, and the therapist asks the client what questions the reflecting team members raised that were of interest to her or him, and which were helpful or not helpful. Sometimes, in a final part, a designated supervisor enters the room along with the reflecting team and asks the client whether she or he has any questions for the therapist or for the team members. This supervisor then raises questions about the therapist's and the team members' questions. One possibility is to raise these questions along some restorying theme that seemed to arise in the course of the interview—something we often find useful.

Guidelines

We have developed a set of guidelines for persons who are going to be on a reflecting team; we hope these will help them respond in ways that will create a reflexive position for the client. (See Appendix A.) Our experience with reflecting team members is that it is most helpful for them to remember to raise questions that address personal agency for the client, specifically in regard to what they have noticed as possible unique outcomes or contradictions to the problem story. If, instead of raising questions, team members express delight or surprise or are otherwise "impressed," the client is less apt to ponder her or his own experience of meaning.

We have often found in our training groups that persons learn the most about being on a reflecting team through experiencing being reflected upon. We discuss this more in Chapter 11. However, we offer an example here to underline how we think about the reflecting process. Once some clients and I (VCD), during a week of intensive training, were being interviewed by JLZ about the process of therapy, and the training group was acting as a reflecting team. Since it was a new group, and the members were feeling their way, I heard a lot of comments and personal reflections from the group and not many questions. Mostly, I found myself not finding that the comments fit my experience very well. They seemed more to come from the trainees' own ideas and experiences—with one exception. One team member raised a question about what I was thinking when I asked a specific question; this member wondered how I thought such a question would be helpful to the clients. I found myself spontaneously reflecting on my own thought process, clarifying for myself a way of working I realized I preferred. Since then, I have been able to return to this specific question and way of working on other occasions. I would not have had this realization had not the team member raised that question.

The following discussion focuses on things reflecting team members can pay attention to in the interview, and ways they can respond to these.

Noticing Preferred Developments

Consistent with our thinking about therapy, we suggest that team members focus on the client's preferred developments, unique outcomes, and contradictions to the problem story as entry points to an alternative meaning. When we ask team members to pay attention to these developments, we find that sometimes they pick up unexpected "gaps" in the problem story that may have eluded the therapist's attention. We suggest to the team that these contradictions have undoubtedly gone unnoticed by the client, so that in their questioning process they might want to focus on making meaning in regard to these possibly preferred developments. This, of course, is very different from simply noticing or commenting on "positives." Remember that unique outcomes are connected to the problem story, in that they are events, actions, or ideas in the client's life that would not be predicted by a telling of the problem story. As the term suggests, they are outcomes that are *unique* in relation to the problem.

The Problem Speaks

I'm going to get into this conversation and mess it up. This is all about "positives." (I have to say this, so they won't expose me.)

The Authors Speak

(*Aside*) Where did he come from?

For example, suppose that the parents in the family experiencing a *rift* had said that they were pleased with their daughter's grades in school. This could have been experienced as a "positive," but it might or might not have been a unique outcome. (It would not have been directly connected with, by being specifically contradictory to, the problem story.) It might, on the other hand, have been an example of an experience leading to more **connection** or **closeness** in this family, but this would have had to be asked about before we would know for sure. On the other hand, when Gary, Judy, and Sharon said that they liked to spend time together, that seemed more closely related to, and contradictory to, their experience of *rift*. Or when Judy said that she let go of **worry,** and Sharon said that she called her parents to tell them what was going on rather than letting **sneakiness** direct her, then those examples were "unique outcomes." They also may have been experienced as positive, but that's not the point.

The Problem Speaks

But if I get you to focus on that, you'll miss the point.

The Authors Speak

(*Aside again*) We thought we had gotten rid of him—or at least changed our relationship with him. We know we now have more power than he does . . .

Being Curious

By raising questions about "gaps" or possible preferred developments, the team members help clients be curious about their own experience—in particular, about what in their own lives may have contributed to these contradictions to the problem story. In this way, clients begin to attribute new meaning to their experience, constructing an alternate story. Again, it is in the raising of questions that this reflexive position is created.

*Asking Both Landscape-of-Action
and Landscape-of-Consciousness Questions*

1. Are these contradictions preferred? Why or why not?
2. Do they have a history? A future? If so, what is it?
3. What different attitudes have they brought forth for the client toward others?

4. Who else might be aware of these contradictions or preferred developments (in the past, present, or future)?
5. What different actions or behaviors have occurred in response to these events?

Questions that address both landscapes have the effect of "thickening" the alternate story, making it bigger in the client's experience than the problem story has been. It is probably important for team members to remember that these events or ideas have probably been neglected, not noticed, or not attended to by the client. They can then remind themselves that they are asking "reauthoring" questions, helping the client make meaning in regard to preferred developments. The team is co-constructing alternative meaning-making possibilities with and for the client.

Responding with Questions and Situating Questions

One team member will raise a question that reflects his or her curiosity about a gap in the client's story or a contradiction that he or she has noticed. This question may show some interest in the occurrence as well as the history or possible future of this contradiction. If the team member makes a comment rather than poses a question, another member may ask what question this comment might evoke. After posing the question, the team member then describes what about his or her experience, education, or thinking has informed the question. If the team member does not situate the question in this manner, another member can ask the questioner to do so. As we have noted above, by situating each question, the team members make it apparent that their remarks are not necessarily right or even helpful for this particular client; rather, they come primarily from the team members' own experience or ideas. This, then, does not privilege the therapist's or team members' ideas over the client's ideas. It has the effect of flattening the implicit hierarchy. Situating remarks may also include why the team member thinks his or her question may be helpful to the client, even though the client may or may not experience it that way.

Being an Audience

The reflecting team's musings become similar to an overheard conversation on which the client can "reflect," picking those remarks and questions that have most meaning and that best fit her or his experience. In this way the reflecting team is also an audience, from which the client experiences an invitation to a continued and perhaps expanded performance of her or his preferred story. This is no ordinary audience; these are participants in a new performance.

Questions about Questions

Since reflecting teams are used most often in training settings, we have found it helpful to include an end-of-session discussion in which a supervising therapist, the reflecting team, the therapist, and the client all come together. During this final part, the supervisor asks the client whether she or he has any questions for the therapist about the therapist's questions, or any questions for the team members about their questions. The supervisor also uses this opportunity to raise questions for the therapist and the team members, with the intent of further situating and making transparent the therapy process. One way we have experimented with doing this is to raise these questions about a theme that seemed to emerge in the interview. This theme may become a title for a counterplot or a chapter title in the client's emerging new story. For example, "A New Hope" might be the theme around which the team members' questions could be further questioned by the supervisor: "You asked this questions about Suzy's taking a stand on what she wanted. As a woman, how do you think this could relate to 'A New Hope'?"

In another instance, in a consultation group setting, the therapist was interviewing a male client about his struggles with **shyness** and perceived **lack of motivation** on his part. The work focused on his reauthoring activities and the steps he had taken for himself and his preferred goals, and the reflecting team raised questions that seemed to point to a possible sense of personal agency for the client. When the supervisor and reflecting team entered the interview room for the final discussion, the supervisor asked the client whether he had any thoughts about what he would like to name this session. After very little hesitation, he said, "Male Sensitivity." Although the supervisor had some thoughts of her own about possible titles, she saw that the reflecting team process had allowed the client to name his own preferred story quickly. She then could easily raise questions for the therapist and the team members, bringing forth this "Male Sensitivity" theme.

The Authors Speak

We now want to demonstrate still further how reflexivity works by making use of a different medium—a one-act play that personifies the problem, the antiproblem, the culture, the client, a significant person in the client's life, and the audience. We think you will recognize this client and the problem she struggles with in her life.

We also hope that you will see how important an audience is in this process.

EXPECTATIONS—REPRISE
(A PLAY IN ONE ACT)

X: (*Entering from stage left and addressing the audience*) Only recently have I been found out! Until then I could hide under **guilt** and a **burden of responsibility.**

MOMMIE DEAREST: (*Walking slowly from stage right*) A "quilt"? What do you mean?

X: No, no! **Guilt.** Surely you know what *that* is.

MD: Well, it's my enemy, so I've tried to pass it on.

X: You've done an outstanding job, I must say.

CULTURE: (*Stage rear, behind MD*) Not without *my* help!

X: (*Stage front*) Yes! You have made this be about *me.* I'm the star of this play. Listen to my uninterrupted soliloquy. I am insidious, intelligent, invisible. I can become very small and sneak inside her head. I can trick her into not knowing the difference between my voice and hers. I take her talents and use them against her. I can reach into every aspect of her life, but I get her mostly when she tries to be a good mother and a good wife. I love that word— "good."

ANTI-EXPECTATIONS: (*Entering from stage left, behind X*) You just think it's about you. I have many strategies that I teach my friends to employ you—strategies to upset your smugness and to help people notice their own desires and wishes. Not the least of which is *naming* you. Surely you've noticed that!

X: (*Turning*) I'm not afraid of you. Strategies—what do you even know about them?

ANTI-**X:** (*Stage center*) I don't mind telling you, because they render you powerless against them. For Dorothy they are **trust, competence,** and **empathy.**

X: She won't even notice those strategies. I am too powerful. I have blinded her to their very existence.

MD: Well, *I* know they're around.

X: Quiet! How could *you* know?

MD: Contrary to what you've made Dorothy believe (and sometimes me, I must admit), I see her strength, and I'm on her side—which, as everyone knows, you're not!

CULT: Quiet! Mothers are the enemy. Not problems!

X: *Yes!* I knew you'd come through.

ANTI-X: We can help Dorothy see through you, **Culture,** and also through your shill, X. Problems are problems, and you imbue them with *your* meaning, making them bigger than life.

X: You think you're so smart. Just how do you think you can help Dorothy? She's my captive.

AUDIENCE: (*Voices from below*) We can help!

X: Who let you in? You're not supposed to talk!

DOROTHY: (*Appearing stage right, next to MD* and addressing X) Ah, but they *did* talk. They not only talked, they asked questions. I found myself pondering the ideas they raised, reflecting on their queries. And I realized that I had already taken some steps toward what I wanted, not what you were trying to put into my head.

ANTI-X: You see, X, those of us who are against you try to find ways to help people notice other things that *aren't* you. Isn't that a clever idea?

X: But, but, but . . . how can you do that? I take up all the space.

ANTI-X: Oh, no, you don't. We have found many, many ways to create space without you by helping people find a way to experience themselves as separate from you.

X: But you turned the audience against me! They've been my best supporters.

ANTI-X: Yes, I did. I asked them to raise questions about what they noticed in Dorothy's experience that not only had nothing to do with you, but that was counter to you—that, in fact, was more about my strategies—and finally, more about Dorothy.

DOROTHY: Yes, I am! I am more about me, about anti-*expectations,* about **trust** and **competence** and **empathy.** And, guess what, X? My mother is on my side! What do you think of that?

X: Argh!

The Authors Speak

The problem has had his say about his tricks and tactics, and we have had our say about some useful problem-defeating ideas. It is time now for our clients to have their say.

PART II

Clients Strike Back

CHAPTER 6

If Clients Talked
Adults Talk about Their Individual Work

HOW DOES THE SONG GO—II

The Authors Speak

We're going to switch gears now and give examples from our clinical work. Well, we're not going to give them—our clients are. Perhaps it is more accurate to say that all of the examples are cocreated. (You decide.) Anyway, we have written this and other chapters in Part II as if clients were speaking about their experience of the work. We have written Chapter 7 from our own experience, but not in a didactic way. We hope it is clear, at this point, why we are using this kind of device to describe this work. We believe that focusing on our clients' experience is more reflective of the attitudes in the work. (Again, you decide.)

A FICTIONAL CONVERSATION AMONG REAL PEOPLE

Cast (in order of appearance):
Vicki: Person raising questions.
Jeff: Person who provided consultation.
Alan, Cindy, Elliot, Karen: Persons who sought consultation.

VICKI: How does a conversation like this start?

JEFF: Anyway we want it to . . .

ALAN: I can't wait. I'm going to start. (*Turning to Cindy*) Cindy, when I read what the problem was saying to you in Chapter 2, I felt it was talking to me too. **Pain, evaluation, self-doubt** are no strangers to my life. **Lack of competence, dependence,** and *fear* have affected me a lot. Looking different, being different, what chance did I have? At least you [Cindy] had two loving parents. I only had one (loving one, that is).

CINDY: Well, how did you manage to begin to escape the problem?

ALAN: The first time I had a serious bout with the problem, I went into the hospital. When I came out, not only were the same life problems around—like family and job issues—but then I was really down on myself. Becoming a hospital patient and being medicated made me feel weaker and made it harder to combat *fear* and *depression*.

CINDY: I know what you mean. I was only in the hospital briefly, after a suicide gesture, but I was treated like a patient for a long time. How can you possibly know what you want, or learn how to handle things your own way?

ALAN: When I left the hospital, I knew I wanted something different. Someone had given me Jeff's name and I called him. It was hard at first to get out of the habit of calling him "Doctor."

CINDY: So what happened?

ALAN: I went in talking about *fear* and *anxiety*, which seriously interfered with my doing anything, at that point. Even though I was still feeling bad when I left that first session, I also felt a little better, too. We had come up with the idea that I was like Rocky—you know, the fighter in the Sylvester Stallone movie? It was because I keep getting back up, no matter what. I saw Jeff again five days later and had my first good day since leaving the hospital. Three days later, when I saw him for the third time, I felt like I was on my way to getting better. Also, I was beginning to trust myself again, to be in charge of my life. At that point, I was ready for once-a-week sessions.

CINDY: I am trying to get a sense of what the problem was. Also, did you ask for sessions so close together?

ALAN: I did. I felt I really needed frequent sessions to stay out of the hospital, which I really wanted to do. I think Jeff thought a couple of times a week was a lot, but when we talked about it together, we decided to play it by ear each session and I would have the option of saying what I needed. What was surprising was how fast I thought I could go to once a week, that I could trust myself again. As for the problem—there were many, including current struggles with my abusive father and the things he did to me, to my sister (who recently died), and to my mother; guilt over things I did as a young man; teasing I received over the years because of my short stature and large head; trying to keep a job. The effect of these issues was to encourage *depression* and *fear*, and the effects of these problems was to create questions about my *competence* to deal with life—something I had faced, to some extent, for some time. We focused more on these last few things (*depression, fear, competence*) than on the specifics of the other issues. At that point *depression* and *fear* were giving me the most trouble.

CINDY: This is making me think about my early work with Jeff—how tackling the "specifics" wasn't helpful at all.

ALAN: What do you mean?

VICKI: I want to ask you about that, too—the "specifics," I mean. Maybe later . . .

CINDY: I first saw Jeff individually five years ago, the summer my parents told me I had to move out. I was 31 years old. I had been in therapy for over 10 years with other therapists. (You can read my comments about this in Chapter 2.) My most recent therapist had just left town. I was extremely miserable all the time and hated myself and my life—what little there was of it. I talked about inadequacy, fear, and feeling out of control. What Jeff finally focused on was the *pain* that these problems encouraged, as well as its pervasive effects on my life.

ALAN: Finally?

CINDY: Well, at first, to use his words, he got "caught in the problem." He tried to help me move out, which was what others in my life thought was right, and when I moved, everything was worse . . . so I moved back. The *pain* around all of this just about did me in. After six months of weekly sessions and many phone calls, we realized that an even better name for the problem was *pressure*, because the problem was invited by my feeling obligated by what others wanted me to respond to, to think, and to do. I was immobilized by it.

JEFF: I really thought it was powerful. I experienced its influence on me in our work in the room, and on the phone with you as well. So what I remember was that the *pain* seemed so dominating, it made it hard to talk about anything else in the session.

CINDY: Or outside of the session.

ALAN: I know what you mean. It was a little like that for me at first. But

I had struggled on my own for many years and had no therapy until I went in the hospital. Maybe that's why I ended up feeling stronger than you seemed to feel.

CINDY: So what worked for you in therapy?

ALAN: I was telling you about my battle with *fear*. Jeff and I looked at *fear's* effects on my life—specifically, how it created habits, how it encouraged avoidance, and generally how it (and the hospital experiences) had affected the view I had of myself. I began to ask myself, "Do I want to be influenced by *fear's* view or *my* view?"

JEFF: Alan, can I clear something up?

ALAN: Sure.

JEFF: In working with people in therapy, I often use that distinction you just mentioned, the problem's view or the person's . . .

ALAN: It's helpful.

JEFF: Thanks. What I am really speaking of when I say "the person's view" is an alternative view or story—one that the person believes will have good effects on his or her life and lead to preferred outcomes.

VICKI: Could I interject something here? Isn't the point you are trying to make that *all* stories are "within" people's experience—that people can choose what stories to influence them from the many possibilities that they have been exposed to in their lives?

JEFF: Yes. There are many possible stories. The problem story has become more dominant, so separating it from the person by externalizing it and making a distinction between the problem and the person makes other possible stories more noticeable.

ALAN: Well, I liked **Rocky** as a story for me.

CINDY: Go on. How did the **Rocky** story help?

ALAN: Well, the **Rocky** story got really filled in when I came back after not seeing Jeff for that first whole week. I was continuing to do better and better, and what we noticed was my strength of will, my ability to concentrate and make things happen. We also talked about how *fear* was depending on certain ideas of being a man. I didn't fit some of those ideas; I tried to fit others, but I didn't have my heart in it, and failed. Despite that, I bounced back and moved forward in my life. I took on some very tough odds and beat them. I kept coming back—like Rocky. When I came to see Jeff the next week, I felt 100% back. And one week after that when I saw him, I returned to work. During those last couple of visits, we focused on my history of mustering strength and standing up to difficult problems at different points in my life. We also focused on some of the special knowledge I had, given my experience. During that week, the problem tried to reappear and I had a chance to fight it off—only one round, and I was the one left standing!

CINDY: Whose idea was the **Rocky** story?

ALAN: Mine, of course. Anyway, at that point, given how good I was doing, I wanted to try it on my own, without therapy. There were big issues left, but I felt strong.

CINDY: How did it go?

ALAN: Okay for about a year. Then the ongoing issue with my dad, and disagreements with my wife, and continued job problems overtook me. I came in for two sessions, and we identified some more of my own resources that I could use. We also began to focus on me being a "good person"—something I can easily forget. Four months later, though, I was in trouble again. **Fear** and **lack of competence** knocked me off the road. **Fear** took over my driving. I could drive certain places, but I had to constantly retrace my steps because I kept thinking I might have hurt someone. I kept imagining I drove too close to people. I had lots of doubt about any goodness I might have. The issue with my dad . . . I thought I could manage it, but it got too big. My wife had very strong feelings about it, and it was hard to disagree. Our relationship began to be affected by this and other problems, and my wife has her own physical problems. I decided to see Jeff again and really tackle the remaining issues this time.

JEFF: Alan, what was your experience of what we worked on this time?

ALAN: Well, I think of it as learning to take charge of the **fear**. First, we began to focus on anti-**fear** practices. These were the capabilities or areas of competence I had, strategies I used, that went directly against how **fear** was directing me. Right from the start we began noticing them, and I began to see the control I had over **fear**—in a more general way than the last time, but also in specific ways around how **fear** was affecting my driving. We also discovered something very important: that I have an amazing ability to plug into an idea or attend to one thing without wavering. You (*turning to Jeff*) called this my "focusing talent." (*To the others*) He helped me notice that **fear** was taking this talent from me and using it against me. We also noticed the possibilities that were created when I used this talent for myself, like focusing on what Alan thinks and wants rather than what **fear** thinks and wants. I began to see even more options for using my abilities in new ways. I remember, Jeff, you asked me if I noticed my own competence and ingenuity, and I did! This helped me erase the doubts **fear** had created, and I began to appreciate myself again.

ELLIOT: How long did this part take?

ALAN: About six weekly sessions. Why do you ask?

ELLIOT: Well, I had a similar problem. I'd had it for years, in fact. I kept it a secret because I was ashamed of it. The rest of my life was good—loving parents, good grades in school, friends, a high standard of living. I was about to start college, and my dad encouraged me to do something about this problem, although he only knew a little. I told Jeff, on my first visit, that what I had heard my problem was called was "compulsiveness." I had to redo many things many times to feel okay. I had repeating thoughts—as often as every five minutes. They told me that if I didn't repeat things, people I loved would die.

CINDY: What did you call the problem?

ELLIOT: We decided on *anxiety*. That seemed to cover all my habits and the way I felt.

ALAN: How long did it take you to deal with this?

ELLIOT: I had four sessions, but I must say that there were no other problems. In the first session, Jeff helped me to notice that I was already able to control the problem—that I could resist *anxiety*.

CINDY: How?

ELLIOT: By helping me see how I *do* break free from *anxiety*: I accomplish things at school and social events, despite *anxiety*. He asked me questions about these things, questions I never thought of, like "What was it about *me* that let me accomplish these things?" I said that I was determined, that I had goals, that I used this to put *anxiety* aside and ignore it. When I returned two weeks later, I had stopped responding to a lot of what *anxiety* wanted me to respond to. I remembered that Jeff asked me what *anxiety* wanted. I said, "To take my life away." I didn't want to let it take my life away. In a way, it was like you, Alan. *Anxiety* was using my determination against me, and Jeff helped me to notice I was beginning to keep it for myself. He also asked me about key strategies. I said that I could remember that if I ignored it, it would stop.

CINDY: Was that it, then?

ELLIOT: No. I returned as scheduled, one month later. Things had gone mostly well, but *anxiety* tried new tricks on me, hitting me with worse possibilities if I did not comply.

ALAN: *Fear* did that to me, too.

ELLIOT: Yes. I began to understand that's pretty typical—*anxiety* and *fear* will have louder tantrums at first to get you back. Anyway, I generally resisted.

CINDY: How?

ELLIOT: Jeff asked me that, also. I remembered that *anxiety* lied.

ALAN: That was helpful to me, too.

ELLIOT: I came up with a strategy that Jeff thought was clever. Any time *anxiety* said, "You are going to . . . ," I changed it to "I am *not* going to . . . " When I returned for my last visit, five weeks later, Jeff asked me lots more questions about how I was managing *anxiety,* what anti-*anxiety* principles I was holding onto, and what that meant about myself. I told him I saw *anxiety* for what it is . . .

ALAN: A liar, an interrupter, a tormentor . . .

ELLIOT: Yes! And I discovered this principle: that if you never enter into it, it can't get a hold on you. I told Jeff (he had asked if I had a guiding adage) that my motto now is "No repeat!" We decided that this suffocates *anxiety.* I had won out with determination!

VICKI: So can I ask my question about "specifics" now?

ALL: Sure!

VICKI: It seems that dealing with the "specifics" about the problem— particularly if the problem is something like *anxiety* or *fear*—that somehow talking about those things "feeds" the problem. Would you say that?

ALAN: That certainly was how it seemed to me. I mean the "issues" were all affected by *fear* and *anxiety* and got me into obsessions, and talking about them made it worse. Once we focused on the effects of the problem and distinguished that from what *I* wanted, we were on our way.

CINDY: Well, when you hear my story, you'll see that dealing with "specifics" actually made things worse.

VICKI: So would it also be fair to say that you and Jeff started focusing on "specifics" when they were about what *you* wanted—sort of paying attention to the details of how you were constructing your lives in more preferred ways?

ALAN: That's a good way to say it.

ELLIOT: Ditto!

CINDY: Absolutely.

VICKI: Great. Thanks. Back to you all.

ALAN: (*To Elliot*) Have you seen Jeff since?

ELLIOT: Well, he called me several months later. He said that a colleague of his had a client dealing with similar problems and experiencing *helplessness.* Would I talk with her? I said, "Sure," and I eventually met with her and her therapist. I was glad I could help.

JEFF: She said you were incredibly helpful. . . . This brings up a question I've been wanting to ask you. What effect does it have on you to be able to share your knowledge with others?

ELLIOT: It makes me feel stronger.

KAREN: I'd like to add something here about that. I have a video of a session I had with Jeff and a group of therapists who were in training in this therapy approach. I also have some letters I wrote. I'm contributing the video and the letters to what Jeff calls the Anti-Anorexia/Anti-Bulimia League. I feel really good about being able to share my knowledge and experience with others. I'd like to share a portion of that session with you all.

CINDY: Well, before you do, what was your therapy like? Was the session we're going to see at the beginning?

KAREN: No, it was the fifth and last.

ALAN: What did you call the problem?

KAREN: Well, there was **bulimia**, of course—bingeing and vomiting, you know. But we also looked at the things that support **bulimia**, like **evaluation** and its friends, **comparison** and **perfectionism**. Another problem that supported **bulimia** was **lack of entitlement.** I used to see my interest in what I wanted as selfish. At first Jeff noticed how I was managing the **bulimia** in some ways, like my saying to it, "Okay, I'll vomit, but I'll decide if I want to or not," instead of just doing it automatically. It also came out that I felt special, was good at things, and had a good relationship with my husband. When I met with Jeff two months later I had taken some more steps to leave it behind, but it had also "counterattacked," as Jeff put it. You (*looking at Alan and Elliot*) both referred to that sort of thing, too. I had come in feeling a lack of self-worth. We talked more about the negative **evaluation** habit, which encouraged me to feel selfish and to feel I must get things just right. But then Jeff asked about something I brushed by at first—those things that I realized I felt pride about. Jeff asked what this reflected, and I said, "Strength." We looked at times I fought off the negative habit and about things I wanted in life—what picture of myself, what desires, and what future.

ALAN: Did that continue?

KAREN: Which?

ALAN: Well, what I would call my **Rocky** story—for you. What do you call it?

KAREN: Interesting you should ask that, because in our third session, about three weeks later, we named it **Karen Power.** This had to do with my putting the binge pattern aside, but more importantly, it had to do with a growing self-appreciation.

CINDY: Self-appreciation—that's still a tiny bit hard for me. What do you appreciate about yourself, and how did you realize this?

KAREN: Well, Jeff asked me questions about what other people, like my husband and coworkers, would notice about me in the different situations we discussed. What I came up with was that I am enjoyable and I enjoy things. I'm thoughtful and reliable. I take the ball and run with it.

ELLIOT: Why **Karen Power**?

KAREN: As a man, you have been encouraged to appreciate your power. As a woman, if I exercise personal power, it's questioned. I am working on being for myself more and noticing that I have the right to do what I want. For example, I'm designing my own life. This was discussed in the session we are going to see. And *I'm* evaluating it more and subjecting it less to others' evaluation.

ALAN: Sounds really good.

KAREN: By my fourth session, which was three weeks later, I had taken more charge of my life. I spied enough on **bulimia** to know the tactics it uses to try to recruit me (I continued binge-free), and when Jeff asked me about this, I was able to share these tactics with him, as well as to share the techniques I was using to manage **bulimia**. I was able to be assertive in several important situations without **bulimia** talking me into being passive (that's not too hard) or feeling bitchy (that's a hard one). Jeff asked me about my own voice, separate from **bulimia**'s voice, and I had some success separating the two. One example of this was that I had even taken time out for fun for myself. When Jeff asked me to come in three weeks later to have a meeting with a reflecting team, I was ready.

JEFF: Let's look at the video. We'll start with the beginning part of the session; then toward the end, we'll hear a reflecting team comment; and, finally, we'll show Karen's reaction to the team.

TRANSCRIPT OF FIFTH AND FINAL SESSION WITH KAREN

JEFF: Catch me up, then, on any developments that have occurred over the last three weeks.

KAREN: I really have tried what we were recommending. It has been overwhelming with the self-improvement barrage I've been under . . .

kind of trying to give myself a break from it, and I have taken some time out for fun . . . but I kind of feel like I'm not getting the same level of return I want to get. I feel like I have plateaued, in a sense. I'm not always reacting the way I want to react or choose to react. I haven't been able to control my choice of things I eat at certain points, although I have been able to control quantity, and certainly I have not gotten into what I consider the "binge" mode for three weeks now.

JEFF: That's a long time.

KAREN: I feel like I'm losing control of the quality of food. I'm afraid it's creeping back. I'm alerted to that. I'm not clear what direction I need to go to fix it.

JEFF: Let me back up and ask you a bit about what you said. You said you've been cutting yourself slack and having fun. I was reading over this letter I copied for you [from the Anti-Anorexia/Anti-Bulimia League archives], and it reminds me of what Kathy said that one of her anti-*bulimic* developments was when she made this profound discovery (*reading*): "When I make the effort to please myself, I feel great." She went on to discuss with David [Epston] the importance of pleasing herself as critical to an anti-*bulimic* direction (*looking at the paper*). She continued to discuss with David the importance of this and the things that pleased her. I'll let you read this. I was curious what you think about this. Do you agree with Kathy that taking care of yourself is an important anti-*bulimic* development?

KAREN: Yes.

JEFF: Why do you agree with her? Why would you say that it's an anti-*bulimic* development?

KAREN: Because I think the things that fuel *bulimia* are not being true to yourself and putting other things in front of what you feel are best for you on a deep level. I think there are different times when I feel like I've sold part of myself and I compromised on something that I shouldn't have, and all that does is lower my self-esteem and make me vulnerable to *bulimia*.

JEFF: You said that in the past *bulimia* was able to get encouragement through your not being true to yourself, and now you are being more true to yourself?

KAREN: Trying to.

JEFF: Trying to. And you've made some—what would you call them? Big steps, or medium steps, in that direction?

KAREN: I think I've made strong steps.

JEFF: Strong steps (*writing*).

KAREN: But I'm not quite there.

JEFF: Not where you want to be yet.

KAREN: I'm sure it's a process, but I'm impatient for more.

JEFF: Do you think that impatience is pro-*bulimic* or anti-*bulimic*?

KAREN: It depends on how I use it. If I use it as a motivator, it's anti-*bulimic*, but if I use it as a criticism, then I think it can be pro-*bulimic*. I'll probably use it as a little of both right now. I mean I continue to try to move forward, so I'm not just saying, "The hell with it, it didn't work out." I'm not taking that stance, but it's causing some internal conflict.

JEFF: So you said you were cutting yourself some slack. Would that be part of using it as a motivator but not a criticism? Does it fit that?

KAREN: Or knowing that sometimes I don't have to be so regimented and I still won't lose control. Or having some more faith in myself— that I'm not that fragile. Because there were times I was superstitious that if I missed one day of working out, that would blow everything, and I think I'm giving myself more credit than that.

JEFF: I would imagine that *bulimia* wants you to think that one day missing it and you've blown it. Does *bulimia* try to tell you that?

KAREN: Oh, yeah.

JEFF: What kinds of things have you used to talk back to the *bulimia*?

KAREN: Well, I think it was—we had talked about being able to differentiate its voice from my own—I've been pretty successful at doing that. I've just been able to respond to it and see the irrationalness of that and be able to respond, "No, I don't think that's true, and thank you for playing."

JEFF: (*Laughing*) Yeah, right. So you've been successfully holding on to your own voice?

KAREN: Yeah.

JEFF: And is that true with respect to *bulimia* and to other things and people in your life? . . .

[Later, Karen and Jeff were discussing Karen's plans to change jobs and move.]

KAREN: I've made steps that are "no-turning-back" steps.

JEFF: How do you account for that? How have you made these steps in the face of *fear*?

KAREN: Stupidity (*laughing*) . . .

JEFF: (*Laughs*)

KAREN: . . . and pride . . . and deep down there must be a *faith* that I can do it.

JEFF: I would imagine there must be that **faith**. Can you see other manifestations of that *faith* in your life, that *faith* in yourself?

KAREN: I think I have *faith* in my life as I continue to try to uncover things. I believe I can handle these things, that the outcome will make me stronger and grow. I have *faith* in that; otherwise I'd say, "Too much pain," and check out. I'd say, "This is not what I want to do."

JEFF: My experience in helping people fight **bulimia** is that this is a situation where **bulimia** would like to come in and offer you an out. It might say, "Come on, Karen, come to me for a while and forget about this stuff." Has it been speaking to you like that?

KAREN: Sure. It's always there, in subtle and not-so-subtle ways. It will use any avenue.

JEFF: It doesn't play fair, does it? Like here's a situation where you don't need any more complications.

KAREN: It plays to win . . . and you know what? It would. It works through me, so I would expect it to be strong.

JEFF: Have you been able to hold on to your competitive edge?

KAREN: Kind of. It has won a few battles recently.

JEFF: So what percentage of the battles do you think you've won?

KAREN: Right now . . . in the past few months, I'd say I've been more like 80–20. Lately it has been 65–35, because of the eating things. But it hasn't been able to stop me from thinking about things and realizing things and discovering things.

JEFF: It hasn't?

KAREN: No, it hasn't.

JEFF: So you've been able to hold onto your own direction in life?

KAREN: I've had successes in my day-to-day life—what I choose to eat.

JEFF: My experience is that **bulimia** likes to try to regain some territory. It sounds like it has regained only some of its barest territory, around food. You've held onto the biggest piece of the territory. Is that right? Does that fit how you see it?

KAREN: I'm really trying to protect my self-image from the bombs that keep coming over the wall. And I'm struggling to protect that, but that's a priority.

JEFF: Do you consider yourself well ahead of **bulimia** because of that, or somewhat ahead of **bulimia**? Where would you put yourself?

KAREN: I'd say I'm further ahead than I've ever been.

JEFF: Would you say you're winning the war, although it has won some battles?

KAREN: Yes.

JEFF: Yes. You know, I wanted to ask you about this. I was interested in *how* you were holding on to that competitive edge. What you said was that **bulimia** wanted to take it from you. We've talked about how this was one of your talents. You said **bulimia** wants to take it from you and turn the tables on you. Yet you've been holding on to that competitive edge. Have you been doing certain things? What have you been up to in order to hold on to that competitive edge?

KAREN: I've been consistent in writing a journal. I've been religious in looking at myself—my focus is not far from that.

JEFF: How does that help you stay ahead of **bulimia**?

KAREN: **Bulimia** likes auto pilot; it wants to take over, and I'm following a path. I'm still on a path and I've got a central focus. It has not been able to persuade me or lure me over to something else.

JEFF: Is this what we've referred to as "Designing Your Life?"

KAREN: Self-improvement—an end in itself. A continuous spectrum. I've defined it as a life goal, and I'm successful if I accomplish it on a daily basis.

JEFF: I imagine that's an anti-**bulimic** life goal, because you've said you're designing yourself and your life on your own criteria. You've said that in the past **bulimia** had you thinking that self-improvement meant cooperating with it—how you look, eat. Do you see self-improvement as consistent with the kind of philosophies you have about how life should be? You've been describing today a process of experimenting and reflecting, experimenting and reflecting. When **bulimia** comes around, you say "Wait a minute," and reflect on what's really happening. And all of that experimenting and reflecting is moving you toward this goal of self-improvement. Do you think it's consistent with any philosophies you have about how someone should live their lives, how you want to live your life?

KAREN: Well, I have a philosophy that we are put on this earth to learn—fortunately I love learning—and I consider that to be an obligation of mine, and in order not to squander it, I should learn as much as I can about as many things as I can.

JEFF: So it's very consistent with that philosophy. Is this a philosophy you've had all your life?

KAREN: Well, I've gotten a lot of rewards from learning, so I feel it has been built over my life. I'm not sure I saw it in terms of *bulimia* or self-improvement before, but I've been able to apply what I've learned in school or in hobbies and things to this, which is really the most important thing.

JEFF: Why do you think *bulimia* wanted to blind you for a period of time to using your own philosophy?

KAREN: It's a strategy that works.

JEFF: What would you say *bulimia*'s philosophy is? If your philosophy is "You are put on earth to learn," what do you think its philosophy is?

KAREN: "I already know the outcome, so I can save you the pain of it—I'll show you the way."

JEFF: (*Laughing*) I see.

KAREN: It's a very "I know what's right" kind of attitude, and to very complex problems: "I have the solution, and I'll fix it for you."

JEFF: I was looking at this letter, and I notice that David [Epston] raised this question with Kathy: "Why is the voice of *bulimia* always gendered male?" And I was just thinking that men were taught to be that way, to think they are always right, so I was interested in how you, as a woman, began to place faith in your own learning, in your own knowledge? . . .

[Later, the reflecting team commented on the session. Here are some excerpts:]

T_1 (VICKI): I wondered what it told Karen about herself that she was listening to her voice and gave herself a reprieve—that she was the architect, instead of submitting to *bulimia*'s demands for no reprieve.

T_2: Why did that stand out for you?

T_1 (VICKI): Competitive edge resonated. I also think of myself as a learner. It's important to me to always stay in front of things, so I have to say to myself some days, "It's really okay that you didn't swim today, Vicki."

[Later, Karen responded to the team's comments:]

KAREN: I thought it was interesting that the question came up—"Why did you think that way?" or "Why did that strike you?"—and they reflected back on their own lives. That's useful for professionals, because everyone brings their own experience into how they view things. I'd like to hear that more from you.

JEFF: Yes, that would be great.

KAREN: I stopped interviewing you after the first time.

JEFF: So we should go back to it.

KAREN: Yes. I found it very enlightening and comforting that professionals were aware of it. I think it's a shift from "This is the way it is," to "That's the way I perceive it," or "That's what I experience." Because when I was in that treatment center, I remember how these people seemed very qualified to make judgments without full information. I think a lot of time they were reacting to other cases or how they interpreted things without that flexibility there. We're all human and bring our biases. I think, however, we'll get a better quality of counseling this way.

LETTERS FROM KAREN

JEFF: Karen, can we add the letters you sent me after the last session with the reflecting team?

KAREN: Sure.

A Conversation with **Bulimia**

I'm not sure that we've ever talked directly. It's strange, since you've played such a major role in my life for so long. There have been times when you've controlled my every waking moment. And there have certainly been times when I couldn't imagine my life without you.

But it has been a while since I've let you play a big part of me. I can't say that I've missed you. I certainly haven't missed the desperation, the depression, the anguish, or the hopelessness that I felt when you were in control of my life. And it's difficult to miss the humiliation, the listlessness, or the isolation I felt day after day. Were you really trying to protect me from the "pain" of living? Couldn't you see what you were doing to me? Couldn't you see that I almost wanted to end it all?

You've always been there to offer a solution to my problems. You've offered me safety, love, and security. You made it all look so wonderful. The trouble is, my problems only get bigger when you're around. In fact, you *inflate* my problems so they appear more powerful than they really are, and you weaken me so I'm in no condition to deal with them. Is this the kind of love you have to offer me? I'm sorry, it's just not good enough any more.

I know that, in some strange way, you've been trying to protect me. I appreciate what you were trying to do—maybe it worked for us for a while. But I've outgrown you now. You don't need to worry. Now I have something much stronger to lean on when the challenges come . . . *me!* I don't need you any more. I can make it on my own.

I guess I should be thanking you. Despite the pain you've caused me, you've also led me to a deeper joy than I've ever known. If it wasn't for you, I wouldn't have been so driven to learn about myself and discover how to relate better to others. If it wasn't for you, I might never have learned how to examine my life and change things that I'm dissatisfied with. I never thought I'd say this, but I believe I'm a better person for knowing you.

But this is where my gratitude ends. I know that you're always lurking somewhere in my mind for the opportunity to reenter my life. I hear your voice in the morning, telling me to stay in bed instead of exercise. I hear your voice when I'm frustrated, hurt, or angry, telling me to eat something tasty to "relieve the tension." You may find this hard to believe, but I actually *want* to feel these things . . . I don't want you to take them away from me any more. These feelings belong to *me,* and *I'll* deal with them! Yes, I hear your voice a lot. But at least I can tell your voice from my own now. That's something I couldn't do before.

So forgive me if I tease or ridicule you now and then. Forgive me when I dismiss you or laugh at your childish ploys. It's just that you don't seem as big as you used to. You used to seem so powerful to me—like a giant. And now . . . you're just a "fair-weather friend" who has lost his usefulness. Like all of the baggage from the past, I have to leave you behind to live a fuller, richer life.

I don't expect you to give me up without a fight. You were made by me, so you have my strength and my stubbornness. Like me, you play to win. On the other hand, since I created you, I am in charge. I can't stop you from creeping into my life, but I can use your energy to make useful choices instead of harmful ones.

You will always be with me on some level. And since we're trying to exist in the same body, we're bound to run into each other. So I'll make you a promise. I promise never to underestimate you and never to stop challenging your "voice." I promise that even if you win a battle or two, the war is far from over. My spirit is bigger than anything I eat or do, so I promise to pick myself back up and learn from my mistakes. Most of all, I promise to let those who can help learn all about you so that they can go about healing others. That's right—you're on trial now! They'll be studying you so future generations of women may learn to believe in themselves and rely upon their own abilities—a lesson I have finally learned for myself.

So this isn't really good-bye. Consider it the beginning of our new relationship—a relationship where I'm in control, and you are merely a "siren" that alerts me when I'm heading for trouble. Again, I want to thank you. Thank you for helping me become the person I am today. Stick around . . . with me guiding you, we can accomplish some amazing things. Work *with* me to design a life that will make us all happy.

A Conversation with Myself

It's amazing! Not too long ago, I wouldn't have known how to reach you. I didn't even know who or where you were. Just a scared, wounded child hidden away deep in my soul, I suppose.

And now you're free! It feels like a miracle, doesn't it? I guess it is. Lord knows, I had my doubts that I would ever really know you. It's a gift I'm thankful for every day. Many others aren't so lucky.

But the real miracle is the person you truly are . . . the person I've come to know these past few months. And I must tell you, you really surprised me! Who knew that you were so strong, so intelligent, so interesting . . . so *funny*? You're very fun to be with. How could I have hidden you for so long?

It's ironic, you know. Ever since I moved to California, I've been looking for a "best friend." And you've been sitting here all along, waiting for me to notice you. I apologize for not looking for you sooner. The fact is, I didn't know how. Now, whenever I'm lonely, we go do something that we both enjoy—see a movie, roller blade, dance. And when I'm scared, we talk. And you tell me that "this too shall pass." And I believe you because I trust you.

Thank you for helping me realize that *I* am the architect of my life! Now I know that no one can make me feel anything I don't want to. No one can tell me who I am, unless I believe it. *I* decide what's true about me. It's nice to finally be "the boss"!

But you and I both know it doesn't always feel that way. Many things are out of our control, and that's a bit scary. I'm glad we've decided not to let the fear paralyze us and keep us from our goals. How comforting it is to know that fear is merely a signal that we're getting to the edge of our comfort zone, and there's something more we need to do so we can grow. I feel better knowing that you'll be there with me—that you'll support and love me along the way.

Thank you for helping me see that things are not black and white, that I'm not a "success" or a "failure" because of one thing I did. Thank you for helping me realize that I'm more than what I do or what I feel. In fact, it doesn't matter what I did yesterday, even if I'm not especially proud of it. If I learn from it, it becomes a useful, empowering experience. Thank you for giving me the permission not to be perfect. From now on, our mistakes won't destroy us—they can only help us improve and grow! And every day is a clean slate to do something new and different. We are not bound by the past. Instead, we're driven by the exciting future that is stretching out before us. All we have to do is have the courage to reach out and grab it. The possibilities are endless!

And thank you for telling me that I don't have to be "on" all the time—that I can take a rest, cut myself some slack. Thank you for reminding me to be *kind* to myself now and then. We deserve it, don't we?

But before we end our little talk, I want to make you a promise. I promise never to hide you away again and pretend that you don't matter. I promise never to sell you short, or conceal the truth from you. And I promise never to shelter you from my feelings, or stuff them down with food. I can't promise that I'll never overeat—or even that I'll never purge again. But let's consider those moments as little "wake-up calls" that there is work to be done, instead of letting them undo all the progress we've made together. I don't want to lose you again! You are my #1 priority. And, by the way, I love you!!

A FICTIONAL CONVERSATION AMONG
REAL PEOPLE (CONTINUED)

ALAN: Wow! How strong you are. You know, I had one question: Did you ever need sessions with your husband?

KAREN: No. Why do you ask?

ALAN: Well, if you remember, before Elliot shared his battles with *anxiety*, I talked about my work to get in charge of some specific *fears* [driving], as well as some general *fears*. After I gained the upper hand on the specific ones, we (Jeff and I) decided to have some sessions to include my wife. I love her very much. I was concerned about what I saw as the effects on her of my problems. She is also a very strong-willed person. She has had to live with the things she has gone through, her physical problems.

JEFF: What I remember was that June [Alan's wife] was overwhelmed when the *fear* took your focusing talent and got you to go on and on.

ALAN: (*Laughing*) and on and on and on and . . .

JEFF: (*Laughing*) Exactly. This seemed to invite what we called a "reject-and-direct" response from her. As a consequence, she stopped listening and "ran."

ALAN: And I tried to follow after her. That was not working very well. I also somewhat resented that she took such a strong stand on the issues about my dad, and money, and other stuff.

JEFF: As I recall our working together, it seemed the more you focused on your life and yourself, the more June worked to create space so that you could take even more charge of yourself. She even put up with your buying a motorcycle.

ALAN: Yes (*Laughing*), that was big, because she wasn't too happy about it.

JEFF: The other thing I remember talking about was an old habit that affected her. We called it "protecting vulnerability," which was in response to a lot of stuff that had happened in *her* life.

ALAN: I really appreciated it when she started to show more vulnerability and face insecurities.

JEFF: And she was clearly thrilled when you began to take more of a leadership role in your own life. "Equal Partners" was a guiding theme.

ALAN: And don't forget **Rocky Heart.** Two years ago when we last spoke, there was very little **self-doubt** affecting me and no **fear?**

CINDY: When you talk about **self-doubt,** it reminds me how it has affected me in my life.

ALAN: Well, let's hear your story. You've heard everyone else's.

CINDY: I already talked about that messy time early on—moving out because my parents wanted me to, and Jeff also getting caught by the problem (**pain** and **pressure**), then failing and moving back home . . .

JEFF: What I remember was helpful was when I stopped trying to lead and instead just responded to the ways **pressure** was affecting you—like "Oh, the **pressure** said that," or "Oh, the **pressure** got you to react that way." After a month or so of doing this, for the first time there was room for you to notice some of what *you* thought, rather than what I, or your parents, or others, or the **pressure** thought.

CINDY: Yes, I started to feel a bit less bad. By spring of the next year, we decided to go to every-other-week sessions, thinking that too much therapy fed the problem. Jeff, I know you had to be careful. If you said too much (or sometimes when you said anything), the **pressure** would take it and use it against me.

JEFF: Yes, I credit working with you as helping to teach me patience. Otherwise the problem would have gotten both of us. I tried to just label what the problem was doing and then to remark briefly on your own agency, like "So you had your own opinion?" or "Guilt influenced you less," or "You made your own decision." If I asked too much about any of this, the **pressure** would attack.

CINDY: (*Consulting her notes*) By early fall or so, we started to call the problem **evaluation.** I had begun to notice, but only in a very small

way, some of my steps—my own decision about a class (that I had
been pushed into by others), my own likes in social activities (despite
what I "should" like), small stands I took (although there was much
discomfort about this), and slack I cut myself (but only a very little).
In October, we were even able to give a title to these developments—
"My Life." In November, *evaluation* really got me, but I also found
I had some values and beliefs that were my own. As Jeff began to ask
about these, they became an important part of "My Life." Christmas
was tough as usual, but I made it through. In January of the following
year, when I saw Jeff, he gave me a certificate (I thought it was cute),
called "Taking Care of Herself in *Her* Way," which reflected my
efforts over the holidays. During the next several months, social
events became slightly easier, and I even asserted myself with Jeff
over an issue, although these sorts of things were tough for me. In
response to Jeff's questions, I told him I saw a "glimmer" of hope and
of possibilities.

JEFF: My memory is that this was the first time you were able to see and
acknowledge any possibility of a new direction.

CINDY: Yes, by that summer my social involvement really increased.

ALAN: So things were good?

CINDY: No, not really. *Evaluation* still shut me down and tormented me.
I don't want to give the wrong impression here. I saw that things
were going better in small ways, but I still felt bad a lot. In spite of
feeling bad, when Jeff asked me where these social steps were coming
from, we were able to look back before the problems—when I was
in high school—and we decided I was "dusting off the old me." By
late summer we began to use "Living for Myself" as a central theme.
Over the fall I noticed more confidence growing, and I could see
even more "glimmers." In December (now the third year of therapy),
when Jeff questioned me about this, I realized *worry* was around only
35% of the time. By January Jeff thought I had accomplished a double
victory over the problem, because, for the first time in recent
memory, I could handle Christmas—and I even noticed I handled
it! In February I thought things went "reasonably well," and in March
I decided to switch to coming in once every three weeks. The theme
we were using was "Endless Summer," because the social direction
that had picked up during the previous summer seemed to be
continuing. I was also feeling less stress and treating myself better. I
had some difficult moments that next summer, because expectations
from the summer before were not being met, so I had a bout with
evaluation, especially given a tough time I had with a dating

situation. I was able to decide it was "okay not to be perfect," and by the fall saw that things were still moving forward, despite some of what we called *self-doubt.*

VICKI: What kinds of questions was Jeff asking then? He commented earlier that he felt nervous about asking too much.

CINDY: He had to be really careful not to say anything that could represent *evaluation,* or even a possibility of it, for me. But by then he was asking questions about how the developments represented preferences for me; how they reflected my values; how they related to ways I had been in the past and wanted to be in the future; what title or chapter heading we would use.

JEFF: Then there were the questions you used to groan at—the ones that went, "How was this different from how you would have handled things or responded two years ago?" and "What developments does this reflect about you or your ability to handle the problem?"

CINDY: (*Laughing*) Yes, I thought, "Here comes that question again!" Recently, it seems that those questions bring up good feelings.

JEFF: That fall we also brought your parents in for a session. In fact, you initiated it.

CINDY: Yes, I remembered a conversation we had during one of those times when the problem got worse for a bit, about not wanting to bring them in during that sort of time. So when things were back going in a good direction, I made it happen!

ALAN: What did you talk about?

CINDY: Well, we all remembered that I had a history when I was in grade school of standing up for myself and saying, "Damn the consequences." This was a very different conversation than I had ever had in therapy with my parents. Around that time it seemed like "Self-Acceptance" became the theme in our work. In the following year, despite my mom getting very sick (breast cancer) and me having a brief bout with *self-doubt* afterwards, things progressed. "Living Life Now" reflected developments, such as taking a class of my own choosing and handling it, taking more responsibility at work, and beginning a relationship (where, for the first time, I participated in a way in which what I wanted came through). "Right for Me" was the theme, as I managed all parts of my life in a way where I was a presence. As I moved out on my own, worked things out with a roommate, and ended a relationship that no longer worked for me, the theme became "Metamorphosis." Soon after, we ended therapy.

ALAN: What an incredible story. And things are good?

CINDY: I never would have believed it was possible for things to be as they are now. I lived too long in horrible, horrible pain and misery, and was sure it would never end. But it got better.

OTHERS: (*Clapping*) Yes, yes!

THE CONVERSATION CONTINUES

VICKI: I have a question for you, Jeff. I've just heard four stories about therapy—with it ranging from once-a-week sessions to every other week to every third week for five years for Cindy, to four sessions for Elliot, five sessions for Karen, and three separate episodes of therapy for Alan. Yet all of these problems seemed to be ones that had a major hold on each of them. How does it get decided how often you will meet and how long this will take? I know it is co-decided, and I think that everyone addressed this issue in some way in the telling of their stories, but I wondered if there was a way in particular that you thought about this?

JEFF: Actually, there is, and it does seem to have something to do with how big a hold the problem has on people and how long it has been around, but not just with that. But I suspect you have some thoughts about this too, or else you wouldn't have asked the question. So let me ask, "Why do you ask?"

VICKI: (*Laughing*) Oh, okay, I'll situate my question. In Chapters 4 and 5, I have related the story of an orthopedic surgeon in his mid-50s, who came in to see me because of a history of emotional abuse as a child, which had devastating ongoing effects of **anger** and **guilt** in his life and which led to obsessive thoughts and compulsive actions. We met for almost four years—once-a-week sessions for the first three years, and then once every other week. Near the end of therapy he would often say, "I am a different person now," and I know he experienced himself that way, as did I. In fact, because he would say those words frequently, I asked him to write a description of *how* he experienced himself in this different way. He did so, and I would like to include that here.

Frank's Reflections

It took me quite a while before I could find a way to put these thoughts on paper. We (Vicki and I) had talked about my experience quite a lot, and I remember when I said that I felt like a different person—that it wasn't just a matter of feeling better sometimes and for a while. It was something that felt solid, stable, consistent. I never thought this would be possible. I told her once that my life was controlled by rules. It was like I was in a little box, one that had existed from when I was a very small child. It was a tight box and limiting and rule-bound, but I felt like I needed it, because my life was too emotionally scary without it. I had a profound experience of freedom and of limitless possibilities, once I could escape that box. And I even let go of *expectations*—of myself, of others, even of my parents. All my relationships felt freer and richer, with more warmth and mutual caring. I couldn't believe how different I felt. Now when I go in to see Vicki and she asks how things are going, I almost always say, "Going well. Working hard." What's more, I believe that my life will continue to go well, and that the hard work is worth it!

I am adding this paragraph somewhat later. When I decided I was ready to end therapy, which was actually only a few sessions after I wrote the paragraph above, Vicki and Jeff had finished this book. So I wanted to put in a final touch: We talked about my ending therapy as a "graduation," a "commencement," and we discussed what my diploma would say. I said, "A Professor of Life." Vicki asked who would come to my graduation party, and I said, "Anyone who wants—everyone." Then she said, "How would you want them to celebrate this commencement with you?" I answered, "However they want." This speaks to my freedom from *expectations,* my desire to be accepting of others in my life. I think Vicki wanted something more acknowledging of me and my efforts, so she suggested that we list all the steps I had taken along the path of becoming "A Professor of Life." I like that. So I think that's what we're up to next.

VICKI: Needless to say, this was a moving experience—having Frank write about his experience of the steps he had taken in therapy. I was very touched by our last session, and remember telling him how glad I was that he had been willing to share his life and his struggles and his accomplishments with me. Also, though, my point here is that we had a number of sessions before Frank began to author his life more in the way he preferred.

To extend this point I want to relate a different story. Recently I met with a woman, Gwen, in her mid-50s, who had been abused by her father between the ages of four and seven. He died when she was seven, her mother remarried, and her experience was one of feeling "outside." Eventually she went to live with an aunt when she was 16. She came to see me because, as she said, "I want to *deal* with these things now." I ended up seeing her for one session. The reason I think we could complete our work so quickly is that I believe, as did she, that she had already "restoried" her life. She wrote some reflections on our meeting, and that is also included here.

Gwen's Reflections

May 25, 1995, 2:20 P.M.

I have had a most interesting day so far. I went off and spent the morning kind of getting ready to see Vicki and start what I thought would be a long series of therapy sessions. Why I thought I needed therapy has to do with how my childhood was very traumatic and abusive, and I have never really dealt with it in a therapy setting. I thought this would be a good time to deal with it because I have never felt better in my life. A month ago I decided to have a morphine pump that was used for chronic pain turned off, and my physical and emotional well-being took a tremendous upswing. I felt that I had reclaimed my body and my spirit. I haven't felt this good in years; although I do continue to have pain, it is *my* pain and I own it.

My mental well-being is good and I am happy. Why did I think that I needed therapy? I think because stuff from my childhood came up a couple of times at an AA meeting. This had never happened before, and it kind of surprised and distressed me. Maybe this was the signal that I needed to work on this stuff. Anyway, I brought it up during my cancer support group meeting; Vicki's name was mentioned; and narrative therapy was talked about. The whole process intrigued me, and I talked about it with the psychologists at work, and they said they thought it might be helpful. I made the appointment and felt pretty good about it. "Time to rewrite my story," is what I thought.

When I got into the office and started talking about myself and my life, I realized that I was in pretty good shape, and came to the conclusion that maybe I didn't need therapy after all. This all came about because as I talked to Vicki, I realized that there was nothing in my life that really needed changing. I am happy and doing very well. I love my work and I have plenty of friends. What is it that I want to change? Life is a matter of trust and following my instincts, which I know are good.

Vicki asked me why I thought it would be helpful to explore past childhood pain. I thought this was an excellent question, and I thought about it as I sat in her office. Why would one want to upset everything when life was going well? I couldn't come up with a credible answer, and I felt lighter and better the more I realized that therapy probably was not the answer. My life is good, and it is my responsibility to continue to keep it good. Therapy is not the answer, but trust in the process of my life is. I have done pretty well up to now, and there is no reason why that should change. I loved it when Vicki wondered aloud if I had already rewritten my life story and did not have to work on rewriting it again. This story has served me well, and I am grateful for it.

I think that maybe I got caught up in the fact that almost everyone I know is in therapy, and they certainly don't have the problems (physical) that I do. I think I thought that I would be better if I went to therapy, but I realize now that I am okay and should be content with how I am. I am in control, and my life is just a series of choices. When I follow good instincts and talk to my friends honestly, I make good choices. When I operate out of desperation and self-pity, I make poor choices. The point is that everything is under control—my life, my mood, and my attitude. I appreciate that Vicki helped me bring all of this into focus and am grateful for our session. Life is good! Thanks.

VICKI: My examples show two people, each struggling with something very difficult from their early lives, and yet one came in for one time only and the other was in therapy for a few years. I think about this the way Gwen and I talked about it: She had already done some considerable work "restorying," and her coming in to therapy was more acting on **doubt** that got pushed up by others. Once she put the **doubt** aside, she could see her own agency in making her life the way she wanted it. With Frank, I participated with him in the reauthoring process, and because the old problem story was so powerful, it took some time for him to separate from it and to reaccess preferred developments.

JEFF: I like to think that all of therapy is co-created with clients (and in some ways with the problem as well). This includes how long it takes. I now try to stay right behind clients, working with their experience and not getting ahead. I also do not want to be so far behind that the problem continues to exert *most* of the influence over clients' experience. The idea is to create with clients what they prefer to have influence them at each step in time in the process. My experience is that it is not possible to put time limits on this in advance. However long it takes or does not take, I hope my clients all would say, "At least we're enjoying the ride!"

STUDENT: Well, I have some big questions before I can continue to enjoy this ride.

JEFF: Go ahead.

STUDENT: Wouldn't you consider some of these people deeply disturbed?

JEFF: Deeply disturbed? No, I wouldn't. However, therapists who use a different metaphor—one that locates the problem in the person and as part of their personality—might. I think of "deep" as inside, and "disturbed" as not behaving like the established cultural picture holds up as ideal, so that consideration doesn't fit the metaphor we are presenting.

STUDENT: Yet these people do prefer to be a different way. They express much pain.

JEFF: Unquestionably, and because they say so. They are facing very difficult problems they would like to separate from, and we, as narrative therapists, would notice some of what other therapists would notice. However, we would understand these things in very different ways, consistent with a narrative metaphor. For example, we might suspect that these people are under the influence of very powerful problems that the ever-present cultural discourse supports.

STUDENT: For example . . . ?

JEFF: Patriarchal structures greatly support **lack of entitlement** for women. Capitalism, as a specified way of operating, defines acceptable performance, correct goals, and so on. Christian beliefs have shaped morals and ethics for centuries. These grand narratives support problems in various ways. These problems often have a strong hold on those people, who might have had "training" experiences that give extra support to these narratives, or whose preferences and strengths fall outside the ones the dominant culture defines as acceptable (but believe they are unacceptable for it). Those people have to work long and hard to separate from the influence of these narratives and reauthor their lives. Probably they have had some experiences that tell them something else is possible, and so they are unhappy with the effects of these dominant stories. For example, in my experience working with women fighting *anorexia*, I find that while these women often have had very oppressive training in dominant ideas for ways women should be, they are also among the strongest and brightest women around.

STUDENT: I think I've got it. You're not trivializing or minimizing problems at all. You're just understanding them differently.

JEFF: You've got it.

STUDENT: I would expect, then, that in different cultures there would be different problems.

JEFF: I believe this is so. Even in our Western, white culture, there have been differences over time.

VICKI: This discussion reminds me of another question I've heard our colleagues raise.

STUDENT: What's that?

VICKI: Do we believe that all other therapies pathologize people, and that only narrative therapy is nonpathologizing? We've had previous conversations about that; some therapy metaphors do see persons as being deficient, but some family therapies certainly do not intend to be pathologizing. I am also thinking about our evolution as therapists and how it never quite fit for us to see pathology in persons.

JEFF: Right. In fact, we were both drawn to family systems theory because we saw that it was a step away from this view. However, my experience is that while some approaches may have pathologizing effects and others may not, often the others aren't exactly empowering of the client either.

STUDENT: Say more about that.

JEFF: As a former strategic therapist, I can say that often I tried to maneuver people toward what I believed were better outcomes for them. Given the metaphor out of which family systems thinking emerged, the therapist can find himself or herself in the position of teaching or directing things toward certain therapist-determined good outcomes. This is in contrast to noticing experiences of clients that support their preferred ways of being. In a narrative approach, the clients own the developments.

VICKI: One of the more helpful shifts for me was when I heard the distinction between "system-determined problems" and "problem-determined systems."

STUDENT: Now you're losing me.

VICKI: It has to do with where different metaphors locate problems (go back to Chapter 1). Earlier family systems theory located problems in the relationship, in the system; therefore, we had "system-determined problems." When I read how Harlene Anderson and Harry Goolishian [1986] were thinking of the problem as affecting the system, that was a beginning for me.

JEFF: And the way we understand a narrative metaphor is that it makes the further shift of locating the problem in cultural meaning systems, as we have been saying here.

VICKI: That is how this approach is more apt to have both a nonpathologizing intent and nonpathologizing effects.

STUDENT: Okay, I think the distinction is clearer. However, I'm still thinking about these powerful problems. You are also saying that narrative therapy is not necessarily a brief therapy. You take the time that the client needs. What about when it doesn't go well? Or when it has frequent ups and downs?

JEFF: Well, my experience *is* one of frequent ups and downs. People take steps away from the problem, then it grabs them back. Haven't you had that experience when trying to leave problems behind? I have.

STUDENT: Yes . . . whenever I make any changes.

JEFF: Some people go through a very long period of being in between—they're leaving something behind, but haven't gotten to the new place yet. The ensuing in-between period can be exciting and uncomfortable [Turner, 1969; van Gennep, 1960]. As therapists, it is helpful to remember this and to help our clients expect this, so as not to think that things are going poorly. These ups and downs are part of a forward direction in a manner that all movement away from habits, problems, or problem identities seems to go.

STUDENT: This fits my experience.

JEFF: As to things not going well in general, this happens in my work from time to time. Often this results from my not carefully following or understanding the client's experience. Sometimes it happens because the problem is powerful and interferes in subtle ways I haven't caught on to. But I don't find this occurs with any one particular kind of problem.

STUDENT: What do you do when this happens?

JEFF: Well, the common idea of consulting with colleagues is a useful one. However, more and more I consult directly with my clients or with clients facing similar problems.

STUDENT: I see—this privileges clients' experience and keeps them at the center. You know, I've realized from this chapter that the clients had good and helpful experiences, but I was still confused about all these other issues.

JEFF: That makes sense to me. You are still being influenced by the dominant ideas in the therapy world and larger culture about what problems are or what needs to be done when they are present.

STUDENT: That brings up one more question. I realize all of a sudden that how you construct the problem, what you make it, is critical. Isn't this a hard thing to do?

JEFF: Students and interns often tell us that this is the hardest thing to learn. Lately, I tell them that the key is paying attention to the client's experience and trying to locate the problem in the cultural narratives that influence all of us.

STUDENT: That still seems hard to do.

JEFF: Sometimes it is.

STUDENT: What do you do when it is hard?

JEFF: First, I cut myself some slack to avoid the pressure of *evaluation* on me. Second, I try to keep talking with my clients, putting words on the meaning I am making of their experience and then asking if it fits for them. I trust we will get there, and . . .

STUDENT: I know. "At least you'll be enjoying the ride."

ALAN: That seems like a good way to end the chapter, but I would like to include the comments I wrote after reading it. Here they are.

Alan's Comments

As Jeff said in the concluding dialogue, I was a co-creator, and that made all the difference in the world. Because of going the hospital route a couple of times (at different hospitals), I saw what the status quo had to offer as far as doctors go. Here is the *Reader's Digest* version:

1. Stone-faced drug pushers who have wrecked people's lives.
2. Others who, just in case you did not have enough *fears,* bring up *fears* you have not even thought of.
3. Others who talk to you in a very judgmental way and point out your faults.

For me, the way I felt is that these people were not on my side. I have no reason to trust these people. I learned to keep my mouth shut so I wouldn't be judged. I thought these people might hurt me.

I have a world of respect for Dr. Jeff Zimmerman. He is a man who puts the patient's best interests first. He is human—but imagine how hard that must be. It's like a mechanic who shows his customer how to fix his car by interactive conversation. When you get all done, you say to yourself, "I can fix this car," and because you came up with the idea yourself, it's a lot more convincing. That's what Jeff does—he gives food for thought to a hungry person, never taking credit. The person learns to feed himself.

CHAPTER 7

Feel Like a Stranger
Work with Couples

The Authors Speak

We have chosen to write this chapter on working with couples from
the experience of the therapist involved in each case. Our way of
working with couples is for the therapist to talk with one member
while the other listens (Zimmerman & Dickerson, 1993a, 1993b).
One reason for this is that each partner has become like a stranger
to the other, as an effect of the dominant stories each is holding about
the other and about the relationship. We could have had each person
in each couple tell the story of his or her experience; however, since
we wanted to write one chapter from the experience of the therapist,
doing so in this one made the most sense to us.

VICKI: Jeff, why did you decide to share your experience about the first
   couple, Brenda and Eddie?

JEFF: Two reasons. First, I thought that their fight to take their relationship away from the problem would be inspiring to others. The work
   was hard, and it took some time, but their relationship is now more
   the way they want it to be. Second (and important for our purposes),
   I learned from it, particularly about more subtle gender issues that I
   wanted to share with our readers.

VICKI: I know what I think about what I'm going to ask, and I'm fairly
   sure what you will say, but it may be helpful to our readers to hear

154

the answer. Why does emphasizing gender seem so important in work with couples?

JEFF: Well, I believe that gender is what couple therapy is about, particularly with heterosexual couples. (We'll talk about our work with same-sex couples later in the chapter.) We've stressed the importance of understanding the problem in its sociopolitical context; thus, the social construction of gender has been one focus of all the work we have presented (with adolescents, adults, and families). With heterosexual couples, male and female gender training affects each person, so that different meaning gets created about various parts of their lives—for example, intimacy, conflict, lifestyle—without their even realizing the different interpretive texts each is using to understand the other. To say it differently, they understand each other in the same way they understand themselves, and it often doesn't fit.

VICKI: Could I interrupt here before you give an example? I actually believe that gender is as influential a discourse with same-sex couples as with opposite-sex couples. It may not be as "visible"—just as gender was pretty invisible in early family therapy work, which was justly criticized for not taking gender more fully into consideration. However, as you show here, we are clearly situating our work in the sociopolitical context of which gender is a major factor; it may be more noticeable because of heterosexual dominance. Nonetheless, we all work a lot with heterosexual couples, so this discussion is necessary. Later in the chapter, I talk more about gender issues with a lesbian couple. This makes me think, too, of how we need to make race and class more visible, as these discourses are also always present. So, moving from the theoretical and abstract, why don't you present your first example?

JEFF: Okay. If you, Vicki, and you, our readers, go back to Chapter 2, the problem talks about what it did to Brenda and Eddie. Their experience is represented as well. If you want to reread that section, it might give you some helpful background. Then I'll tell the details of the story.

BRENDA AND EDDIE
Jeff's Story

I met with Brenda and Eddie for 26 sessions over about a year and a half—the longest I've worked with any couple. My sessions with couples and families last 80 minutes, with a session usually every other week. This arrangement allows for more focused and intensive work in the session, and then for time between sessions for developments to occur that I can raise questions about. As therapy proceeds, sessions occur even less frequently. I try to do what makes sense: to schedule sessions closer together when the couple is first beginning to attack the problem, and then further apart when developments are occurring that are necessarily slower-moving, which require more time as well as continued effort by the couple. Toward the end of therapy, with anyone I've seen for some time, we spread the sessions out. In my sessions with a couple, I talk with one member while the other listens (the other, I hope, is thus in a reflexive position). I firmly establish this direction in the first session. When the problem loosens its grip somewhat, I may relax this structure.

When it was Eddie's turn to tell his story in our first session, he related that when Brenda became pregnant, he experienced their resulting marriage as an obligation. He said that he felt he was on the spot all the time, and he also didn't like conflict; both of these experiences had the effect of encouraging *withdrawal.* He felt pushed to be "move involved" in the relationship; he didn't like the pushing, although he very much wanted the relationship. When Brenda told her story, it included a "rough start," as well as her efforts over the years to make a peaceful home and to gain acceptance for herself. After many years, she decided she couldn't live with the lack of input she got from Eddie—about anything (her, the relationship, him)—so she finally began to care more for herself than for the relationship. The effect on her of being neglected was *resentment,* which encouraged *coldness.* They both agreed that their relationship was affected by an *up-and-down pattern* in which they first seemed more involved, then they drifted apart (as when *withdrawal* affected Eddie). Brenda eventually responded with *coldness* or *anger,* and then Eddie fought the *withdrawal.* When this happened, Brenda slowly let down the "wall" that had been encouraged by *resentments.* Brenda was tired of this pattern. Therapy was to be the last chance, although she was frank that *hopelessness* made her believe that nothing would help (they had been in other therapies). Eddie wanted to push himself to be more involved, but didn't really have a picture of how this would occur. Despite the problem pattern and the way it worked with both of them, Eddie was able to notice some of what he liked about being involved with Brenda, and Brenda said (when asked) that she had glimpses of what it could be like during those periods when they were more connected.

When I next saw them, Eddie had taken some anti-*withdrawal* steps, which included speaking his mind and talking directly about his needs and feelings. We discussed this at length—how he managed this, whether it fit for him, and why. Brenda remained understandably cautious. She struggled with whether to respond to him on the basis of her positive feelings, since she was still affected by a lack of trust that any change would last. Over the next two sessions, we discussed the developments centering around Eddie's attempts to let himself be better known to Brenda and to take responsibility for some of the emotional and social aspects of the relationship. I attempted to place this in a context of gender, including how men (most certainly including myself) are taught to keep to themselves, to react to conflict with withdrawal, to expect that women will care for them and for the relationship. If responsibility is not just work-related, as we men have been taught, but relationship-related as well, what might we do differently?

In the meantime, Brenda and I continued to look at *resentment*'s effects on her. I believed that *resentment* was an inevitable consequence of the things Eddie did or didn't do. I saw Eddie's responses as not intentionally hurtful, but as gender-affected blindness. In addition, Brenda's gender training had encouraged her to feel responsible and to work very hard for the relationship for many years; this fed *resentment* as well. I paid attention to and raised reauthoring questions about Brenda's efforts to make herself feel satisfied, instead of only or mostly working to make the relationship more satisfying. Another important development involved Brenda's saying what she wanted and not just going along with things to keep the peace.

In the fifth session, an incident occurred in which Brenda confronted Eddie directly, and Eddie "hung in there." Along with the training Eddie had received in how men should be, he also shared some additional training he had had in *withdrawal*. *Fears* of rejection and abandonment had gained influence over him earlier in life, and these *fears* encouraged *withdrawal*.

In the sixth session, Eddie described continued success in sharing his thoughts and feelings with Brenda "more than usual," and he also felt better about doing so. He said very strongly that it was "time to speak my feelings"—both the angry ones and the ones that made him feel vulnerable. Brenda continued to take care of herself, although she did say that she let the "wall" down some.

Eddie attended the next session by himself. He called about this, and I said "Okay," with the condition that anything he revealed I could feel okay about bringing up in later joint sessions. He agreed to this, as nothing he had to say was a secret.

The Authors Speak

VICKI: What if he hadn't agreed? Suppose he had an important secret and wasn't comfortable about your potentially bringing it up? I know you usually say you most likely won't bring something up, but you like to reserve the right to do so.

JEFF: I'm more flexible than I once was about this. I play it by ear now. It depends on what it is. I might like the opportunity to have a conversation about the effects of whatever the secret is with the person. It also may contain critical content—for example, abuse. In this case, Brenda couldn't make it to the session, and Eddie wanted the time. There really wasn't a secret.

VICKI: This is a tricky issue. Other than the possible "secret" issue (which I think we both handle in the way you mentioned), meeting separately will have certain effects on each person and on the relationship. Thus, I am not much interested in meeting with members of a couple separately. I sometimes will do so if one or the other cannot come in at the last minute for some reason, and I do find in such cases that the time is well spent, often in exploring more extended personal meaning systems that may be affecting the person. I tell the person, though, that the same work could be done with the other in the room, and often with more substantial good effects. The reason is that the other can be in a reflexive position, if there is enough separation from the problem, and can then begin to notice different aspects of the partner's experience that might be preferred. I find when couples have this experience, they want to continue in this way. Anyway, let's get back to the story.

Eddie shared with me his concerns that Brenda's needs were not being met, that she wanted things from him, and that he sometimes responded to this pressure by "turning off." I asked him whether he knew what he wanted from her or from the relationship, separate from what she wanted. I thought that **withdrawal** and the **up-and-down pattern** might have him attending to what Brenda's picture of a relationship was. What did he want that was worth pursuing? This turned out to be a revolutionary question for both of us. For Eddie it was a novel idea; as a man, he knew one got married and had kids and worked outside the home. The presence of a family to do things with, to come home to—that's what it was about. What did he personally want beyond that? He said he needed time to consider what his needs might be in a relationship. Before, he had only considered what he might personally want in matters separate from the relationship. For me, it helped me realize that men really don't think much about this question. A relationship means stability, home as castle, sex—but more than that?

This question became an important theme for Eddie, and also something I began to attend to more regularly in all my work with couples.

When I saw this couple three weeks later, Eddie had been asking himself that question a lot, and it was helping him be more present in some of the ways Brenda wanted. Now he truly decided he wanted some of the same things she did. Brenda's experience was that there were "deeply good" moments on a couple of occasions, which she contrasted to Eddie's absenteeism in the past. However, this created some confusion, as she wasn't sure which direction she wanted to go in. She could depend on herself consistently, but not on the relationship. The effects of the past, and her wish for a future that was definitely different, led to some impatience, some analysis, and some caution.

While I asked Eddie more and more reauthoring questions concerning his own wants over the next couple of sessions, Brenda continued to question what she wanted even in the face of these developments. After the 10th session, Brenda sent me a note saying that she had found herself quite upset when she left the last session. My consistent responding to Eddie's small, slow steps toward his preliminary picture of what he wanted had the effect of heightening frustration for Brenda, given how much time she had already put into the relationship. What was more important was that when I questioned her reactions to Eddie when he was trying to talk to her as possibly having the effect of discouraging him, it had the effect of again making her feel responsible for the relationship. When she thought I meant she should create space for him, she said, "I'll be giving in order to receive?" That experience invited a **bad-person picture** to overtake her: "If I had just been different, a bit more perfect, put a clamp on unreasonable expectations, accepted a more complacent role, acquired a 'thicker skin,' everything probably would have worked out just fine. I just wasn't good enough, smart enough, deserving enough to be loved." I realized that, in effect, my comments had replicated the dominant culture. How could I have been so blind? Was it the remnants of my previous systems-based thinking? My enthusiasm for Eddie's steps? Or my being a man, with its concomitant effects of seeing entitlement from the point of view of a man's experience? I could only be pleased that Brenda was willing to send me this note and return to the next session to discuss it; this indicated that I had somehow accomplished creating that kind of space in our work together. I am eternally thankful for the lessons that I learned here. I translate them into the following:

1. Therapy, from a gender perspective is not necessarily or usually "balanced." It goes in phases. Often this means that the man takes steps first, while not much is expected right away from the woman for the relationship.
2. As therapists, we need to give women constant validation (given the culture) that a relationship orientation can be resumed at

their own time and pace. Years of neglect and mistreatment, even if these were the results of ignorance, can't be wiped out by several months of steps by the man. If we attend to a man's steps enthusiastically, we need to be overt about what these steps mean for the woman, which often translates into "Not anything, necessarily."

3. Expecting a woman to do anything concomitantly, or even to attend to the man's experience and not her own, may have the effect of bringing back the burden of responsibility. The experience of the woman may be that once again she is being asked to make the relationship work, despite her having tried to do so for years.

These comments are not meant as rules for all situations, but as important aspects to attend to, particularly for male therapists. If these ideas prove helpful, our readers should thank Brenda and some other women I have worked with who have helped me to appreciate their experience.

The Authors Speak

VICKI: Jeff, I find it interesting that you say "particularly for male therapists." Although I probably agree with you, I also find that I inadvertently cooperate with the dominant culture's injunction that women should be responsible for the relationship. In fact, because that discourse also operates on me as a woman, I find as a female therapist that it tells me this: Not only must I be responsible for how the therapy goes; I must also help the woman in the relationship do *her* job better. I have worked hard at noticing this influence and am trying hard to resist it. One of the ways that it is most apt to come up for me is when I find myself following one of the old adages I learned as a family therapist—that is, to work with the member of the couple (family) who is most interested in change or the easiest to help change. Isn't it interesting that we have most often thought it is the woman who fits that category? By catching this tendency, I have focused more on trying to help the man notice that he might like to take his share of responsibility for the relationship.

JEFF: I'm glad you added that here. Would you say some more about how, as a female therapist, you might run into some difficulties with the male member of the couple? I've heard you say that you don't find it so easy to invite men to act more responsibly—that doing so as a woman can seem problematic.

VICKI: I've learned a lot from you, from our colleague at MRI, John Neal

[1996], and from Alan Jenkins [1990] about how men are usually not interested in doing things that have harmful effects on their partners or the relationship. Their preference is to participate in a loving, nurturing way. However, male training has not been very rich in providing men with ways to do that. So I find that I talk a lot about preferences and interest in acting responsibly, and we do a lot of work on noticing specific instances in which they are already acting in preferred ways—not unlike what you did in your work with Eddie. Because I am respectful of their point of view, nonblaming, and validating of their intentions, I find that the work goes well. I do think, however, as I believe you are also saying, that men must take the first step. Given the power differential in every heterosexual relationship, it cannot be otherwise.

JEFF: You know I agree with you here. I wonder whether our readers will find this provocative.

VICKI: Let me add one thing. I really like the question you asked Eddie—about what was *his* picture of the relationship. I suspect it would be helpful to include that question regularly. I know I'll be more intent on making sure I ask it now.

JEFF: Thanks. Let's go on with the story.

Anyway, after I apologized and took responsibility for the effects of my comments, over the next couple of sessions Brenda and I talked about the **bad-person thing**—how the culture encourages this, and what the effects on women typically are. We continued to notice the effects of **mistreatment** on her attitude and her reactions. She persisted in saying she did not believe the relationship could work out. Eddie continued to take steps, despite questioning whether it was worth it, given where Brenda was. He decided it was worth it because he was learning to be how he wanted to be in a relationship, and no matter what eventually happened, he valued these developments.

Our 14th session was with a reflecting team and was videotaped. We include some excerpts.

Brenda and Eddie: Some 14th-Session Talk

Sequence with Eddie

EDDIE: I'm beginning to get a picture of what I want, what I need. So it makes me feel stronger.

JEFF: Stronger. Has this had effects on other parts of your life directly? Or will it?

EDDIE: Yeah (*laughing*). I feel it will have positive effects on all aspects of my life. I feel a lot more connected to my kids. I feel a lot more stable at work. Things come and things go, and if something happens it's not the end of the world. I have a bigger picture of things. They're not going to throw me out of my house if something goes wrong there. I think it has positive effects on all aspects of my life, because you have that good base to come from.

JEFF: That base of yourself, your own sort of ideas. This has only been in four months. What about . . . ?

EDDIE: Well, there have been a lot of turning points. Okay. We started focusing on what the real problem is. But I think it really started when I quit drinking.

JEFF: Right. I guess it would. When was that?

EDDIE: Three years ago.

JEFF: So that was really the first major step.

EDDIE: And I did it for all the wrong reasons.

JEFF: I remain unconvinced of that.

EDDIE: (*Laughing*)

JEFF: I know we had this discussion—you said you did it for Brenda. And I said I couldn't imagine it was possible you only did it for Brenda. You must have had some of your own reasons for it.

EDDIE: That's true.

JEFF: Even if they weren't the most obvious ones.

EDDIE: Right. But being able to do that forced me to take a look at what is the path I want. I mean I didn't focus in on it like I did four months ago, but I had the inkling that was the direction I needed to go in, because I couldn't keep drifting along—which is the way I felt like the first part of my life.

JEFF: So what do you think you did during those three years that prepared you for having this revelation? I agree with you, it probably wouldn't have happened if it wasn't for whatever happened during those three years.

EDDIE: Well, it was kind of a big revelation—maybe not so big. Before I quit drinking, everything was focused on me. All the blame in our relationship was heaped on me, and the fact that I wasn't taking responsibility and that I was irresponsible and drinking, and "If you only would stop drinking, everything would be okay"—which I didn't buy for the longest time. I got to the part where a series of things happened that made me want to stop drinking. But everything wasn't hunky-dory or beautiful and wonderful. And we didn't live happily ever after. But what did happen was, I was forced to take a look at our relationship realistically. And it was much more a couple's problem than Eddie drinking too much. It was a lot of things that needed to be worked on to get the air cleared. We needed to find out where we stood with each other. It wasn't the sitting down and saying, "Here's your thing and here's my thing." It was a long progression of pain and anger and all of that stuff. It's not like I sat down after I quit drinking and said, "Okay, that didn't work; let's go on to something else." We said, "This isn't working; now what are we going to do?" And we went to a therapist and I went to a therapist, and you know some things were working and some things weren't. And I look back and say I've been heading in the right direction, but like that (*makes a zig-zag line with his hands*), not like that (*makes a straight line*). It's not like I saw the goal and went for it. It has been like this (*makes the zig-zag line again*). I've been stumbling around in the dark, punctuated by these little revelations: "Oh, yeah, this is what I need to work on," and you stumble along a little while and other things come up. It's not like I can see the end of the tunnel and I'm going right for it . . . you know, "In four months I'm going to be okay" (*laughing*).

JEFF: Right. You know it's not my experience that it happens that way (*makes a straight line*). People do stumble along.

EDDIE: Right. I look back at the last three years and I realize I'm heading in the right direction. I'm happier than I was three years ago.

JEFF: That's some proof of that.

EDDIE: I feel better about myself, my interactions, our relationship. It's not perfect. I don't know that it will ever be perfect. I'm hopeful that it will be even better than it is now.

JEFF: Like, do you have a glimpse of that? If it's in another three years—if I ran into you in three years, what steps will you have taken? Can you imagine what they'll look like if this progression keeps going? Even if it goes through the . . . you know . . .

EDDIE: Winding road . . .

JEFF: The winding road. You can see what you've left behind, it sounds like. I'm curious . . .

EDDIE: I still catch myself doing things I did three years ago. Like stuffing feelings or not saying anything when something comes up. And maybe the next day saying, "Yesterday when you said this, or three days ago when you said that, it kind of made me angry." I would like to be able to do that (*snaps fingers*) when it happens.

JEFF: More in the moment.

EDDIE: Sure, more in the moment. And I find myself holding back. I realize it's going on, but it doesn't explode out of my mouth. It doesn't come out very free. When it comes to intimacy, I wish I was more verbal. I wish I could get into that easier than I can. I wish I could speak those romantic, "I'm close, I love you"-type things easier than I do now. It's still very much of a struggle to verbalize that. It's not easy for me to ask for things. "I need this; please, can I have it?"

JEFF: So in three years those things might be happening more (*snaps fingers*) like that. We picked those three years as an arbitrary figure— that would be the end of the road you headed down. And now you're in the middle. You realize these things when they're happening, which you didn't three years ago, and you get some of them out at some point. And that's different from a year ago . . .

EDDIE: From four months ago.

JEFF: So what do you think when you look back three years from now, as to how you got from where you are now to where you are then? What steps do you think you will have taken?

EDDIE: I don't know what they'll look like. It's a matter of practicing those things.

JEFF: (*Writing*) Practicing.

EDDIE: Those things.

JEFF: Keeping practicing. Like shooting a lot of layups.

EDDIE: (*Laughing*) Yeah. Realizing you are feeling something and verbalizing it, whether it's anger or love or confusion—the things I used to ignore. Now I'm even starting to realize, to see inside, to get them out [gives examples]. Yeah, you're right. It's like shooting layups. Practicing.

The Authors Speak

With these questions, Jeff was attempting to develop a timeline of landscape of action for Eddie's new story.

Sequence with Brenda

JEFF: It's easy to get into "What's wrong?" and "Why is it taking so long?" So I'm trying to understand that.

BRENDA: There are times when I feel impatient. I haven't felt the need to express that since I saw you last. Things have been generally pretty good. But I might feel frustrated, not so much in terms of the relationship . . . but I do feel frustrated that the relationship as a whole . . . is this going to work? When Eddie is finally at that place where he is able to say and do what he is feeling, is it going to be mutually satisfying to the two of us? Is it what both of us will want when we get to that place that we haven't come to yet? So that does occur to me.

JEFF: And do you think that . . . I would think that has something to do with the effects of some of the experiences over the last 20 years, being in doubt. Is that how you understand it?

BRENDA: Uh-huh.

JEFF: And I was wondering about where you were with respect to that. I haven't actually caught up with you in a long time on that. Have you shifted one way or the other? You were being cautious. There were a lot of questions about whether you would want to continue in it or not, regardless. I don't know if it has shifted or not. Does seeing where this might lead to . . . does this have any effect, or not? That's what I'm curious about.

BRENDA: I'd have to say that my feelings really fluctuate. The past three weeks have been reasonably pleasant, so I haven't spent a lot of time and energy dragging up some of the old **mistreatment.** A lot of that hasn't really occurred to me, because it has felt relatively good in the last three weeks. But I need to be honest, too, and say I don't know where we are going.

JEFF: Right. I wasn't meaning to imply you could possibly know at this point. I was interested in how much of this **mistreatment** thing is hanging around. Has it gotten any more or less?

The Authors Speak

Jeff was intentionally wanting to continue to go at her pace—something *she* had called his attention to, if you remember, after the 10th session.

BRENDA: I'm probably still cautious. I probably observe very carefully what is said or what isn't said, or what is done or what isn't done. I'm still a keen observer. I felt my observations in the last three weeks— because things have been generally pleasant and Eddie has been very supportive—have been less critical, or where they've been cautious I haven't had to drag out some of that old stuff and say, "Yes, but." And it's nice not to have to dredge that up. It's unpleasant to do that.

JEFF: What I'm interested in is, lots of time when there have been *feelings of mistreatment*—no matter what happens on the other side—it is difficult to give up "Yes, but" and caution. I wonder a bit about what you've done to put them aside. I know it seems they've just not been around. My experience is that this is not necessarily a given when the other person is taking some steps. It wouldn't have to happen—it's not a given. So my belief is you've actually done something to loosen the grip of those *mistreatment* memories. Somehow. I don't know what you've done; I just wonder about that.

BRENDA: I don't know that I've done anything. I really don't. I'd like to accept some of the responsibility for making it different, but largely Eddie is the one who has made the overture, and I have noticed it. It's not like I'm getting into that thing where we were for so long, where I'm making him responsible for the relationship. That's not how I see it. I see a successful relationship as having a mutual sort of exchange. And my feeling is, he's beginning to know how to exchange and I'm responding to it.

JEFF: So maybe what I'm paying attention to is that you are noticing and responding. And given these *feelings of mistreatment* . . . I've known situations where *feelings of mistreatment* have stopped people from noticing and responding, despite what was happening on the other end. That's what I'm paying attention to. You are noticing and you are responding.

BRENDA: And I think that's real important too, because there have been times in this relationship when we've come through a really hard time, and I would feel mistreated or feel that the kids were neglected or whatever was going on, and Eddie would come home with flowers and I would just as soon throw those right in the toilet.

JEFF: Like "How dare you?" Right?

BRENDA: Yes. I'm sorry, that doesn't fly. You're not in jail one week and bring me flowers the next, and all is forgiven.

EDDIE: I'll stop bringing you flowers.

BRENDA: (*Laughing*) No, that's not what I'm saying.

JEFF: (*Laughing*) Let's be clear about that.

BRENDA: But it has taken me time when we're going through a really bad period to let go of something that has been said or not been said. To forgive that. And to see, okay, this is a sincere effort. These are not just some posies to pacify you—isn't everything okay now? I have required more than that to be convinced. Because it has been too long.

JEFF: Yeah, it's inevitable it would go like that. This leads me back to what I was curious about, that somehow you've been able to shake all those *feelings of mistreatment* and respond, even if you are still cautious.

BRENDA: (*Chewing a piece of gum*) It's so cold in here, that's why I'm chewing.

JEFF: (*Getting up*) I know what we can do about that. When you first came in here, it was stuffy.

BRENDA: I didn't think so, I thought it was just right. (*Eddie says something to her.*) Eddie thinks it's just right now also. He's comfortable.

JEFF: I'm more like Eddie.

EDDIE: (*Laughing*) It's a gender thing.

JEFF: (*Laughing; to Brenda*) So you are able to notice and respond and not let these *feelings of mistreatment* blind you? That's what I was paying attention to.

The Authors Speak

It was important to Jeff here to continue to focus on her agency in this regard.

BRENDA: I think so. It has to do with the place I'm in when he does something that I might notice or respond to. I might be in a place where I don't respond, as I have the last three weeks. That's bound to happen, depending on my mood.

JEFF: Sure.

Jeff's Story (Continued)

After this session, Eddie continued to take steps, having to fight *fears*— of abandonment, of Brenda's "reactions"—although this was an awkward time for him, given what was going on with Brenda. The next seven sessions (over a four-month period) were used to help him continue to fight the *fears,* to be more the way he wanted, and to develop a new story about himself. One content topic involved Eddie's efforts to approach Brenda sexually in a way that fit better for both of them. Mostly, though, these sessions involved more intense work for Brenda, as she now had to decide whether she wanted to "open the door" again. (This was an issue the team raised.) What were her wants? How did the problem's history affect her attitude about getting what she wanted in this relationship? How did her experience as a woman affect what had happened and what might happen? We agreed that fear and guilt were not good reasons to stay involved. I asked her what percentage of love was left. She said, "20%." In what seemed to be a useful decision for our work together, we decided to focus on this 20% rather than continue to debate the question of her future involvement. Working on the 20%, we focused on what she considered were current intimate interactions (Weingarten, 1991). In a couple of sessions she came up to 50% (50% a chance for the future and 50% a waste of time). As Eddie took more and more substantial steps that Brenda was on the lookout for, Brenda saw more and more possibilities and increased her openness toward him. We also kept staying clear about what wasn't her responsibility, fighting the cultural ideas that tried to recruit her into the **bad-person thing**. Questions about her own acceptability dropped to 10%. At our next session (22nd overall and eighth after the meeting with the team), Brenda reported that she was "feeling better" about opening the door, so we worked on separating the everyday-type stuff that occurred with all couples from the influence of the "20-year bag," which had her strongly reacting to any hint of some unwanted direction. Eddie said that he felt closer to her than he had in a long time, and that he was holding on to his feelings and tolerating conflict.

The Authors Speak

VICKI: Can I interrupt? I'd like to make something clear. These weren't your goals, Jeff, or some idea that relationships require this?

JEFF: Absolutely not; this was their picture. Back to the story.

At the same time, Brenda said that she noticed "a difference in the relationship" and that it "felt pleasant." We decided to have the next session in a month. When they returned, Brenda said she felt closer to Eddie than she had in a long time; she was setting realistic standards; and they were starting over and were "new people." Eddie said that they were talking more and appreciating each other, and also that he had more self-esteem. On their visit one month later, they reported that these developments had continued. Two months later we had another session with a reflecting team. We include more excerpts.

More with Brenda and Eddie: Some 25th-Session Talk

Sequence with Brenda

BRENDA: The time we do have together, I'm feeling good about. We're both investing and invested in what's happening. That feels good to me.

JEFF: I'm interested in how you've noticed Eddie invested in ways you appreciate.

BRENDA: There is still a real sense of freedom, I think—where we both feel free to go and do, and we established that a long time ago. We both need to have that. But at the same time, the time we've had together has so often been . . . and not even any of the ugly times, the sort of plain times . . . has been so absent of any, I don't know . . . has just been absent. We're both in the same room, but somebody isn't there. There has been so much of that, that I really pay attention to the time that we're both home. I don't want to be clingy, nor do I want to be clung to, but it feels really nice to be heard when I have something to say.

JEFF: So now people are home. They're home when they're home.

BRENDA: And the kids are, of course, really home when they're home . . . of course, I'm speaking about Eddie and me . . . and the time that we're physically, actually home can't be very much, but when we are, we're both there a lot more of the time . . . if that makes any sense.

JEFF: It makes a lot of sense.

BRENDA: That's something that I know—that I've come to realize is very important to me, as with a very, very close friend. I want not only to be heard, but I also want information put out there that I can listen to.

JEFF: Right.

BRENDA: There's less of that. I want more of that, but certainly it is coming right along.

JEFF: (*Writing*) Coming right along.

BRENDA: So I'm feeling, and I'm really working on not allowing this euphoria—"Okay, it's vacation, everything's wonderful"—to sneak in there. I'm trying to have as clear a perspective as I can, to look at things for what they really are. And for those mediocre times—it's okay, there are going to be those times. I just don't want to be stuck there all the time. I'm feeling less stuck in it. And Eddie has been very sweet and considerate and present.

JEFF: (*Writing*) Sweet, considerate, and present.

BRENDA: And we looked at the old tape about the flowers.

JEFF: I remember that.

BRENDA: I'll never forget it. I don't want flowers.

JEFF: What has taken their place?

BRENDA: They didn't . . . they never worked anyway. So I don't want to start off with what has taken their place. But I think the fact that Eddie and I are working on this—honestly, sincerely trying to do something with this relationship. When that's happening, there isn't—flowers are lovely, but they don't replace something that's missing.

JEFF: You don't need flowers when you have a relationship that you can feel.

BRENDA: One that feels good.

JEFF: Yeah.

BRENDA: One that's a bit more equal . . . with give and take . . . yeah.

[Later in the session:]

JEFF: What difference does that make . . . since the last tape . . . to that old history, to how you are thinking about things? I mean . . . I have a list here that is a different list than you might have given me on the last tape. You are being heard more. Eddie has been sweet and considerate and present in a way that not only replaces the flowers, but gives you more of something you want. You are being listened to. What difference does that make to your thinking about the relationship and your picture of it?

BRENDA: Well, I'm feeling like there is a choice for us. I'm feeling like this could work. It's not something I felt very strongly about for a long time.

JEFF: Yeah. I think that has been a more recent thing than the last tape. I don't know if you would have said that then.

BRENDA: I don't know if I would . . . on the last tape. No, I wouldn't have. I may have said it on the last visit, but on the last tape . . . no.

JEFF: Sometime in the last couple of months?

BRENDA: That is a new sensation. And it's exciting. Yes, this could really work. We could be happy, and we could be grandparents together, and that is very exciting. Now a large part of the time, contrary to my feelings just one year ago, I'm that way more often than the other way. It's reversed.

JEFF: In a major way, reversed.

BRENDA: Yeah, it is. I mean there was so far to come. I never really . . . I always said what I'd like would be this . . . but to really feel like it was happening . . . I couldn't imagine it. So that has been really nice (*looking misty-eyed*).

JEFF: Have you been sharing this with other people? Is this something you talk to Darcy [a friend] about?

BRENDA: Darcy and I haven't had much time. This is the first time I've had time with Darcy in a year, other than a quick phone call. We tend to get down into the depths when we do get together. You know she asked me last night, when it was just the crickets and the creek, "You and Eddie are doing pretty good, aren't you?" And I said, "It feels really good, Darcy." And that was it . . . Darcy is one I would trust to talk to. I do it in here. I have this friend, a mutual friend, from almost as early as the time Eddie and I met. She is coming out to visit in August, and I will catch her up. Why were you wondering who I talked to?

JEFF: Oh, I was less wondering who exactly you talked to, and more interested in whether you've been talking about the relationship in a different way. My thinking behind my question was that I imagined it would be a bit scary to be out there with a whole different story than you have been previously. You've been cautious and stuff, and I was just wondering about what it meant that you were ready to share things with people—what it said about how far things had come.

BRENDA: I haven't lost all my cautiousness, but I don't think about it every single day—and I was thinking about it every single day: "I don't know if I want to give this because . . . " I mean it's just how it was. It's still there, but it has changed; it's not all-present like it was. It is a little bit scary to begin, not boasting, but because you know there's always the "Who knows where it's going?" And a year from now, I don't want to be whining to Darcy and have her say, "It was good last year!" I'm trying to just . . . I don't want to color it, but at the same time I want to appreciate it for what it is, and it's far more colorful than I imagined it would be a year ago.

The Authors Speak

These questions invited Brenda to redescribe the relationship and circulate it to a wider, relevant audience.

Sequence with Eddie

EDDIE: I felt like I was participating a lot more. Brenda had this recent problem with her mom, and it was a lot easier to give my opinion about what I thought. In the past I would hold back and just go,

"What do you think?" or say, "Maybe they think this," but I would always be so obtuse about it, and now I was able to say, "Here's what I think," which is kind of a change for me.

JEFF: Right. So how would . . . ?

EDDIE: So it became more of a two-way thing, rather than me just listening and making a couple of comments. It was me listening and then making a couple of comments, and then she listened and made some comments back. And I made some comments back. It was more of a dialogue as opposed to a monologue, which is the way it used to be.

JEFF: So what do you think about that? Have you enjoyed that?

EDDIE: Yeah. I have enjoyed that.

JEFF: But what have you enjoyed about that?

EDDIE: I've enjoyed having my point of view validated, I guess. Not really validated—that's too strong a term. Having my own view accepted. Being able to put out my own view without, you know, I guess, "Maybe this isn't what she wants to hear," which is what I used to do a lot. Not only with Brenda, but with a lot of other people too.

JEFF: Has that voice been quieter and your voice louder? What's the balance between the two?

EDDIE: I think the voice that allows me to speak my own mind is becoming stronger, rather than the voice that says, "Watch out." It's really interesting. Just a small little aside about that: Over the weekend we were up at the cabin, and I was talking to somebody— actually, it was Sherry; it's a long, complicated story—but she was saying one of the reasons that she was really crabby last year at the same time was that her husband was being a jerk. And, you know, normally I would go, "Yeah. . . . " This year I just kind of said, "That's interesting—what your husband does affects the way you feel and how you act." She just looked at me with that funny look and smiled. (Giggles)

JEFF: (Laughing) So she was surprised to hear what you have to say about that?

EDDIE: (Laughing) Yeah, because normally I wouldn't say something like that. I would think that's pushing my nose in her business, or pointing out one of her weaknesses. It would be a faux pas kind of thing. I just treated it like a regular comment: "Oh, what he does affects how you feel. How long . . . ?" (Laughs) You know I was just kidding around with her about that . . . normally I wouldn't have done anything like that . . . but it felt okay. The world didn't come to an end. She didn't stomp off in a huff and never speak to me again, or any of those weird things you might imagine.

JEFF: So when you can do something like that, what difference does that make to your feelings about yourself? When you can let your own . . .

EDDIE: That really is the whole difference, how I feel about myself. I mean that's where the biggest change is that has happened over the past two years—how I feel about myself, how I value my opinions, and how I interact—am beginning to interact—with people in a different way. Because of the way I feel about myself, not only in this relationship, but in business. I have things where normally I would roll over when something negative happens, but now I speak up and say, "Wait a minute; you know this isn't right." It's not a comfortable thing to do. It's much easier to roll over and say, "I'll do this or that." But it feels better. I'm not relishing the conflict, but I'm getting used to the conflict.

JEFF: So you're realizing you can handle the conflict?

EDDIE: Yeah, that I can handle it, and it's not the end of the world. And it's better to speak up and speak out how you feel—it makes me feel better at the end of it, even though it's uncomfortable at the time. That the results are better after it's all said and done. I mean it's a scarier thing, but just with Brenda and me, what has happened over the last six months or so, when I do speak my mind or give my opinion—yeah, it's scary, and "Oh, God, what is she going to think?" and that kind of stuff. But a dialogue is much better than the one-way rule.

JEFF: When you are able to do this, is this more consistent, I'm assuming, with certain ways of being and handling things that you value? I mean, is this handling the conflict and taking a direct approach to it—is that more consistent with what you wanted to see about yourself, for yourself?

EDDIE: I don't think I ever really had a clear vision of how I saw myself—you know, "Here's the goal" or "I want to be that way, that's how I want to be." I didn't have a goal like that. I just knew it wasn't working like it was and that I wasn't getting what I wanted.

JEFF: So what do you think about that now?

EDDIE: I think that I'm starting to get more of what I want. I don't know if you ever get everything you want.

JEFF: If you figure out how to do that, I'd be happy to come and take lessons from you.

EDDIE: Conscious optimism. You can't get all your wants, but you can have some of it.

JEFF: I think there's a song like that.

EDDIE: So, yeah, it feels a lot better now.

JEFF: Now that you've tried this on, does it seem to fit more for you?

EDDIE: It fits more for me.

JEFF: That's what I'm trying to get at.

EDDIE: Yeah, it really does.

JEFF: So, you're seeing differences in all parts of your life?

EDDIE: It has affected more than just . . . it has really affected Brenda and me, that's obviously the starting point that I began with. I see it affecting interactions with friends, in business; I see it affecting a lot of different things . . . even my kids.

The Authors Speak

These questions attempted to connect the steps Eddie took with his preferences, his values, and his new descriptions of himself (landscape of consciousness).

Jeff's Story (Finale) and Conversation

Our last session was six weeks later, when we finished our work together. About one year after that, I was invited to a ceremony in which Brenda and Eddie renewed their marriage commitment to each other.

VICKI: I can see why you chose that couple. It certainly illustrates some important issues regarding gender. I do, however, have some questions for you.

JEFF: I knew you would.

VICKI: Is this a typical starting point for you—looking at both ends of a pattern? It's really more of a **withdraw–withdraw** pattern than the more frequent **pursue–withdraw** one I often see affecting couples.

JEFF: My usual starting point is a pattern, with each member of the couple grappling with his or her own end of it for his or her own reasons. In other words, the way each is responding to the other doesn't fit each person's preferred picture, as they described it to me when I raised this question. With this couple, problems affecting them had been around for a long time. I imagine that if I had seen them any time up to 10 years ago, or even 5 years ago, the pattern would have looked more like *pursue–withdraw.* Given the gender instructions Brenda responded to for many years, some form of *pursuing* was inevitable. Women feel responsible for the relationship and work hard to make it happen. When they are feeling stressed, they have been taught to affiliate. *Pursuing* is the only thing that makes sense, given gender "requirements." On the other hand, men have been taught to expect to be cared for; to have their wants met; to be right all the time ("What do you mean, this is my opinion? It's true!"); to have work needs dominate all other issues; and to engage in "not thinking" about relationships, only about themselves. When any of these "rules" are violated, men feel stress and often experience a sense of inadequacy and do what they've been taught to do, which is to isolate themselves. When there is any stress, and particularly couple stress that affects both people, then each member wants the opposite of what the other wants. A pattern can develop that often has more far-reaching effects on the relationship than whatever the stress or issue was that got them going in the first place. As Gottman's research suggests [see Gottman, 1994], after the *pursue–withdraw* pattern has been around for a long time, the woman tends to give up, and what develops is a *withdraw–withdraw* pattern. Gottman suggests that this is the final phase before the relationship falls completely apart.

VICKI: This is what you had here. Is that why it took a long time?

JEFF: Yes, because the problem had been around since the beginning of their marriage (20 years), and because the *withdraw–withdraw* pattern had them close to the end. It also took a long time to help Eddie take the steps he took, to help him keep taking them, and to firmly establish a direction. Then, and it couldn't happen concomitantly (remember?), it took some time for Brenda to decide whether she still really wanted the relationship, as well as to separate slowly from the effects of 20 years of not getting what she wanted. With some couples, once developments occur—each partner taking separate steps or even relationship steps together—therapy could end more quickly. I've seen some couples as few as three times, after which things have progressed well without more therapy. As with kids, adolescents, adults, and families, it depends on how long the problem has been around and how much of a grip it has on them. It seems important for our readers to notice that with Brenda and Eddie, despite the problem's strong and lengthy hold on them, they kept some good feelings for each other—an amazing victory for their relationship! This said something to me about the foundation of connection they had. My theory is that this is what made it possible for them to do their work both separately and together in rescuing their relationship from the problem.

VICKI: Can we summarize this? We usually start with a pattern, externalizing each end of the pattern for each member of the couple—in a sense, a separate problem affecting each of them, such as *pursue* or *withdraw*. We note the effects for each. We question them about whether this way of responding fits their picture of how they want to be in a relationship. We note unique outcomes and make meaning of them. Then, in subsequent sessions, we focus on developments . . .

JEFF: Right . . .

VICKI: We both have a strong commitment to situate the problem in its sociopolitical context. (I'm repeating myself here.) In this case you attended to the context of gender, and very secondarily to family-of-origin issues. The problem seemed to evolve toward capturing more cultural and personal meaning systems. For example, you talked with Eddie about *fear* of abandonment, which encouraged *withdrawal.* With Brenda you addressed the effect of the history of the problem itself, as well as gender-encouraged conclusions, such as the *bad-person thing* and entitlement issues (her wants). These meaning systems or stories then are responded to with the same process—externalizing, deconstructing along the experiences that produced the meaning (history of the problem, gender, family issues), noticing effects, looking for unique outcomes, and following developments.

JEFF: Yes.

VICKI: How long do you think you spend, on the average, with couples?

JEFF: About half as long, in terms of both time and the number of sessions, as I did with Brenda and Eddie.

VICKI: Could you give our readers and me some other examples, with other couples, of how things go?

JEFF: Sure. In the next chapter I describe some work I did with Natalie, an eight-year-old girl. Here I want to tell you about my work with her parents.

IRENE AND ANDY

JEFF: When I had my first session with Irene and Andy, the problem was so big and so overwhelming that I ended up constructing it as *anger.*

VICKI: Not separate ones for each?

JEFF: When couples come in with an extreme situation, in which they are uncomfortable all the time and so focused on the misery in the relationship, I find it more useful to start this way. The pattern with its individual aspects doesn't seem as compelling as the dominant affective experience, such as *anger,* that is overshadowing the relationship. *Pain* is another problem I commonly construct as affecting couples when they report their experience in this way. Certainly, I look at specifics and at the different habits that might support *anger.* For example, in this case, Andy didn't pay much attention to his wife, didn't seem interested in what was going on with her, often came home late, ate separately, and let his strong ideas dominate. Nor was he as responsive to Natalie as he could be. He saw that *anger* encouraged all of this, and that many of his seemingly uncaring responses were *anger*-influenced. None of this fit his picture of how he would treat someone he loved. Irene saw how *anger* got her to interfere with Andy's relationship with Natalie, and what effect this was having on that relationship. She could also see how *anger* got her to conclude that Andy wasn't interested in her or the family. Since, after all, *she* tried to make it work, what else could she conclude?

VICKI: This is a good example of what we discussed in an earlier chapter—that people make up stories to justify how they are responding, when they know they are not responding as they "should" or perhaps even as they would like to. I suspect that Irene knew her intentions toward the relationship and toward Andy were good, so she must assume, if Andy was behaving as he was, that his intentions must be bad. This view of his intentions then affected all the interpretations she was making. And the view was inevitable, given the way *anger* (and, I assume, other problems) were affecting both of them. I would guess Andy was engaged in a similar process of storying his experience with Irene.

JEFF: Yes. I find that bringing out these stories is useful in all the work I do, but particularly with couples. Helping them notice how problems create a view of the other person's intentions is a useful step in opening space for them to consider or notice other possibilities. Thus, I sometimes ask whether they have noticed any things that could reflect other intentions, or whether, given a new statement about the other's intentions, certain events that have occurred might be viewed in new ways. This kind of process can also be a springboard toward a conversation that makes distinctions between intentions and effects. Many men, particularly, don't pay attention to the effects of what they do; they are not used to thinking about the other person's experience, only about their own. If problems encourage a view that the other's intentions must be bad, then each confronts the effects by attacking the other, who, of course, defends herself or himself because each knows that her or his own intentions are good. On the other hand, if we can help couples get curious about effects or can comment on them in a manner that separates them from intentions, the effect of the comment can be quite different. That is, it will be heard differently and more constructively.

VICKI: How did the work go with this couple?

JEFF: After the first couple session, I was able to notice and make meaning about a number of significant developments. For example, Irene stopped interfering with Andy's relationship with Natalie, and Andy made significant efforts "to be pleasant," which Irene even noticed; she commented, "He's trying to be nicer," and indicated that this was a happy surprise. These developments, combined with what I noticed in the first session—cooperating with each other, despite *anger,* in putting Natalie back to bed—allowed each to begin to see new possibilities for the relationship and to acknowledge a new direction.

VICKI: Here's an instance where one member of the couple noticed the efforts of the other. In my experience, this doesn't always happen so quickly.

JEFF: Not in my experience, either. This is another advantage of talking to one while the other listens. Each person can report his or her efforts, which the problem has probably stopped the other from seeing. Being in a reflexive position can help each attend more easily to what the other is saying and to the therapist's response to this. Despite the problem's efforts to blind them, this process can help each begin to notice "another story." If the partners talk too much to each other, they'll talk under the influence of the problem, which I tell them they can do at home without my help. Usually I ask each partner to catch me up on her or his own efforts; of course, when one partner has already noticed the steps of the other, I am very interested.

VICKI: So, with this couple, you kept looking for anti-*anger* developments.

JEFF: Two sessions after the first one, given that things were moving along nicely, we began to look at "big issues." With this couple, instead of evolving to more individual specific meaning systems, we focused on a major *anger*-supporting issue—Irene's discontent at being moved to the area from her birth country by her husband, and the effects of this immigration on her life. Irene felt that Andy was able to hear things about this that he hadn't heard before.

VICKI: I assume you addressed the gender context—that men feel they have to fix or do something, and not just listen when issues are presented.

JEFF: Yes, and we also looked at another gender-related issue—entitlement. When I asked Andy, he said he believed that things should be equal and they should each have an equal say in how their likes went, but Irene felt that it hadn't worked out that way. We (myself and the couple) were beginning to understand Andy's response in a context of men and work. Andy's work needs became the frequent reason that Irene couldn't have what she wanted—for example, the space to develop her skills or to move. We men have been recruited very powerfully into evaluating our success as men and as people by our accomplishments and our standing at work. This can have us clinging to any rights that support this endeavor and to give all else, including what our partners might want, a lesser priority.

VICKI: As a woman, I find it hard to confront that one with men . . .

JEFF: Even as a man, I find I have to do it very carefully. I believe it is critical to stay with the man's experience and work slowly toward helping him to notice how the culture has led him (us) down that road, and what effects this is having on his (our) life.

MARILYN AND KARL

VICKI: I gather you have one more example.

JEFF: Yes, I picked this couple because I was able to tape our first session and I wanted to share some of the transcript with our readers. I've already shown transcripts from the middle and near the end of the work with Brenda and Eddie, but people seem very interested in a first session. This couple is also a good example of another extreme; that is, Marilyn and Karl didn't come in with great **pain** dominating the relationship, but instead felt mostly good about the relationship and about each other. They thought there were a few small problems interfering with things' being even better.

VICKI: So here you used one problem also. I know we both use the pattern affecting the relationship, and thus two problems, when a couple comes in with each person presenting the other as the problem. My experience is that "the other is the problem" presentation is the one that occurs most frequently.

JEFF: Yes, that's my experience also. That's why I find myself often constructing some variation of the *pursue–withdraw* pattern. But Marilyn and Karl were more together, and they presented a relationship
problem. What I like to do in these instances is pit their relationship
against whatever problem we construct. In this situation, the problem
turned out to be *rules of giving.* Let me share some part of our
conversations that led to that construction. But, first, let me catch you
up on what has happened in the sessions so far.

Jeff Situates

I had just spent about 30 minutes meeting with Marilyn and Karl and
talking with Marilyn. She had presented "communication problems," and
then when I began to ask her "effects" questions, we started talking about
the problem as *avoidance*—how it minimized her concerns or stopped
her from sharing her reactions, and how it had each of them running from
conflict and protecting the other. I was thinking that women in general
are coached in this by *lack of entitlement.* Men are often influenced by
withdrawal when it comes to relationship conflict, but what Marilyn was
saying suggested that Karl's responses were not shaped by *overentitlement,* as with many men. When it was Karl's turn, he said he was fighting
this tendency to give and give and give, and he proceeded to give
examples of this across his life.

Excerpts from First Session with Marilyn and Karl

KARL: I figure if I give so much, nobody can say anything bad about me.

[A little later:]

KARL: My problem is I'm not happy with myself.
JEFF: You're not happy about being enslaved to this *giving* thing?

The Authors Speak

VICKI: Jeff, what made you choose *giving* and not *self-hate* or *self-ques-
tioning?*
JEFF: I thought that *giving* was more present and evocative for him at this
point. It also had the potential to be something affecting both him
and the relationship.
KARL: Yeah, because I do it in our relationship.

JEFF: But that's what you're unhappy about? I'm just trying to sort this out.

KARL: It feels like I carry so much baggage here that I feel like I'm going to explode.

JEFF: So the effect of this *rule of giving* ends up drowning you, interfering with what you want to accomplish . . .

KARL: Oh, yeah, here's a classic example. [He proceeds to give an example from their relationship: Marilyn reacts to something he feels is picky.]

JEFF: What does the *rule of giving* have to say about what Marilyn wants?

KARL: [After some musing out loud] I feel she doesn't tell me exactly what she wants to do and when she wants to do it, because of some reason—she's afraid I might get mad or whatever.

JEFF: So this *avoidance* thing I talked to her about makes some sense to you?

KARL: Oh, yeah.

JEFF: And this *rule of giving* has you bending over backwards doing things you think she wants, or know she wants, or imagine she wants, or all of the above?

KARL: That I hope she'll see, but I think it's kind of just gotten to the point where she's either blind to it or she doesn't care about the things I'm giving, or that I'm maybe doing this just for myself, like a self-satisfaction thing. I'm doing all the things that I can afford to or feel like giving and . . . just so I'll . . . and she knows that. It's obvious I'm not doing the right thing, that's for sure.

JEFF: That's the conclusion you've come to?

KARL: Yeah, yeah. [There is some discussion of this and how he doesn't end up doing some things for the relationship he thinks would be good.]

JEFF: I think this *rule of giving* is a real important thing.

KARL: Yeah.

JEFF: So I'm just trying to figure out all the ways it affects you, get at its intricacies. That's what I'm trying to do here. One way the *rule of giving* interferes with your relationship with Marilyn is that it has you doing lots of things both out of the house and in the house. It eats up a lot of your time.

KARL: Oh, yeah.

JEFF: It's harsh about its specifications about what you ought to do, and that takes time away from some of these things you said you might like to do, like call her up for lunch. The *rule* says, "You can't call Marilyn up for lunch because you haven't put enough, or you could put a little more, finishing touches on this house (*Karl nods*)—because you ought to do that. So don't think about calling Marilyn up, think about painting another design." Something like that? Is that one way the *rule* interferes? Is that right?

KARL: Yeah.

JEFF: Something like that. I know it's kind of odd—if *rules* could talk, what would they say?

KARL: That. And I would be worried about what people . . . maybe I'm dirty that day or something. I don't want to go into her office; it's nice and pristine. I'm worried about people thinking maybe, you know, "Why doesn't that guy have a real job or something?"

JEFF: (*Laughing with him*) Gee, I always thought you guys had the real jobs, and we didn't. I always think, "Maybe I should get a real job." (*All laugh.*) So *evaluation* plays a part in these *rules?* It's bigger than even *giving.* You have to look a certain way . . . [There is further discussion that helps Marilyn and Karl to ally themselves together against harsh *rules.*]

JEFF: I have a pretty good beginning picture of how these *rules* affect you—how they interfere with what you want, how they interfere with how you feel about yourself, and how they even interfere with what you might do for the relationship. Do these *rules* interfere with how you talk with Marilyn? Do they affect that at all?

KARL: Not all the time. [He proceeds to give examples of when they have and when they haven't.]

JEFF: So are you saying sometimes these *rules* have the effect of weighing you down, shutting you down?

KARL: Oh, yeah. My mind will go over and over, regurgitating stuff before I feel I can put it out.

JEFF: It stops you from being spontaneous.

KARL: Oh, totally. [He gives examples of how *rules* push the "shoulds" and interfere with what he says or feels he can do.]

JEFF: I was wondering if these *rules* say something about what Marilyn should and shouldn't do.

KARL: I'm starting to see if I quit going beyond the call of duty, in my point of view, and quit giving so much, and start taking a little bit—I can see how it would affect my business. Now in my personal life, I can see it having the opposite effect. All of a sudden I become this guy who—maybe I'm telling her exactly how I feel about everything all the time, maybe good or bad. I am just (*stutters and is at a loss for words*). I'm guessing her point of view on this would be that I turned into some evil character.

JEFF: Oh, I think you are saying that these **rules** make you come to the conclusion that you shouldn't tell her everything that is on your mind.

KARL: No, I'm asking you. I don't know. Maybe I would become a better husband, a better person, a better everything. I don't know.

JEFF: Well, I don't know, but I imagine it would make some difference in the communication thing.

KARL: Yeah, we'd be talking all the time. I'd be telling it like it is all the time.

JEFF: Well, you'd be telling her like it is for you.

KARL: Right.

JEFF: And if she could get past the **avoidance** thing, she would be telling you like it is for her. Do you think that would be a good state of affairs, or a better state of affairs? Or not?

KARL: I think it would be worth a try if we both understand what we're both doing.

JEFF: I would imagine that could make quite a different direction than it was with the problem you came in here for. (*Both Marilyn and Karl nod strongly.*)

JEFF: So I don't know what the effect will be. I don't have a crystal ball—we'd have to see.

KARL: [Gives an example of what he does to make Marilyn mad.]

JEFF: So these **rules** have you organizing yourself by thinking what would make her mad and having you react. They have you saying and doing some things and not saying and doing others—using the threat of her being mad against you. Is cooperating with the **rules** having a good effect? Are they telling you the truth? Is cooperating with them leading to a better relationship?

KARL: Well, I can only assume it would make my job easier.

JEFF: If you could escape the **rules?**

KARL: Oh, yeah. [There follows a conversation of the **rules'** effect on the relationship.] I'd like to try it. [He begins to discuss the pain of following the **rules,** then says they're his enemy.] I have tried to exorcise them lately at work.

JEFF: These **rules** haven't completely put you in jail and thrown away the key. You've had rebellious moments against the **rules.**

KARL: I'm fighting them. I just haven't tried it at home. I'm dying to.

JEFF: [A conversation follows about how the *rules* won't let Karl go so easily and how he will fight back.] The *rules* will say, "Karl, if you do that, you're . . . " [more conversation]. I'd like to go back to Marilyn before we run out of time. [I then summarize how *rules* and *avoidance* interfere with their taking the relationship to the next level.]

MARILYN: Well, I have a lot of these same *rules* . . . I have the opposite reaction. I don't do anything.

JEFF: So they immobilize you.

MARILYN: [Gives an example of Karl's reaction to her comment when she tries to say something, and how she feels she has to be "careful."] I want him to realize—these aren't my *rules*. I want you (*to Karl*) to tell me what you want! [Later:] We like each other so much, we feel we have to be careful. I realize this isn't working.

Jeff Summarizes and Workshop Participants Question

The rest of the session was spent talking about the *rules* and how Marilyn and Karl's relationship was good, with the *rules* being a limiting factor. I spent time at the end summarizing the effects of the *rules* on the relationship, the unique outcomes I gathered from each of them in relation to the *rules,* and how their relationship seemed to have so much they liked. I wondered whether the things that they liked might allow them to pit their relationship against the *rules* and continue the developments that were already occurring.

We shared this tape in a workshop we did at the Narrative Therapy Conference in Vancouver and, as we always do, we asked participants to write questions for our clients. In a sense, this returns the favor our clients have granted by allowing the tape to be used for teaching. Also, since we ask workshop participants to focus on unique outcomes, their questions are reauthoring ones, so they become a kind of reflecting team for the clients. We'll share here some of the questions the participants wrote (primarily for Karl).

1. Are there times that you can remember, with Marilyn or at work, when the *rules* didn't seem to be around or interfere—when you were just spontaneous? What was it like?
2. What does it tell you about yourself that you have been able to stand up for what you felt you deserved in a work situation at least once before?

15

3. What one thing do you think you will be able to accomplish in your relationship with Marilyn that the *rules* have been keeping you from?
4. How could you rewrite the *rule of giving* so that it would benefit you and your relationship with Marilyn?
5. As you continue to put the *rules* behind you, how will your new levels of energy improve your relationship with Marilyn?
6. I am curious about how your relationship will develop as you openly challenge the *rules.* I wonder how you and Marilyn will join forces in doing this.
7. I am curious about what a *rule*-free life would look like to you, and what would be the difference between this and your present life?
8. As you free yourself from the *rules,* how might this affect your relationship with your son?
9. As you begin to break or "exorcise" some of these *rules,* what effect do you think it will have on how you see yourself as a person, as a husband, as a father?
10. As you win more battles against the *rules,* how will your life look in the future?
11. Who do you know who would be least surprised to hear about this new version of yourself—one not dominated by these *rules?* What would you tell him or her about this new version of yourself?
12. If you were to share these new possibilities with family or friends, with whom would you do it and in which way?
13. Now that you have a plan of action regarding the *rule of giving,* I wonder what you would call this new way. I am also curious about who would appreciate this new learning. Is there anyone you both could tell this to? Or how would you think about honoring this new experience?

PLAY IT AGAIN: MORE CONVERSATION

STUDENT: I want to make sure I've organized what you have said. A couple comes in, and you ask each person separately to tell you what is his or her view of the problem or problems affecting the relationship. In the most frequently occurring situation, one partner presents the other as the problem. Umm, well . . . I thought you said you externalize separate problems for each. But how do you do this when each one says the problem is the other?

JEFF: I ask, "What effect does it have on *you* when your partner does [whatever each says the other does]?"

STUDENT: I see. What the other does becomes the invitation to some habit that supports the problem pattern. This habitual response becomes the specific problem affecting the person speaking. Okay. Do you sometimes name the pattern?

JEFF: Often, toward the end of the session, I might ask, "This pattern, supported by **pursuing** on one side and **withdrawing** on the other—what effect does it have on your relationship?" Maybe the response will be something like "Distance." So we have **distance,** with its allies **pursuing** and **withdrawing,** interfering in these people's lives.

STUDENT: Okay, I've got that. Now you also said that sometimes, if the relationship and the life in it is presented as bleak—an unpleasant, affectively dominated situation—you would externalize one thing affecting the relationship.

JEFF: Yes. Eventually this could evolve into different stories or meaning affecting each one—for example, **lack of entitlement, abusive habits, fear of rejection.**

STUDENT: That's true from whatever type of problem you construct at the beginning?

JEFF: Yes, that's how our work often goes.

STUDENT: And the third starting place is also to construct one thing— but in this case it is a more narrowly defined problem affecting the relationship, one that the relationship has enough "something" to combat?

JEFF: To get at that "something," we ask about what is happening in the relationship they prefer. In this kind of case, there is often a lot the partners notice regarding their preferences. We can then raise the question about how they can use these preferred aspects of the relationship they have constructed to help support each other against the problem.

STUDENT: So a general way to organize this is to follow the partners—if they present the relationship, go that way; if they present each other, go the other way. Now I also gather you think it is important to ask about what are the ideas, beliefs, stories, views of the other the problem has coached each person into.

JEFF: Yes. In this way, we can work with the meaning about the other that is influencing each person.

STUDENT: You also ask each person to take his or her own steps, to work to a way of being each one prefers for himself or herself. I guess you ask about what that is—what ways each prefers, right?

JEFF: Right. Each person is encouraged to head toward that view without reference to or expectations for what the other is doing. In this way, when the other doesn't reciprocate (I tell them this most likely will happen in the beginning), then each person can appreciate what he or she did as a victory for himself or herself. It's a no-lose situation. If the other eventually reciprocates, then great. If not, they have each gotten back to how they want to be and can take that into another relationship if they so desire. Of course, in the third type of couple presentation we've discussed, where the couple is collaborating against the problem, then encouraging just individual steps is not as useful a direction. Wherever we start, when we get to the point where the problem has been pushed aside enough for the partners to collaborate—when they have more interest in collaborating with the other—that's the direction we want to go.

STUDENT: And in your work, the problem is constructed in its cultural context. I guess that means mainly gender?

JEFF: Yes. But, depending on the couple, it could also mean age or race or class—or, with same-sex couples, perhaps the context of hetero-sexual dominance.

VICKI: As I said earlier, gender is more visible now in working with couples, whereas race and class are also always present, but more invisible. I think heterosexual privilege is another invisible cultural specification. What I find is that I turn to the people with whom I work to consult with me about their knowledges. If they are too strongly dominated by the problem, then I often ask someone else who may have some specific knowledge to consult with me. For example, as I discussed in Chapter 3, I was working with a lesbian couple in which the partners were mutually struggling with the effects of *blame* on their relationship. We had done a lot of work around the pattern that supported the *blame,* as well as the personal stories that had developed, given their life histories. But it still seemed as if something was missing. I asked a colleague, a therapist who was a lesbian, to consult with me on the case; I wanted to know whether there was something about lesbian culture that would shed some light on how I might work more helpfully with this couple. What she told me was that within a context of heterosexual privilege, what often operates on same-sex couples is a belief that all their needs must be met by the relationship. Along with this, the female gender training that this lesbian couple had received had also recruited the partners into believing that each must be always "there" for the other. When neither of these things occurred—that is, all needs were not met and each could not fill all the perceived needs of the other—then the context became ripe for the development of *blame.*

STUDENT: It sounds like there are many contexts and cultural effects to attend to . . .

JEFF: Yes, contexts or discourses that have been encouraged by cultural and personal experiences.

STUDENT: So the work evolves when . . .

JEFF: As we respond to developments, different kinds of problem examples may be given, or broader definitions pop out—like *fear of abandonment* as a more encompassing meaning system than *withdrawal,* as we saw with Eddie.

STUDENT: And I suppose these "bigger" meaning systems are also affected by the larger cultural context.

JEFF: You've got it. But . . . can I ask you a question now?

STUDENT: Sure.

JEFF: In this chapter and in the preceding ones, did you feel we used descriptions that were more favorable to women's experience than to men's?

STUDENT: Well, I didn't really notice. Being a woman, however, maybe this made sense to me.

JEFF: Why would it make sense?

STUDENT: So often in the world, it's the other way: Women are defined in relation to men and men's experience. If you lean it the other way a little, more toward women, then that too addresses the sociopolitical context of patriarchy—by not replicating it. And I think challenging it means constructing problems for men that label the operation of power they are engaged in.

JEFF: Well said. That reminds me of a newspaper headline I read: "Woman Nags Man to Death" [Jenkins, 1990].

STUDENT: Let me guess—it's about a man murdering his wife because she was nagging him. It's a good example of what we were speaking about.

JEFF: I wonder what our male readers are thinking about this? Can they see it as one way of taking responsibility (historically) for men's effects on women's experience? Or are they affected by male discourse in a way that blinds them to certain operations of power they are engaged in? If so, I recommend Alan Jenkins's 1990 book, or a 1992 article by Michael White.

CHAPTER 8

Just Let Children Talk
A Child's-Eye View of Problems

OH WHERE, OH WHERE HAVE THOSE PROBLEMS GONE?: GROUP THERAPY FOR DEPWESSION, PART 1

ATTENTION DEMON: I feel so weak. I can't get Sandy thrown out of school very much. I used to be able to get him all the time.

RED DEVIL: I'm such a slimy, yucky monster, but I can't get Larry to play with the other boys I get into trouble *no* more.

FEAR: I used to keep Natalie out of her room. Now she plays in there all the time!

ALL: We're so depwessed!

THERAPIST: Calm down, now, fellows, calm down.

FEAR: Calm down?! I'll scare you, I will. You won't be able to play in your study.

RED DEVIL: And I'll twick you into twouble.

ATTENTION DEMON: And I'll take you over and get your mom and teachers and friends not to like you.

THERAPIST: Okay, okay. I know you're hurting.

ALL: Hurt! Hurt! Hurt!

THERAPIST: Now I know what Michael White means when he wonders, "Is there a therapist in the room?" Do you guys want help, or what?

RED DEVIL: (*Crying*) I want Larry back.

THERAPIST: Tell me what the problem is that's getting you.

HYPERNESS: I'm **hyperness.** H-e-r-e I come . . . I don't get depwessed. H-e-r-e I go . . . I'm gonna do this the whole time. Like with kids!

THERAPIST: What was that? Go ahead, **Red Devil,** tell me your story.

Red Devil's Story

I am the **Red Devil.** I like to get children into trouble. I make them mad and I make them not listen. I put bad things in their heads. Larry was one of my favorite toys. He's so smarty-warty that when I got him, he did really good bad things. I made him think that what he wanted was what the teacher said "No" to. I used to like to get him to do what Danny says, 'cause I've been telling Danny what to do for a really long time, and Danny acts like he's Larry's friend. And Danny has lots of bad ideas I help him with. After I got the teacher to yell at Larry, he felt really scared, and then he listened to me some more. When the teacher called his mommy, then his parents talked to him. He liked this, too, even if he felt more scared. So he listened to me more. Now I don't get any attention from him. What did I do wrong? I'm so sad and lonely.

THERAPIST: This loneliness thing . . . Do you think that the recent movement to marginalize problems—to see you as the problem and not kids—do you think this has something to do with the isolation you feel?

RED DEVIL: (*Crying*) What?

THERAPIST: How will loneliness affect you in the group? Will it get you to listen to the **Attention Demon?** If you do, will you feel better then?

RED DEVIL: Maybe yes, and maybe no . . .

The Authors Speak

Our idea in letting the problems that affect children speak is to try to imagine, with our readers, just how children experience problems. The specifics for the **Red Devil** and the others have been taken directly from what children have told us.

This raises another question: Do we care if problems have problems? Do kids? Do adults? Maybe we could ask.

INTERVIEW WITH LARRY
(SEVEN YEARS OLD)

INTERVIEWER: Larry, when did you start getting rid of the **Red Devil?**

LARRY: After everybody fussed a lot.

INTERVIEWER: When you saw Jeff?

LARRY: Before.

INTERVIEWER: What did you do?

LARRY: I started trying.

INTERVIEWER: How?

LARRY: I didn't speak to Danny or to no one like that during recess. I listened more. I did things faster.

INTERVIEWER: So Jeff didn't help?

LARRY: Jeff made me see the **Red Devil.**

INTERVIEWER: He called it that?

LARRY: No, he asked me what its name was, and I called it that.

INTERVIEWER: What else did he do?

LARRY: I drew some pictures of the **Red Devil** getting me and me getting the **Red Devil.** Jeff asked me which one looked better to me. I said the one of me getting the **Red Devil** felt good.

INTERVIEWER: And the other?

LARRY: Both good and bad.

INTERVIEWER: In what ways?

LARRY: I told Jeff bad 'cause I got into trouble, and good 'cause I got attention from Mom.

INTERVIEWER: What happened at home after your parents heard what you said?

LARRY: Well, I got a little more attention from my mom—she's busy with my little sister—but only a little. My dad started helping a little more.

INTERVIEWER: Do you think that's what helped you get rid of the **Red Devil?**

LARRY: Not really. I already started before I saw Jeff, and in the first session Jeff had me list the ways I already was fighting the **Devil.**

INTERVIEWER: What happened next?

LARRY: When I saw Jeff the next time, I remembered the score, 'cause he asked me. It was **Devil** 2, and Larry 18. I got an A! I told Jeff this was good, and that I wanted to keep doing it.

INTERVIEWER: How did you do it?

LARRY: Jeff asked me this. I said I ignored some kids—like Danny—and I was able to think before I did stuff. Every day my mom asked me what the score was, and this helped me remember. One time, instead of jumping into a fight, I tried to get other kids to stop. When Jeff asked about this, I said I liked "peace, not war."

INTERVIEWER: Since you've been taking these steps, what have you seen in your teacher's face?

LARRY: What?

INTERVIEWER: Has your teacher seemed pleased?

LARRY: Very.

INTERVIEWER: What about your parents?

LARRY: Proud. I talked to them about what I did. My dad seemed to listen more, too. But they didn't get an A like I did. I told Jeff all this stuff, too. He gave me an award.

INTERVIEWER: What kind?

LARRY: A "Beating **Red Devil**" award.

INTERVIEWER: Jeff, I'm curious about one thing. What's the relationship, in your mind, between the developments Larry showed and the reactions of his parents?

JEFF: That's a really important question.

INTERVIEWER: You must think so—you wrote it!

JEFF: Yes. Well, coming back from this postmodern divergence . . . my experience was like Larry's. In our first session, I noticed that he had some ideas and was, occasionally, taking steps against the **Red Devil**. It wasn't most of the time, but it was some of the time. We did notice how the **Red Devil** was using the bait of Mom's response to help keep its influence strong. Larry's parents had recently immigrated; in addition, his father was consumed by work and his mother was consumed by taking care of Larry and his younger sister (who was three years old) and working at her part-time job. These factors had effects and provided the context in which the problem developed. Yet, in the month between sessions, Larry was able to turn almost completely away from the **Red Devil**. He did this mostly by seeing the effects of it on his life; by accessing his skills and his values, such as "peace, not war"; and by getting just a little more support from his parents.

The Authors Speak

These transcripts are fictional, but they are based on our notes and on our child clients' responses to the questions we ask them in sessions. We hope to illustrate the usefulness of bringing out children's experience.

HYPERNESS: But *I* interfere with kids' experience. I just make them *go*. No thinking with me!

GROUP THERAPY FOR DEPWESSION, PART 2

THERAPIST: *Fear,* why don't you tell us your story?

Fear's Story

I first told Natalie I would come and get her at night in her room. She believed me! Then I made it hard for her to play alone at any time in her room. Then I made her nervous about some other rooms, and even started on the bathroom at school. I told her she better not be alone!

> Once I made it hard to sleep,
> Into her life I did creep.

I made her tired during the day and began to get her to call home from school. I made her dad real mad—he didn't understand why she couldn't just go to bed. I got him, though: He ended up in her bed and she ended up in his! I made her mom cranky, too, because she had to stay with Natalie when she tried to go to sleep. Natalie's parents don't get along too well, anyway, so it was easy to get them to fight even more over me. That made Natalie even more scared. But now Natalie is seeing she can be brave, that she is bigger and stronger than me. Now she's going to bed in her own room and talking about tricking me into the ocean and burying me. I'm so afraid.

THERAPIST: What does **Fear** do when **fear** gets him?
FEAR: I go to sleep, of course. I'm a real coward.

INTERVIEW WITH NATALIE
(EIGHT YEARS OLD)

INTERVIEWER: Natalie, can you remember when **fear** was getting you?
NATALIE: Oh, yes, it was very bad. I told Jeff all about it and drew him a

picture of *fear* getting me and me getting it. Wanna see it? (*Shows pictures.*) Here's one of me burying *fear.* He didn't like that at all.

INTERVIEWER: You could imagine burying *fear* the first time you saw Jeff?

NATALIE: Well, after Jeff asked me about how the *fear* was affecting me—at night, at home, at school—he asked me if the *fear* was getting me to grow down or up. I said, "Down," and Jeff asked me what I thought about this. I said I didn't want the *fear* to get bigger and me smaller. Jeff asked me where I was still bigger, and I said I played in the playroom by myself. Jeff asked me what I called that. Did I think it was "bravery"? I said, "Yes." Then I realized I could play alone in the kitchen, in the piano room, and in the living room in the morning. *Fear* hadn't taken all my bravery from me. This helped me know I could get *fear* rather than it getting me.

HYPERNESS: I made Johnny grow down, also.

INTERVIEWER: Ignore that. **Hyperness** likes to annoy and to interfere. What else did you and Jeff do in that first session?

NATALIE: We came up with a plan. I said I wanted to take *fear* into other rooms and *punch* him. Then we decided that after I punched him, I would lock him up and take him out of the house and hang him in the garage. I also came up with the idea of taking the door off the closet so I would know *fear* couldn't hide in there. Oh, and I hung my picture up in my room—the one that I drew where I was burying *fear.*

INTERVIEWER: What about your parents?

NATALIE: They each were going to help me with part of my plan. Jeff also said something about them figuring out a way to pull together, but they thought they were too mad at each other. They do fight a lot . . . They agreed to notice how the *fear* gets them to fight more, and said they would talk about their problems next time.

INTERVIEWER: What do they fight about? You?

NATALIE: They do fight about me. Mom doesn't think my dad treats me right or pays enough attention to me. But they fight about lots of stuff.

INTERVIEWER: Does *fear* have an easier time getting you when they fight about you?

NATALIE: Not especially about me, but when they fight about anything.

INTERVIEWER: Now I know you went out of the country for a month. What happened to *fear* when you were gone, and then when you came back?

NATALIE: Well, I pretty much left it behind. Actually, I tricked it on the airplane, and it fell in the ocean.

INTERVIEWER: Did that work?

NATALIE: Pretty much. I slept in my own bed most of the time. I felt a lot bigger, went more places, and was less tired. The people around me had a—how did Jeff ask it?—bigger picture of me then they would have had if *fear* had colored it.

INTERVIEWER: How about when you came back home?

NATALIE: I went to sleep in my own bed. One day I told my mom, "Go away. I want to be by myself." Jeff wrote down the day and said out loud, "Natalie sends a message to *fear* on Monday, May 8, 1995." I even asked to stay home alone while my mom ran a quick errand. I can beat *fear* and don't need my mom or dad to hold my hand all the time.

INTERVIEWER: What was left?

NATALIE: Well, at home I do get up in the middle of the night and go into my parents' bed. I think I'm sleepwalking. I told Jeff I was ready to do it all on my own, like on vacation. Jeff asked me what I thought my parents should do if I'm sleepwalking, and I told him they should take me back to bed. Jeff asked my parents if they could put *anger* aside and help me with this, and they said they could. Jeff made another appointment to work with them on getting *anger* out of their relationship.

INTERVIEWER: Now, Jeff, isn't this really a classic family systems case?

JEFF: Any case is "really" what you make it to be—haven't you been reading this book? But let us both respond to what we imagine you are asking about.

The Authors Speak

Did Natalie's *fear* reflect, metaphorically, what was going on in her family and in her parents' relationship? Were her parents fighting their fight through her? Could her mother more easily confront her father on issues regarding Natalie than she could on issues for herself? These are all ways that family therapists, including ourselves, have thought about a problem like this; in the past, we found this thinking helpful and useful in our work with families. But we don't think that these kinds of problems represent evidence that functional hypotheses are "true" or exist anywhere but in therapists' constructions.

From a narrative metaphor, we would explain the problem and its effects differently. We could view the *fear* as affecting the parents' relationship with *anger,* and then using its effects to alienate the parents further. Situating the problem in the culture, we might notice how gender role specifications encourage Mom to stand up for her daughter's needs (and not her own). At the same time, gender specifications might have encouraged the husband to worry only about family income and his own personal needs, rather than to be concerned about his wife or daughter's needs. Once *fear* grabbed the daughter (as it does all kids, particularly at night from time to time), then *anger*'s effects on the parents could be such that *fear* could use these effects to gain even more influence—getting the parents not to stand together, with Natalie, to fight *fear.* Once *fear* gained influence, it took on a life of its own and became its own problem. The point we are trying to make is that a problem doesn't have to be thought of as "causing" another. Therefore, a problem can be taken on and pushed aside without other problems' necessarily going away. Constructing the problem in this manner allows persons, separately or together, to take steps away from the problem and toward their own preferred ways, without muddying the waters with talk about what a problem "truly" signifies. Talking about different problems and their effects on people in the system, as well as the problem's effects on other problems, may be cumbersome; however, we find that people experience it as liberating. By contrast, functional hypothesizing, with the notion of causality inherent in it, depends on all parts of the system to change, and some people experience this as restraining.

So in this case the parents took a stand at night against *fear* for and with Natalie, despite the influence of *anger.* And, as we have seen in Chapter 7, they also worked together to rescue their relationship from *anger.*

GROUP THERAPY FOR DEPWESSION, PART 3

Attention Demon's Time

It's about time I got to talk. I've had my way with Sandy for a long time. After all, how else would he get anyone to pay attention to him? Not that he realizes I am around. I stay pretty much invisible, getting him to react to situations in such a way that everyone notices him. I have to admit, though, Sandy was a pretty easy mark. In the first couple of families he lived in, nobody really wanted to have anything to do with him except when they wanted someone to yell at or beat up. That was like food for me—lots of rage training. When parents and relatives treat someone in these ways, I become the kid's only hope. And it's fun for me—when I get kids to react and to develop annoying habits, they get yelled at and hit more, and I get so powerful! I followed Sandy into some foster homes, where adults tried to like him, but I got under their skin. Now he's living in another home, and I've been working him hard there, and in school I get him endless consequences that he can't get out from under. I was even getting him thrown out of class. Of course, no one in class likes him. Who would like someone I can get to act that way?

The best part is that, while Sandy looks obnoxious, inside all he wants is to be hugged and touched. He misses his birth brother, who lives in another family. He wants some more time with his most recent parents, who adopted him, but they are really annoyed by him. And he believes he is "bad," because he does everything wrong. That's how his parents, his teachers, and the other kids treat him—the way everyone has treated him all his life. It has been so easy to convince him to do silly stuff, to show off and have tantrums. Besides, he's so bright I can get him to think of especially annoying stuff to do. Now, all of a sudden, he is beginning to reject me—that ungrateful pup! He's controlling himself at school and at home more. He's even considering putting me aside with other kids. Doesn't he understand I have feelings, too? I was there for him when he needed me. Why should he just begin to reject me? How fair is this? Why . . .

THERAPIST: Okay, I see you're feeling a bit lonely, like the others.

ATTENTION DEMON: A bit! Can't you see the pain I'm in? Can't . . .

THERAPIST: If you don't stop, I won't talk to you.

ATTENTION DEMON: (*Puts claw over own mouth.*)

INTERVIEW WITH SANDY (13 YEARS OLD)

INTERVIEWER: Can you tell me about this **Attention Demon?**

SANDY: Whaddya wanna know?

INTERVIEWER: From what it said, you were badly treated growing up . . .

SANDY: I don't wanna talk about that. I just wanted to be touched and hugged.

INTERVIEWER: What did the **Attention Demon** get you to do?

SANDY: The teacher was mean. The other kids ignored me. I guess I would show off or act silly. Everyone gets tired of me—even my adopted parents.

INTERVIEWER: It sounds like you were in a bad spot. How did you get out of it?

SANDY: I began to use my own abilities, my own powers, for myself.

INTERVIEWER: What do you mean?

SANDY: I am strong-minded. And I can listen and remember things. So I can attend to what I want and not let the **Demon** get me going.

INTERVIEWER: Have you always been able to do this?

SANDY: Well, when Jeff helped me to notice what the **Attention Demon** was doing, I said it got to me 95% of the time. Later on in that same session, I changed it to 90%, because I realized that I could entertain myself by reading or doing schoolwork. I could also have good conversations. Jeff asked about this the second time we talked (the first time we met with my parents), and by the next time I was 30% in charge. I felt proud, because one time I started to make noises and stopped. When Jeff asked me about this victory, I said I felt stronger. I even did something someone else wanted me to do, without a fuss—and this felt good. I paid a little more attention to what the teacher was saying, and I controlled the **Demon** on the bus. It felt good to be more in charge of myself. I told Jeff I was listening to myself and to others more and to the **Demon** less. I was using my abilities for myself to fight the **Demon,** instead of the **Demon** stealing them and using them against me.

INTERVIEWER: Was this hard work?

SANDY: I guess.

INTERVIEWER: Did the **Demon** just go away?

SANDY: No, stupid. What do you think?

HYPERNESS: I don't go away at all!

INTERVIEWER: Well . . .

SANDY: I got more and more in charge. Looking at Jeff's notes, by the third session I was 50% more in charge at school and 20% at home. I was listening more to the teacher than to the **Attention Demon.** I told Jeff things went better when I did this, and I felt better about myself. I was using my ability to strongly listen and remember. Jeff asked me about the future that I now saw, and I said it was good. Maybe play the sax. Maybe be a scientist. I wanted to act properly and be polite. I was growing up more. Even my mom noticed that I was.

INTERVIEWER: Did things keep going in this direction?

SANDY: At school, as far as the teacher went, it did. Three weeks later I was up to 75%, even after the **Demon** got me in big trouble one time.

INTERVIEWER: Did you and Jeff talk about this trouble?

SANDY: Not much—only what I did the rest of the time to have so many victories. My mom told me she saw that I was making strides.

INTERVIEWER: Does your mom sit in on the sessions?

SANDY: She usually comes in for the last 10 or 15 minutes. Once in a while my dad and she both meet with Jeff. Recently I did some work with my adopted sister, too.

INTERVIEWER: So you put the **Attention Demon** aside and get in trouble less, especially at school. Were there other problems?

SANDY: Well, Jeff got my parents to notice how the **Demon** works them, by getting them mad at me and pulling away. We also talked about what Jeff called "outdated survival tactics," like lying and stealing—habits I got into when I was younger. That summer I worked on some stuff, but I only saw Jeff a few times. I had fun at a camp I went to—I got along with the kids better than at school. Jeff asked me what they noticed about me, and I said that one boy thought I was "fun" and that a girl thought I was "cute, cool, and smart." When school started, the **Attention Demon** was still getting me with my sister—it got her with me also. We also talked about another problem, **arguing and reacting habits.** It's hard to do everything my mom wants. Eventually I told Jeff I was scared to let go of these habits or else I'd have no control. And they pop out so fast. Worst of all, they get my mom to think I'm mad at her, like I'm doing it to hurt her. Jeff and she worked on that. I struggled with these habits through Christmas and into the winter.

INTERVIEWER: And the **Attention Demon?**

SANDY: I kept him under pretty good control as far as the teacher went. But it still interfered with making friends. It was hard to keep working on this stuff. Sometimes it made me feel bad just to bring it up, even with Jeff and even though we only met every other week. I've had so many therapists and parents and teachers . . . I told Jeff this in February.

INTERVIEWER: Did it get easier?

SANDY: Well, in March, I did something that really got my mom down on me. I was really scared and down on myself. Jeff and I talked about **fear** getting hold of me, telling me that I was unacceptable to anyone. I just wanted to hide out. I said I thought I was weird. I told Jeff I wanted to be cool and calm and act less silly around kids. Jeff talked to my mom alone that day. He told me that he thought the problem was getting to all of us, and he wanted to help get her back on my side again.

INTERVIEWER: Is that how you would say it, Jeff?

JEFF: She told me that what happened made her feel "like dirt." We discussed how these problems wanted her to be mad at Sandy. If they could recruit her into feeling "like dirt" and then treating him "like dirt," they could influence him even more powerfully. We acknowledged together how strong these problems were, and how they had followed Sandy from his early living situations into this one.

SANDY: After that, things got better. I told Jeff at our next session that my mom put her arm around me, and I felt cared about. Jeff and I went back to work on how the **Demon** was interfering with my relations with other kids. This was hard because I hated to think much about this when I was with other kids. I learned that this was a **Demon** trick—"not thinking."

SANDY'S MOM: It looked like things were really coming to a head, as the **Demon** was fighting back at him as hard as it could . . .

JEFF: To "not think" . . .

SANDY'S MOM: Yes, but I wasn't letting it get to me any more. When he was upset, I tried to put the problems aside and put my arms around him and connect.

SANDY: I really want to be rid of this problem before school next year. Dorky behaviors will really get me mistreated by other kids in middle school. My end-of-the-year report card was five A's and a B, but I thought I could do better. I still hadn't beaten the **Demon** with other kids at school much, but I did begin to have victories at the swimming pool. School is hard because I'm interested in stuff that the other kids think is nerdy, like science. Something else really good happened early that summer. My sister and I worked on what Jeff called our "sister- and brotherhood." We developed a plan to work together on lunches and my Mom agreed to stay out of it. And it worked! We called it a "nice and cooperatable (we made up the word) sister and brother-hood." We'll have more fun and likeableness now. My goals for camp are to act "regular" and watch out for the **arguing habit,** and for any dorky or weird behaviors the **Demon** might invite me into.

INTERVIEWER: I think I've lost control here!

JEFF: Well, those **control habits** are hard to break. It does take some trust and some time. . . . In working with Sandy and his adopted parents, we were addressing the effects of prolonged physical and mental abuse, without speaking much about them directly. This was Sandy's preference, and I used his wishes and comfort level to guide me. There were some dramatic developments at first, and some major growing in preferred directions that everyone noticed. Some of those subtler, harder habits are taking more time—in part because of the effects on our relationship of issues of fear and trust, and in part because his adopted parents have to work hard to stay on his side. Recently, there seem to be bigger developments occurring again. It seems most important to let Sandy be in charge of the pace and letting me know what he needs. We have to spend time in sessions making sure we're together on the goals and that they are what Sandy wants, not just me wanting them and him responding.

Just the other day I saw Sandy when he came back from camp. He reported, "At camp I became a different person," and he said that he had stayed that different person at school this year. When I asked him what he meant by that, he said he was acting "regular," and if you remember, this was his goal. So the developments continue . . .

HYPERNESS: It takes a long time to deal with my effects also!

JEFF: (*To hyperness*) I think everyone is tired of your disruptions, interruptions, having to give special attention to you . . .

HYPERNESS: That's what I do when I get kids to behave the way I want: I wear parents down. And if they try to challenge me, I make things worse. Kids, they can fall more and more behind and feel worse and worse about themselves. With their parents more alienated, feeling more ineffectual, and just trying to keep things together, I can crush the family.

JEFF: Well, I'm not intimidated by you. And my experience is that once families stop being intimidated by you, a lot can happen. Take Johnny, for example—if our readers want to reread something about him and his story in Chapter 2, we'll hear now what he has to say.

INTERVIEW WITH JOHNNY (10 YEARS OLD)

JEFF: I wanted to do this interview myself, because I know sometimes it's hard for you to answer questions. We've had 13 sessions over seven and a half months, and all of them have been with you and your family. Even your brother has come to many of them. At first, just naming it *hyperness* seemed to make a difference. You began to be able to let your parents know when *hyperness* was around. This seemed to help.

JOHNNY: Yes, it helped.

JEFF: Do you remember how you did it?

JOHNNY: No. I just noticed it getting me.

JEFF: And you said so . . .

JOHNNY: . . . to my parents.

JEFF: We discovered some situations where *hyperness* didn't get you as much.

JOHNNY: Like in the car.

JEFF: Are your parents still taking you for rides?

JOHNNY: Yeah. I like that.

JEFF: It give you some nice *hyperness*-free time with them.

JOHNNY: I think it's good.

JEFF: We also worked on your "growing-up chart." Could you go over what is in it so far?

JOHNNY: Okay. Here's where I took charge of my nighttime stuff—like brushing my teeth and getting ready for bed.

JEFF: I remember an even earlier step when your parents put you in charge of staying in your room and getting yourself to sleep. I mean they came to say "Good night" and spent a bit of time with you, but then they expected you to entertain yourself.

JOHNNY: Yes, I find things I can do myself.

JEFF: Okay. What else? Doing homework longer and by yourself. Beginning to take charge of the morning routine.

The Authors Speak

VICKI: Jeff, you seem to think this chart was helpful. Can you say something about that?

JEFF: Well, it seemed that one effect of *hyperness* was not to let Johnny have a picture of the past or the future. Reviewing the chart helped him to really visualize the direction he was going in and to have a sense of growth and movement. Incidentally, I believe it helped his parents as well.

VICKI: What happened with them?

JEFF: We looked at how the *hyperness* created a lack of independence for Johnny, with concomitant lack of independence for them, particularly his mom. This encouraged *frustration* and *anger.* Johnny's increased independence began to encourage a more relaxed connection between him and his mom. His dad said he was beginning to accept the limitations of the effect he could have, so that he was just letting solutions "happen" more.

VICKI: Why did this occur?

JEFF: I believe it was the result of witnessing the small steps Johnny started making when we put him in charge of deciding what to do and how to do it. His parents also could see that he was making some effort and how hard it was. Oh, and they also felt free from feeling like they were responsible. This made a big difference in the amount of pressure they felt and the space they could have.

VICKI: I imagine for everyone to begin to see the problem as separate from Johnny made a big difference also.

JEFF: Yes, his mom said she felt less critical.

VICKI: And his brother—you worked with him, too?

JEFF: Yes. We looked at how the **hyperness** invited **resentments** to overtake him. And these **resentments** encouraged feelings of **helplessness**. These feelings of **helplessness** affected his dad as well. With the brother, particularly, this problem got him to distance himself. This had the effect of inviting Johnny to try harder to get attention and made him vulnerable to **hyperness**-encouraged tactics to try to get his brother to respond.

JOHNNY: You forgot about **shyness**.

JEFF: That's right! It was the last thing we worked on before you took off for the summer.

JOHNNY: I remember after we talked about it, I went into a new store by myself. That made me feel a lot bigger.

JEFF: I can't wait to hear how you managed on your family's trip this summer, and what you did when your parents went off by themselves and left you alone.

JOHNNY: We'll see . . .

KIDS HAVE THE LAST WORD:
ANOTHER CONVERSATION

STUDENT: What's a typical interview?

JEFF: Usually we have spoken to the parents on the phone, so we have some clues as to their ideas about the problem. As we do with teenagers (which we'll discuss more in the next chapter), we like to ask children to go first, helping them if necessary or sometimes having their parents prompt them. (Of course, this is after we try playfully to connect with them.) However, if this is too difficult for them, we quickly back off. We believe that responding seriously to

clients' experience is as important with children as it is with adolescents or adults, and may be a more novel experience for children. We
come up with a description of the problem that uses their language
and metaphors, and then we ask them some more about it (i.e.,
externalizing questions). We often ask children to draw the problem—perhaps to draw the problem getting them and them getting it.

While a child is drawing, we speak to the parents, using the
descriptive language of the child. Parents seem to see the value in
this, particularly after witnessing the conversation with the child.
We become interested in how the problem might be recruiting the
parents or how they may be *inadvertently* playing into its hands. If it
is relevant to do so, we help note how the problem may be dividing
them. We ask whether this fits their preference for responding to the
child and what their preference might be. We get them to describe
some time when they are able to act more according to their preferred
ways. We then return to the child, review the drawings with him or
her, and show particular interest in the one where the child gets the
problem. We ask more about how he or she currently gets the
problem and might continue to get it in the future, as well as the
(potential) effects on the child when this occurs. We may also show
interest in some special talent that the child might use or is using
against the problem—an idea of David Epston's.

In some situations [White, 1984, 1985], we all may construct a
plan to fight the problem. As therapists, we have some ideas about
what has worked for other kids, but we work closely with each
individual child, getting a great deal of input from him or her. Mostly,
we let children supply the specifics, including novel strategies they
have already developed.

If the child whom the problem is directly affecting is young and
has a younger sibling, we may wonder how the problem makes use of
the younger sibling or the parents' relationship with her or him.
Often, if the sibling is present, we can see this happening in the room.
If the sibling is older, we ask how the problem affects the relationship
between them. With older children (10 and up) and older siblings,
we ask them each about the problem, giving equal time and space for
each child. Sometimes parents need to be encouraged to bring the
siblings, but we have found their presence to be very helpful, particularly as we ask questions about the problem's effects on relationships.

STUDENT: Parents, usually mothers, call and want therapy for their
children. Why is this? What do you say to them?

JEFF: We live in a culture that says that the individual is the center of all
meaning, that each person is like a container with responses pushed

into it. Parents inevitably think this way about their kids. Of course, they blame themselves for creating this—particularly mothers, who have been told they are responsible for everything about their children and what their children do. They harbor a fear that we will blame them, too—something that does occur in some therapies, as a consequence of the way therapists have been taught to think about problems. What we say on the phone is that we want the whole family present, because when problems grab a child they tend to affect everyone. We tell them that we think the other family members could most likely be a great help to the child in fighting off these problems. Not that they created the problem, but that they could be a part of the solution.

STUDENT: Do you see kids individually?

JEFF: Sometimes yes, and other times in combination with parents or the whole family. With Larry and Natalie, all interviews—in each of their cases, only two—were done with the whole family. Sandy was seen with the family, with his adopted mother, and also alone. With very difficult problems like *anorexia,* or problems that have been around a long time (like the ones affecting Sandy), we use various combinations at different times. We use "what makes sense" as a guide, but regardless of whom we see, our thinking is always the same. For example, with Sandy, problems like "The only way to get attention is by . . . " or "The only way to have control is by . . . " or "You're bad and so you must . . . " had gained their meaning through experience and thus had a strong hold on him. However, these problems affected him in a social context (and were developed in one), and so working with him, his mom, his sister, and his family were all ways of addressing the effects of these problems, as well as getting everyone to notice other developments and to respond accordingly.

Also, with children like Sandy, a focus on their talents and abilities seem particularly important. David Epston [1993] has developed a whole interview schema around this. Because these children have been in so many conversations focusing on their defects, a focus on their special talents is refreshing and powerful, in that it helps all (kids and parents) to begin to notice completely different things. Another example would be children like Johnny with so-called "ADHD." Those who work with these children know that they have much greater creativity and imagination than other kids. Perhaps whatever doesn't allow their brains to focus on things also has the effect of opening their minds up in ways that allow more possibilities for them than for other children.

STUDENT: One more question for you: Why is this chapter so short?

VICKI: I want to jump in here. Jeff asked me this, too, and when he did I said, "Because work with kids is short." We tell our other students that working with kids is often the best way to learn this work, because they seem to respond to it so quickly.

JEFF: Right. The work does go quickly, especially if, as the therapist, you keep straight to the point—and let the kids do the talking.

STUDENT: Okay. So now I have some questions for the kids you asked to be consultants. (*Turning to the kids*) What do you think a problem is?

STEPHANIE (10): It's just things.

MEG (7): Things that get you into trouble.

STUDENT: What do you think happens when a problem gets you? What do you do?

STEPHANIE: You get frustrated.

AUTHORS: And what should we do if the problems have problems? If they get lonely?

STEPHANIE: Is this a "stupidity quiz?" What kind of a question is that?

MEG: I don't care about that. They deserve it!

AUTHORS: (*To the problems' group therapist*) The children have answered. Let the problems be lonely!

CHAPTER 9

Dissing Separation
Adolescents (and Their Parents)
Tell Their Stories

RE-MEMBERING: SLACKERS ALSO TALK
A Room with a View

The streets were empty in this part of town, and the sky was exceptionally black. Not even a star was blinking through the cloud cover. As they drove slowly along looking for the address, the light framed in the far window looked warm and welcoming in the darkness.

"That's probably it," Sharon said.

They'd decided to get together at Marcy's house, because they could spread out, be comfortable, and not be disturbed by others' comings and goings. Even though Marcy lived in an apartment with a friend and went to the nearby community college, she often spent time at her parents' house, and this was one of those times. Her parents had even stocked the refrigerator, which made her laugh, but she was glad. Joe and Becky were coming together later, though they didn't know each other very well. Becky had her driver's license, but her dad still didn't like her taking the family car at night. Oh well. Sharon knew that Becky wasn't exactly resigned to this, but they had talked about how getting mad certainly hadn't helped.

"How did we all meet?"

Greg was so startled, he visibly jumped.

"I'm sorry . . . I was just thinking . . . "

"Well, don't think out loud while I'm concentrating!"

"Did we meet at that summer class at the community college?"

"I think so. It's funny. We were all so different and at different ages, too, but something seemed to click when we started talking about our experiences in high school."

"There it is. See Marcy at the front door?"

Marcy decided to open the front door and look for them. She knew her house was hard to find, so she had turned on all the lights that faced the street. There was a car coming toward her. It was them! "Hi," she yelled out. "It's here!"

The room was spacious and comfortable—little furniture, but lots of pillows and places to stretch out. Marcy went to get cold drinks for them, and when she walked back into the room Sharon was saying, "It made a lot of sense to me. I don't know why. It just did."

Greg turned to Marcy. "She's talking about that time in therapy—you know, the *rift?*"

Marcy laughed. "Oh, *that* time, when you actually *agreed* with your parents!"

"Yeah, *that* time!" Sharon said, also laughing. "Actually, what the therapist was saying back then when I was only 15 made a lot of sense. At least the questions she was asking helped me realize something I hadn't thought about before."

Greg said, "You are both so flipped out. Now I don't have any idea what you're saying."

"Okay, okay. Listen up."

"Right, Greg. Pay attention. I mean, I finally got that I didn't want to be fighting with them and sneaking around and all that stuff. It didn't make sense. It was too much trouble. And besides, I *like* them."

"Your parents?!" Greg and Marcy exclaimed in unison.

"Of course. Don't you like yours?" asked Sharon.

"Well, I guess I do," responded Marcy. "I mean even more so now than I did two years ago. And I thought we'd be fighting for years. Gosh, I'm only 20, and everyone told me we wouldn't be able to talk until I was 30, if then. I mean, people were predicting we'd always be enemies."

"People told me that, too," Greg added. "Especially since my mom got remarried and they had another kid and all that. Everyone said it was hopeless. And boy, was I feeling that way last year before I left for college!"

"Yeah. I know what you're saying. My parents' friends had me as the world's worst juvenile delinquent. You know, I was stealing and then lying about it. I didn't graduate from high school. I blew it when I did move out. Whew! The next thing you know, I was going to come up with repressed memories." Marcy giggled.

"And never have a chance to do what you really wanted," Sharon added.

"You mean . . . what do you mean? . . . do what I wanted?"

"Yeah—like get along with them, for one thing, and decide what you wanted to do for yourself, for another."

"Hey, isn't that the doorbell, Marcy?" Greg said, thinking this was getting way too heavy.

"It must be Becky and Joe. They finally found it."

The room quickly took on the frenetic energy that Becky brought with her. As Marcy left to get more cold drinks, she thought, "I bet Greg and Becky would be good friends. Either that, or not at all. They both grew up so well trained in *anger*." Then she laughed at herself for thinking about it that way. When she came back to the group, she could hear Becky holding forth.

"I really didn't get it for a long time. The pressures were too great—my dad having that psychiatric diagnosis, and my family's belief that I was still 'grieving' over my mother's death. And then when my dad remarried, I really *liked* my stepmother, but I knew I wasn't *supposed* to. The funny thing is a that couple of years ago, when I was only 14, the therapist helped me see it was okay. In fact, it was more than okay; it helped me relate to my dad better, even today."

Joe joined in. "Yeah, well, being the first-born son and having all those *success pressures* were hard on me. For girls, staying connected—at least to others—is considered okay. Guys are supposed to 'get out there' and 'just do it.' Let me tell you, it was tough realizing that it was just fine to want to stay close to my family—and not only tough for me, tough for them, too. Both my parents kept pushing until the therapist—I guess it was her—opened the door for them to think differently. But it took a couple of times around."

"You got it!" Greg said. "I'll tell you, my mom was having the hardest time with me going away, and I couldn't let her know it was hard for me, too. My new stepdad kept pushing for me to 'just go.' I couldn't believe that our therapist seemed to understand my wanting to stay close. Do you know, that's what helped us—my mom and me—have that great talk on the long drive to college. I think we'll always look back to that conversation as a foundation we can stand on for the future, no matter how much *anger* gets between us."

"Yeah," answered Joe. "Well, coming home for me, after flunking college the *second* time, it was something knowing my parents were going to be there for me. It took a while, but the whole idea that I could think about what I wanted to do and pursue my own goals, with my parents there to support me . . . that made *all* the difference. I mean, I'm not there yet . . . I'm still in school, and living at home besides, but I've got a job and I'm getting good grades. *And* I like what I'm doing!"

He paused for a few seconds, pondering something, and then continued. "I remember what seemed like a turning point. I had gone to therapy when I was 16, and we talked about *lack of effort*. It sort of seemed to fit—at least my parents and I got along a little better. But then I went to the community college and didn't do so well. My parents got royally pissed off and told me to move out. Then I started drinking and barely making it. Finally, they helped me look for a college I could get into that they thought I might like, and away I went to the middle of Tennessee to study music. I really tried to make a go of it—if nothing else but to please them—but that turned out to be my undoing. When I came home after the first year, barely making the grade, I went back to therapy . . . "

View 1

VICKI: This *success idea* seems to have been around for quite a while.

JOE: I think it was around when I first started to see you, when I was 15 or 16.

VICKI: So maybe **lack of effort** was tricking you into thinking *that* was the way to find your own way. I say that, because finding your own way can be a good thing, but it sounds like **lack of effort** got you to find no way.

JOE: Right, now that you put it that way. But you know I really have to make this work. My parents are going to get tired of paying for my education.

VICKI: What do you think this *success idea* is telling you about their paying?

JOE: What do you mean?

VICKI: Well, I wondered if it made it harder for you to figure out what you wanted for yourself.

JOE: I really don't like my classes, but I don't know what else to do.

VICKI: Would you say that the *success idea* has somehow blinded you to your own ideas and interests?

JOE: I just don't know what I want.

Review 1

No one could speak. Joe's story sounded vaguely familiar to all of them. Finally, when the clock's ticking and everyone's breathing filled the room with silence, Greg ventured forth with what they all were thinking: "This sounds so much like what happened to me."

"Whew," they all gasped.

Greg continued. "My mom thought my going away to college would solve all my problems. In fact, she even said that. She thought it would make me grow up." Then he turned to Joe. "I don't get how this was a turning point for you."

Joe thought about it for what seemed like another interminable period of time. He knew what he thought, but he hadn't spoken it out loud before. Finally he said, "I realized that the *success idea* was overriding any ideas I might have for myself, and that my worry about my parents' financially supporting me was somehow tied into what I thought *they* thought. Once they came into therapy to talk about this with me, I realized *they* weren't pushing me; the *success idea* was."

Another gasp. Joe couldn't believe his own ears. He had been so well trained in nonthinking, in non-reflected-upon activity, he didn't know he could be so eloquent. Well, at least, it sounded eloquent right then.

But he had little time to celebrate his newfound thinking and speaking voice, because Greg was starting to think and speak, too. "Well, I already told you about my turning point, but what led up to it was . . . "

View 2

VICKI: So how does this **quick to anger** get between you and your mom?

GREG: It does, a lot. We have trouble talking about things. But I don't like it, and I'd really like not to have so many fights with her. I'd like to get this taken care of, so that when I come home from school over holidays and things, we can get along.

MOM: I think going away to school will be good for him. He'll have the structure of college life and the safety and security of a dorm. Maybe he'll grow up.

VICKI: (*To Mom*) So you think that college will provide structure and security? Somehow that seems strange to me, especially having heard lots of kids come back from college saying how unstructured it seemed to them.

MOM: Well, I know he feels structure and security here at home, with me . . .

VICKI: How do you think the **quick to anger** has blinded you to the closeness you and your son have?

MOM: Well, I get sad when I think of him leaving. I would like for us to stay close.

VICKI: So you don't like it that the **quick to anger** pushes you apart?

Review 2

It was dawning on Greg that he had thought about this before, but he hadn't reflected much on it. Maybe the therapy experience had opened up more than he thought. He found himself telling the group, "That did it! I didn't like the **quick to anger** and neither did my mom. I went away to college, but like I told you, we had that great talk on the trip there. Not that the **quick to anger** is completely gone, but we at least know we can talk things out."

Marcy was bursting. "Come on, you guys! Give us a chance. Isn't that just like guys—taking up all the space?!!"

Sharon laughed. "Usually, but thankfully, these guys listen to us. Right, guys?"

Greg and Joe fell over each other with mock humility, softly chanting, "Yes, yes, yes!"

"So, you were saying, Sharon, before we got so rudely interrupted . . . "

"Well, only that I found that talking with my parents was something I wanted to continue to do, no matter what was going on in my life—like you, Becky."

Becky had been thinking about what Greg was calling *quick to anger*. It felt a lot like her experience. They didn't call it that, though. It just seemed like a long history of *anger*. She came out of her musing to hear Sharon's comment and found herself saying, "Right! It was hard with my dad. We had such a long history of *anger*, so it was tough, because the *anger* came out so much. But starting to talk with my stepmom helped, and realizing that I had some solid relationships with other adults—my aunt, for one; some teachers, for others; and my therapist, who listened, but also questioned my ideas. I remember one time . . . "

View 3

VICKI: So what you're saying is that there is a history of *anger* in this family . . .

DAD: Well, it seems like every time I open my mouth, she gets upset and walks away or picks a fight with me.

VICKI: And this *anger* pops up whenever you try to have a conversation.

DAD: We *can't* have a conversation. She won't listen to me!

BECKY: What do you mean, *listen* to you? All you ever do is lecture me and tell me what to do or what not to do.

VICKI: (*To Becky*) So the *anger* gets between you and your dad . . .

BECKY: I can be rebellious if I want!

VICKI: The *anger* tells you you can be rebellious?

BECKY: All teenagers are that way!

VICKI: All teenagers are that way?

BECKY: That's just the way it is.

VICKI: Do you like that—the *anger* coming between you and your father, telling you that it's okay to be rebellious? Is that okay with you?

Review 3

Becky came out of her musing to say to Greg, "So you can see why I thought of this. It sounded pretty similar to your experience. But with you, the therapist asked your mom about her 'college' ideas. She asked me about my 'teenager' ideas. No one had ever asked me anything like that before."

Sharon jumped in. "So I can guess what you thought."

Marcy flashed on her first family therapy session two years ago. She added, "Me, too. Funny how we have had similar experiences. When we went to therapy, my parents talked about my *slipping* . . . "[1]

View 4, Part 1

VICKI: I'd like to ask each of you what the problem is that brought you here. You may have different ideas about that, so I'd like to ask about each person's perspective separately.

MARCY: Don't look at me, I have to think about this.

DAD: Okay, I can start. I feel that she is slipping—not so much "slipping away," but slipping in her schoolwork, her attendance at school, her feeling that she would like to be a part of the family. I think she's slipping away with that. I understand that's a normal part of growth—to want to get away and to want to break out of the nest. But there have been some instances that have been more than disturbing. [He then relates a tale of Marcy's taking money, quitting swimming, getting poorer marks at school, and answering her mother back—all of which bring up an experience of "hurt" for Dad.]

VICKI: Is all this a part of the *slipping* you're talking about?[2]

DAD: Yes! I feel it's *slipping*. The idea that she doesn't want to go to a four-year college. She's been accepted to four or five, and she would have been accepted to a lot more if she had made a little effort. There has not been any effort whatsoever.

VICKI: So the *slipping* seems to have taken away some of the effort and some of the discipline that you saw before?

---

[1] The previous "transcripts" are fictional. What follows here is an actual transcript of portions of a first session. This conversation begins after the initial "joining" or getting to know each other. The family members have read this chapter and given their permission for the inclusion of the transcript. It is rather long, but we hesitate to interrupt it with comments about our thinking. As a compromise, we make our comments in footnotes, so that our readers can decide whether to let the conversation flow somewhat seamlessly or to check on the footnote text. We also include some of our ideas in a dialogue between ourselves and a "student" a little further on. Finally, Mom makes comments herself on the therapy at the end of the chapter.

[2] Dad's use of the word *slipping* became a focus for the multiple "problems" he was describing. It made sense to talk about it as *the* problem, an "externalization" of what he was experiencing as the problem.

DAD: That's right. It's a boredom at home, a boredom at school, a boredom, period. And then, again, the straw that broke the camel's back was taking the money and lying about it. That hurt deeply.

VICKI: The **hurt** that you experienced was mostly in response to the stealing and lying; I'm wondering what your response was to the **slipping** in general.[3]

DAD: I think it's all one. You know, that she can do better, that she can progress, that she can produce. And you see this gradual "I don't care." It's **hurt.** I know what the consequences are, after 50 years. And she should . . . (*Chuckles*) I was going to say, "She should listen to me."

VICKI: That's usually the idea that we have as parents.

DAD: Right, right.

VICKI: It sounds like the **slipping** gives you the idea that she's not listening to you. . . . [4] (Dad nods.) So who's next?

MOM: (*Pause*) I think I'm here because I see a real failure in us as a family, and it's just terribly disheartening. I don't think we're communicating properly. I think that's why I'm here. There are a lot of negatives. I'm a very strong-willed, hard-working woman. I've worked for everything I've achieved, and I've been a real plugger. I want only the best for Marcy. And somehow she has resented a lot of things. I've bent over backwards. What I see with Marcy that has me concerned, along with us as a family not communicating, is she's 18½ and she should now be motivated or concerned about her future or seriously working toward something, and I don't see her doing diddly. I see her managing her day. I don't see her with a goal. I see her standing still. I see most of her close friends are excited about their future; they have made their decisions and they're going. I see that she has lost her self-esteem. This "slacking" started her freshman year in high school.

VICKI: This **slipping** or **slacking** that you and Jim [Dad] have talked about . . . [5]

MOM: I think it has been coming a long time. I think that maybe I didn't discipline her properly.

VICKI: So when you see this **slipping** . . .

---

[3]My (VCD's) interest here was to understand the effect on Dad of the **slipping**; I was thinking that whatever the effect was, it might hinder him from working *with* his daughter to counter the **slipping.**

[4]By now, **slipping** seemed to fit as a useful externalization of the problem.

[5]I picked up on **slacking** as similar to **slipping.** I also wanted to think about the problem as having less to do with what Mom might be interpreting as **blame** (of herself or others).

MOM: It reflects on what I did or didn't do.

VICKI: So the *slipping* gets you to feel bad about yourself?

MOM: And you talked to me the day that the stealing happened. With all this *slipping,* I thought we had at least the honesty and integrity . . .

VICKI: So the *slipping* took that away, too?[6]

MOM: I questioned my memory. I attacked myself to protect her. I wasn't letting myself see it.

VICKI: So when Jim says his response was one of *hurt,* what would you say yours was?

MOM: Tremendous distrust.

VICKI: Has this *distrust* continued?

MOM: Since the event? Sure. I can't handle another lie.

VICKI: Are you also seeing this stealing as a part of the general *slipping?*

MOM: Sure, I think it has to do with the kinds of people she's associating with. I see her *slipping.*

VICKI: So it sounds like the *distrust* extends to friends, companions.

MOM: Doubt—all the way across the board.

VICKI: So that *doubt* is not only getting you to distrust your daughter, but also getting you to distrust your own parenting?[7]

MOM: Sure. And I have a tendency to analyze my parenting skills, which are from my past, my own mother, and my education. You know, I was a child development major. What it was 30 years ago and today are totally different. But I'm not going to allow my age difference to be a part of it, because I still think that I've stayed in tune, and her dad and I have. I may have a generation gap in terms of her interests, but I shouldn't have in terms of values, concepts, beliefs.

VICKI: Sounds like even though the *doubt* has gotten you to analyze all that, you still have some confidence in your own knowledge.[8]

MOM: You got it! Absolutely.

VICKI: There's still some *confidence* there?

MOM: Sure. That's the reason I'm here. If I didn't have the *confidence,* I wouldn't have called you. I would have maybe said to Marcy, "You need to find another home next year."

---

[6]This is simply an example of staying with the problem as the problem.

[7]**Doubt/distrust** was the effect on Mom that might prevent her from helping her daughter proceed toward preferred (for all of them) ways.

[8]I wanted to see whether there was a glimmer of a unique outcome here.

VICKI: So what does that **confidence** tell you?

MOM: I'm not giving up.

DAD: (*Interrupting*) All of these things, both our comments, are pointed and very negative, but there's still a tremendous love. I can say there's **hurt,** but you know, I have . . .

VICKI: The **hurt** hasn't taken away the love.

DAD: No. The love for her is never-ending, and the love for her mother is never-ending. Therefore, we're here.[9]

VICKI: (*Pause*) So, Marcy, did you put it together in your head how you want to talk about the problem?

MARCY: Well, not really. First of all, I'd like to say this year was my growing year; this was the year that I just completely changed. I broke away and I found out what kind of person I want to be. I've thought about a lot of things . . . the kind of person I want other people to see me as. I've thought about my values, I've found out about a lot of things. My self-esteem is very high right now, actually. My mother sees my self-esteem as low, because I'm getting bad grades and stuff, but I know I can do the work. I'm so sick of school; I'm so ready to just leave. I've made new friends about twice this year, and the first time I was just hanging out with these people, and everyone was fake, and I couldn't be myself, and I said, "No, I don't want this," and so I went out and I made new friends, and with them I can be myself and they really understand me. You know, that's made me feel really good about myself. And they really motivate me, too, and . . .

VICKI: It sounds like you're pleased with it.

MARCY: I am pleased. I'm not pleased with my grades. That is one thing.

VICKI: So you're not pleased with your grades, but you are pleased with some of the other decisions you've made.

MARCY: I'm pleased with my progress that I am making in school.

VICKI: So you're telling a very different story than your parents are experiencing. They're seeing **slipping,** but you wouldn't call it **slipping.** It sounds like you have a very different experience.[10]

MARCY: No, it *was* **slipping.** It was, but just recently in about the past month, I've slowly been doing better, and I can see it . . .

---

[9]This was a poignant moment in the room. Both parents were teary-eyed.

[10]I was wondering whether Marcy thought there was a problem. Sometimes kids protest that there isn't one. I also wanted to see whether **slipping** was a way to talk about the problem that captured *her* experience.

VICKI: Well, talk to me for a minute—I mean I want to hear about the last month, because I think that would be really important—but would you talk to me for a minute about *slipping,* because that would help me see—fill it out a little.[11]

MARCY: Well, before, things were really hectic in my house, and I was seeing Jerry [boyfriend], and I was questioning that, and my friends were starting to not talk to me any more because I was moving away from them, and school was just boring to me. I'm a senior, and I want to leave, and I think I should move out and get a job and be making my own decisions. I just felt like I was ready to leave, but I had to stay.

VICKI: So part of the "growing year" had sort of a built-in transition. You're getting ready to leave high school, and there's some boredom around that. So that would look like *slipping* to your parents?[12]

MARCY: It kind of looks like *slipping* to me, too, because I really should be concentrating on doing my work and stuff.

Review 4, Part 1

Marcy couldn't believe her own words of two years ago. She interrupted the sequence: "This is so weird—to look back at this conversation now. Of course, there was *slipping,* but not 'slipping away,' as my dad said. The *slipping* had to do with all those expectations from the culture that got translated into what I thought my parents wanted and my teachers wanted, and even what others my age seemed to want, and it got me to think that the only way I could make it would be to leave home and be on my own. I really needed my folks' help. It was interesting where this all went."

"I think I had a similar experience." Sharon said. "But I was younger. I mean you were a senior in high school; I was just a freshman when we went in to talk about the *rift* in my family.

So what happened next?"

View 4, Part 2

VICKI: How do you think the *slipping* has affected your relationship with your parents?

---

[11]If I had stayed with her story of improvement, I feared her parents would have felt that I was discounting their experience. Besides, Marcy did say it *was slipping,* and we believe it is helpful to map the field of influence of the problem.

[12]It occurs to us that Marcy's comments here speak to the complicated effects of a "separation" metaphor, which we have commented on previously and comment on more later in this chapter.

MARCY: It hurts me to have them see me like some juvenile delinquent, like I'm not going to accomplish anything. Because I have goals.

VICKI: So you think it's hurting your relationship?

MARCY: Well, yes, obviously, because it's hurting me, and it holds me back further from them.

VICKI: So the *slipping* has led to some hurt.

MARCY: And it gets me angry.

VICKI: So, it has affected communication, the way that your mom sees, and your dad sees.

MARCY: They don't like my schoolwork; they don't like how I go upstairs all the time and sit in my room. They think that I don't tell them the things that are happening in my life. Nothing really is happening. They don't like my friends.

VICKI: So you think this going up to your room and not talking to them is something that you're just not doing, or do you think the *slipping* has made you less interested?

MARCY: No, I know the reason I go up to my room is that my mother and I can get into a fight about almost anything. So, I'm just trying not to.

VICKI: So it's really a way that you're trying to keep the fighting from happening?

MARCY: Well, I guess. Yeah.[13]

Review 4, Part 2

"Looking back on this, I can see that I really wanted for me to be able to talk to them, and for them to be able to talk to me. But we were all caught up in those cultural expectations that told me I was supposed to be independent, and that I wasn't supposed to be learning from them, but was supposed to be breaking away from them," Marcy commented thoughtfully.

Sharon said, "What do you mean, 'cultural expectations'? You've said that a couple of times now."

"I wasn't thinking about it that way then. It was later, when we had more discussions about the successes I was having and following my own ideas, that we referred to those expectations. But I could see that the *slipping* was telling me I wasn't 'doing it right.' Listen to what I said next; it's so interesting to hear this now . . . "

---

[13]It wasn't clear what meaning "going to her room" had. Was it the action that fit the construction of "adolescent separation," and/or was it an act that Marcy actually initiated to promote "connection"—that is, to keep from fighting?

View 4, Part 3

MARCY: They want me to find a job and be motivated and go to school and do my work and get better grades, and I just said, "Well, actually, that's what I want to do, too."

VICKI: You wanted the same thing?

MARCY: And I never really thought about that, 'cause, you know, 'cause I never sort of think about the same things my parents do.

VICKI: Let me see if I've got this straight. The things that your parents may have wanted for you, that the *slipping* was kind of in the way before . . . it sounds like now you're saying that you want some of those same things too?

MARCY: Uh-huh. And . . . I know I started doing it, and things got better, and I started feeling better about myself. And all of my friends see this happening to me, and they keep saying, "You'd better go home right now and do your homework." It's kind of funny, because I've never had friends who've said things like that.

VICKI: You know, this experience is a month old, you said. It sounds like you're taking steps to go more the way you want to go, and even more the way your parents want you to go. Sometimes things that are only a month old don't get noticed by other people. Who else do you think is noticing it besides you and your friends?[14]

MARCY: Well, two of my teachers. I think three or four of my close girl friends, and two of my guy friends. Well, they sort of noticed it, but I started explaining it to them, and they said, "Okay."

VICKI: So you're telling them about it, too? It's not just that they're noticing it, you're telling them more about what you're thinking about, what you want.

MARCY: Right. I say, "Hey, you guys, push me, help me." It's easier to have your friends push you instead of your parents (*laughing*).

VICKI: So when do you think your parents will start noticing that you're doing more of what you want, and it also fits what they want?

MARCY: I think in about three years.

VICKI: Do you think it will take that long? You don't think they would notice it quicker, huh?

MARCY: No. Well, there would really be no way that they would notice it right now.

---

[14] I was thinking that perhaps Marcy's parents might be affected by **distrust** here, so I was hoping to broaden the context of others noticing.

VICKI: Really? Why? Do you think that the *slipping* has gotten too big?

MARCY: Yeah. It definitely has. I'm having to dig myself out of this huge hole. It wouldn't be noticed until maybe, like, after the first year that I'm in college.[15]

Review 4, Part 3

"Whew," gasped Sharon. "Those expectations are really big, aren't they? I mean, they get us to believe, and our parents to believe, that we have to go away to college or get a really good job or move out and be independent, to finally be doing what we're supposed to be doing."

Joe reminded them, "I told you that was my experience. I know my parents see it differently now. Thank goodness, because it has gone better for my younger brother and sister. But what's sad is that it doesn't have to be this way."

"Ditto," said Greg. "I'm glad we talked about it *before* I left for school."

"Well, you haven't heard the end of my story yet," said Marcy.

"I want to hear," Becky responded. "Maybe it will help me."

"What's clear to me now is that the *slipping* story was so big and so powerful that it had gotten my parents and me to believe that I couldn't be successful. So in some ways I was right when I guessed they wouldn't notice the steps I had taken until after the first year in college. But in another way I was wrong, because I think this discussion and a couple of others like it helped pave the way for them to notice my efforts. You see, I didn't go away to college, not right away. I went away eventually, and I had some difficulties; but, wonder of wonders, they supported me, they saw my side. So when I was wanting to take a step back and consider my future, they were there to help me. We joined together as a team. And that helped me eventually decide to do some things for myself—with their help."

"You know, as you talk about this, I'm really glad we went to therapy when I was only a freshman in high school," said Sharon. "The *rift* hadn't gotten too big. We still could notice how connected we were, so we could escape the *rift's* influence fairly quickly."

"Well, we escaped *slipping,* too," rejoined Marcy. "But, it did take some time."

Becky entered in. "The *anger* is still big between my dad and me, but at least I see it. And I'm no longer interested in being 'rebellious.'" She laughed. "You know, like 'all teenagers are'!"

Greg joined in. "Me, too. It's so easy to blame society or our parents or 'the divorce.' Sure, things like divorce and remarriage and school difficulties and stuff

---

[15]Again, we believe these comments by Marcy reflect the sociocultural metaphor that supports "separation" as necessary; that is, only after kids "separate" and go away can they be successful.

affect us. But what I got to see is how I could pay attention to what *I* wanted, what I *and* my mom preferred."

"Well," Joe added, "I don't need to repeat myself. Being the old man of this group, I can say, 'Been there, done that.' But you know what? I keep learning all the time, and keep paying attention to my own preferences. It's not easy, believe me. The pressures, especially the **success pressures,** are so strong. And the expectations. I know what you mean, Marcy. It's great that we've all met each other. We can be a community of support . . . "

"But you know what else?" added Marcy. "I don't think what we're saying is all of it. I think what you just said, Joe, is really important. I mean, I think that **slipping** and the **rift** and **quick to anger** and **anger** and **success pressures** are still around, and that they're somehow really big. I mean, my friends all experience something similar here. Why is that?"

The Authors Speak

What about what these young people are saying? They said they had learned to pay attention to their own ideas, and that often these ideas were not different from their parents' ideas for them, but that sometimes they didn't fit cultural expectations. We know about this. As teenagers we didn't follow mainstream prescriptions ourselves, and we're pleased about the results. As therapists, what do you readers think is "mainstream"? Only you can decide!

"Separation": A Reflection

STUDENT: How do you decide what to call the problem, given that it comes in many disguises? I mean, **slipping, rift, anger**—it seems so confusing. This seems to be a really difficult aspect of this work.

VICKI: We find it most useful to pick a name that captures people's experience, and one that allows us to address those "expectations" the group of teenagers referred to. In the case of Marcy, her dad's use of the word **slipping** became a focus for the multiple problems he was describing. It made sense to talk about it as the "problem."

STUDENT: But when adolescents in particular hear that you are calling the problem by a name their parents suggest . . . what then? And what about the ideas I've heard the two of you present—the effects of this "separation" metaphor? How do you address this?

VICKI: We find that the clients' experience of the problem is often similar for parents and adolescents, but the reasons they construct to explain it are very different. As we said earlier, this usually involves a story about the other. For example, with the **slipping** presented here,

Marcy's mom seemed to be going in the direction of **blame** (self- or other-blame), and also toward **doubt** and **distrust**. For her dad, it was more about Marcy's having some difficulty in accepting the next steps in life. And for Marcy it was a "growing-year" story and about her parents' not understanding.

But the point we really want to get to here is this "separation" thing. We have become interested in how it affects families and kids, what it tells them, how it gets them to experience themselves in ways so that kids actually *are* bored in their last year in high school and think they need to move out of their homes to make it in the world. You can see that Marcy's comments reflect the sociocultural meta-phor that supports separation as necessary. We want to know how this metaphor gets parents to think they have to pressure their kids to make "independent" decisions, and that when they don't act "responsibly"—according to somebody's idea of "responsible"—then there is something wrong with them. When we ask about these things in the therapy room, kids and parents can move toward a clearer understanding of what their preferences are.

STUDENT: Let me see if I understand the implications of all you have been saying. "Stories are constitutive" means that a "separation" metaphor would be constructing kids and parents' experience of themselves in a way that separation becomes an inevitable direction for families with adolescents. When kids get to be teenagers, they think they should rebel; when they get to be seniors in high school, they experience a "need to get on with things." If kids don't rebel or rebel too much, according to the culture, then something must be wrong (either with the kids or with their parents). In the past, pathological stories have been constructed by therapists (biological for the kids and/or "bad parenting" for the parents) to explain these results, just as when Mom attributed the problem to self-blame and self-doubt or to Marcy's low self-esteem.

VICKI: Yes, and we think many problems can be understood this way. For example, in some families, men respond to culturally constructed notions about power in a way that has problematic effects on the rest of the family. Yet we persist in calling these families "dysfunctional." If one follows the culture, that can be called "dysfunctional," and if one rejects the culture's specifications, that is called "dysfunctional" also.

We believe when we talk about "dissing separation," we are getting to the heart of the problem for teenagers and their families, because it addresses a cultural process that seems to have a lot of negative effects on families and often invites them to pathologize themselves.

ON THE LINE OR ONLINE:
PARENTS TALK, TOO
Being There

"Well, since our kids got together . . . I guess they're not 'kids' any more, are they?" said Gary, Sharon's father, as they all met for the first time. "I'm really glad you agreed to come together when I contacted you all by e-mail."

Marcy's parents nodded. Jim said, "Makes sense to me. Plus, we have the room here, so why not?"

They all stood around awkwardly. It could have seemed like a strange gathering, but they knew they had something in common. Judy, Sharon's mother, voiced it when she said, "It seems like all of us have had the chance to realize how our connection with our children is so important, and that we don't have to lose it when they become teenagers."

"Hooray!" responded Ginny, Marcy's mom. "Let's sit down and talk. I know *I* have a story to tell. Anyone want something cold to drink?"

As Ginny came back into the room, Jane was describing what it had been like for her as Becky's stepmother—wanting to connect with her, but also realizing *she* wasn't going to be the answer to the **anger** that had such a strong history in that family. Bart hadn't been able to come to this gathering; he was doing his usual business traveling. Jane laughingly announced, "Becky and her dad are getting along better, because now when he comes home, he just wants to spend good time with her. There's less chance for the **anger** to make an appearance." She added, "I'm not saying he doesn't work on it . . . and Becky, too."

"I think that's the most noticeable thing in our family," Ginny chimed in, "that we're all really paying attention to how we want to work together. We're not at all interested in anything even remotely looking like **slipping** entering into our lives again. In fact, Jim called our old therapist the other day, letting her know how things were going in a good direction."

"Well, she's not really *old*," laughed Jim. "That would make me a dinosaur. But I wanted her to know that the effort paid off. And she even called us back to offer her congratulations."

Joe, Sr., and Patty had been very quiet. After Jim's remark, Joe volunteered, "We thought we were on the right track with our son after we went to therapy when he was in high school. But, you know, looking back, I think the **pressure** was just too great. We didn't mean to add to it, but we so wanted him to experience success in his life. When we understood that **success** was in itself a pressure . . . "

"I think we're on the right track now," said Patty, and Joe agreed. "But tell us, Ginny and Jim, how did *you* all get things going in a good direction?"

"I remember the end of the first family therapy session. We had a reflecting team, and I was raising a possibility after we got back together in the room with our therapist . . . "

Online 1, Part 1

GINNY: I think very often 18-year-olds or 19-year-olds think of themselves as leaving home, and *boom*! I like to think they think of themselves as having a family. They have their own life. There's no question. But they do have a family.

[Later:]

GINNY: Sometimes these changes that occur happen in college for most people . . . I've been told . . . if young people *do* do this at home, at least they have a support system, hopefully; that they're not alone, away at college.

VICKI: They have that context of caring.

GINNY: Uh-huh. Just that huggy feeling of knowing you're home. When you're out there, and you've got those changes . . . it's not the same.

VICKI: You see it as a good thing that Marcy is going through these things now?

GINNY: If it's meant to be . . . sure. I'd like the muddle to be gone . . .

Reply Post 1, Part 1

"So you can see what I was thinking . . . I really wanted us to stay close, and Jim did, too. But when Marcy seemed so confused (what we were calling *slipping*), it just seemed like it was better that it was happening when it was, when she was home and knew she still had our support."

"Yeah," Jim added. "But I think it took some time before *she* realized she had it."

"Why do you think that was?" Gary asked. "I know that has been really important in our family."

Ginny quickly replied, "I think the *slipping* was too big. And we got really discouraged when we didn't turn it around as fast as we thought we should be able to. In fact, listen to what we discussed at the end of the session when that other therapist, Jeff, was asking questions . . . "

Online 1, Part 2

JEFF: I have questions for everybody—for the team, anyway . . .

GINNY: Sure.

JEFF: I'll tell you how I thought about all of this. I thought this was a story of *reconnection,* and what I mean by that is that stories of *reconnec-*

tion for people Marcy's age usually start with stories of **slipping,** because to achieve **reconnection** requires some **slipping.** The thing about **slipping** is that once **slipping** gets a hold, it could just take off and keep on going, and there's never a guarantee that there will be a use of that toward **reconnection.** But it seems clear here to all of us that there's a **reconnection** occurring already, at least from where I sit. It may not feel that way to you two, as parents.

[Questions were asked of the team at this point, and then:]

GINNY: May I ask a question? Does everyone slip in life in order to develop? I mean, define **slipping** for me.

JEFF: Well, it's unique. People seem to do that in unique ways. But we also think that there's not much out there to help young people grow up without **slipping.** That's unfortunate, because perhaps it isn't necessary. That's something Vicki and I have talked about. Because of the world we live in, that seems to be the option that seems most open to most people. But something about our society maybe could be different. Some of what has been left out is some context for young persons to go forward without some of that **slipping.** But right now, that doesn't seem to be there. But as parents . . . my children are younger, but as a future parent of a future teenager, part of what I'm beginning to think about is what I might do, knowing this—what I might do to create something like that . . .

Reply Post 1, Part 2

Ginny continued, "I've thought a lot about that, and looking back, it almost seems inevitable that we went through another couple of years before we got to the **reconnection** place. I was angry for a while, because the whole process was so painful. And I thought the therapists thought we were already there, and I knew we weren't. But our therapist did hang in there with us. So I can look back at those remarks now and see how they fit."

"Don't you also see, dear," said Jim, "how you really understood what was going on, even back then?"

"Agreed," added Joe. The others smiled and nodded.

Ginny said, "Say more what you mean."

Karen, Greg's mom, responded. "I remember thinking college would be 'the answer' for Greg. There was so much **anger** between us. I just thought he needed to get away. I know our therapist questioned, perhaps even challenged, that idea. You talked about wanting your daughter to know she had a family, and about how important it was to give her support."

"I know, I know," answered Ginny. "I guess I didn't know how much I knew. Maybe if I had listened to myself more, rather than to *self-doubt* . . . I mean, I even questioned whether *slipping* was necessary."

Jim thought about what she said and remembered how he had talked about their "tremendous love," and how one of the other therapists had raised the question on the reflecting team about the "history of that love." He said, "It was probably the love that got us through, because, no doubt about it, the *hurt* was big. It's good to look back at this now, and know we got through it!"

"Hooray!" responded the group, again.

Gary had been pondering what was being said, thinking about how he and Judy and Sharon had held on to their connection with each other, when Judy joined in. "I remember a discussion we had. It was about me as a parent. I didn't know how to respond, but it helped me really value what I brought to the family and to our sense of connection."[16]

Online 2

VICKI: So when you first came in here there was a lot of *fear,* subsequent to the accident [i.e., the car accident Sharon was in]—fear of potential danger. How did you overcome the *fear?*

JUDY: Well, you asked me a question, which has been resonating with me for the last month. You asked me a question in the last session: "Is it okay with you that Sharon makes her own decisions when they turn out to be choices that you wouldn't necessarily make for her?" I thought that was a key question. I really thought about that a lot. I had to come to the conclusion that I either trust her to make her own decisions and to deal with the consequences or I don't. And there isn't any gray area. It's just . . . I really needed to face that. And, yes, I do want to protect her from negative outcomes, but I can see that I'm just not going to be able to do that. And so . . . I mean I just looked at it very logically, and thought if I continue to be anxious and overbearing, it's just going to continue to drive her underground and keep her mad at me and all of the negative things that were starting to escalate.

VICKI: And not lessen the danger.

JUDY: And it doesn't lessen the danger. I mean, I thought if it could impact the outcome then I might have a justification for continuing down that road. But it doesn't lessen the danger; in fact, in some cases I think it might even increase it. So . . .

---

[16]What follows is another actual transcript that the family members have read and given their permission to reproduce here. Gary, Judy, and Sharon, of course, are the family described in Chapters 2–5.

VICKI: (*To Sharon, who is nodding*) And you think so, too?

SHARON: Yeah.

VICKI: So, it sounds like, Judy, that one of the ways you handled the *fear* was that you made a decision that you wanted to operate more out of *trust.* Is that what you said?

JUDY: Yes, and I think the other way that I've been handling the *fear* . . . because the *fear* doesn't come up in me as much as a couple of months ago . . . one of the things I've had to settle for myself is that, in my heart of hearts, I really trust Sharon's judgment. I can go really crazy when I think about what's out there in the environment that she's exposed to. But I've had enough conversations with her, and I know that she thinks very logically, that she's a clear thinker, and she's pretty discerning. I have to go with my own feeling that I know my daughter pretty well, and I trust her.

VICKI: So the *trust* is a bigger experience for you than the *fear?* . . . And you went to that as a much more solid sign of your relationship?

JUDY: Uh-huh.

VICKI: Can I pursue this one further question? I have this idea that people's parenting changes as kids get older—that the quality of *trust* changes because the dangers are bigger or the context is broader, as you said, all those things out there. So I wonder . . . I'm going to ask you this, Judy, but you, too, Gary . . . what does it tell you about you as a parent that you could put your cards in the *trust* arena rather than *fear?* What does it tell you about you?[17]

JUDY: I think it's just a much more positive approach. And I think it communicates a whole different message to your child . . . than to be driven the other way by the mistrust and the expectation that they're actually going to make bad decisions that are going to end up in negative outcomes. Of course, they still can, but I think it's the attitude of the parent. I've had that attitude with Sharon, a lot of "My God, I'm so afraid that you're going to screw up," which communicates to her, "I don't really trust that you're going to make the right decisions about yourself."

VICKI: It gets you to pay more attention to the "screwing up" than to the good decisions.

JUDY: Yes.

VICKI: Because there will be both.

---

[17]We're always interested in helping people access preferred ideas about themselves as persons—although we often find (as you see here) that people have trouble answering these kinds of questions.

JUDY: Right.

VICKI: So when you said it's a much more positive approach . . . yes, I'd agree with you . . . but I wonder: What is the shift you see in your parenting as Sharon has gotten older?

JUDY: Well, the thing that comes to mind is, I feel like I'm shifting the responsibility for her behavior and her actions and her attitude more to her. [Judy then tells a story of watching Sharon play soccer and not recognizing her at first because she looked so grown up, then realizing how grown up she really is.] It was a shock. Here is this person who looks like a 17- or 18-year-old. It was just a physical taking in of "Judy, you have to let go; she is a young woman; she is not this little girl that you carry around in your mind." So it was one of those moments of "getting it" as a parent and seeing your child as a young woman. It was a tender moment.

Reply Post 2

Judy took a deep breath and put her hand over her heart, recalling those words. Then she said, "So, you see, I could answer the question about parenting, and it was really helpful for me to think about those changes. But the question about me as a parent, as a person—that was hard. Even now, I don't know what it means."

Ginny nodded. "Later in therapy, I remember being asked questions like that, too. Questions like 'What was it about me as a parent, or as a mother, or as a person, or as a woman . . . ?' And I hadn't thought of my part so much. But now, looking back, we can see that we've known all along how important we are in our relationships with our kids. Like you said, just trusting them can have profound effects on how they begin to trust themselves."

"Well," responded Judy, "I also saw that the *fear* was contributing to the *rift,* and that *trust* was the antidote to that—it was the way toward increased **connection.** I suspect you saw that, too, as your family moved toward **reconnection.**"

"Right," said Jim.

Ginny nodded again, remembering how she held on to her confidence in herself as a mother and, together with Marcy, opened up lines of communication between them. "I don't know . . . I don't think we're there yet. I guess we, as mothers, need to trust ourselves, too."

"I would hazard a guess that none of us are ever *there,*" said Patty, "although what you said about trusting ourselves would probably help. It has been up and down, back and forth, for us. We keep checking in with each other to make sure we're going in the direction we want."

"That's just how I would say it," added Jim. "In the direction we want . . . "

More Reflection

STUDENT: That's a big word—"Direction." It seems that all of this work is about shifting the direction in ways clients prefer.

VICKI: Yes. Our experience is that when things are moving solidly in a desired direction, therapy can end.

STUDENT: I was interested in that question, "What does it tell you about you as a parent . . . ?" I noticed that Judy found it a lot easier to answer the question about herself parenting than about her as a parent and a person.

VICKI: We're always interested in helping people access preferred ideas about themselves as persons. Even though we often find that people have trouble answering these kinds of questions, we still ask them, because we believe that doing so opens up the idea of "personal agency." We believe this idea promotes persons' making choices that fit better for them than those that are encouraged by the problem.

STUDENT: So what happens to young people when they're in their early and mid-20s—you know, after college, or after they move out of their homes. The world out there is pretty tough. What about these young so-called adults?

VICKI: Our belief is that "connection" is still the key metaphor here.

STUDENT: Well, okay, then what about even younger people? What you're discussing here fits for 15- to 20-year-olds and older, but how about a 12-year-old? And everybody knows that boys and girls "mature" differently.

VICKI: Actually, we are going to address issues for younger adolescents in the next chapter—that is, how young girls in early adolescence are prone to "lose their voice," and how young boys, at about the same time, become strangely influenced to become nonreflexive and nonthinking.

STUDENT: What about other races, other ethnic groups, different socio-economic classes, nontraditional families? You've been showing white, middle-class families here.

VICKI: You're right. That's what we have illustrated. We do think we have underattended to other races, ethnic groups, social classes, and family forms. We are currently exploring ways to extend our thinking and our consciousness to those groups, and we are interested in how to be accountable to them, making certain that we can be responsive in ways that fit for them. We believe that narrative ideas have wide application, particularly because they take nothing for granted and challenge subjugating practices of the culture, whatever that culture happens to be.

STUDENT: Have you any experience here?

VICKI: Some, but not as much as we'd like. You might be interested in knowing that part of our exploration in disassembling the metaphor of "separation" was to look at other races and other ethnic groups. Our colleague Lisa Berndt did some research and wrote about how some indigenous people and those of other ethnicities regard what we call "adolescence." You might check it out [Dickerson, Zimmerman, & Berndt, 1994].

STUDENT: I have another question. What about multiproblem families? You know, the ones whose kids end up at departments of social services, in juvenile courts, in alternative schools, and in residential treatment centers.

VICKI: We have experience in social agencies, at teaching hospitals, and in consultation to residential facilities, where these "multiproblem families," as you call them, have been clients. We have seen the application of narrative ideas work well. In fact, "multiproblems" have real effects, and it is in our exploration of these effects with families, kids, social workers, case managers, probation officers, and teachers that we find the alternative histories and the unexamined resources, and we work to make these apparent. Often these families have been marginalized by the culture (and now are being further marginalized by the mental health culture), and we find that they respond quite well to an approach that doesn't pathologize how their lived experience might stand outside traditional norms.

STUDENT: Okay, so what's next?

VICKI: The next chapter!

A Final Word

GINNY: I'd like to have a final word here.

VICKI: Sure, that makes sense.

GINNY: When you sent the transcript to me and then called and asked what I thought, I had several ideas, and I wanted to share them here . . . for other parents, other families with teenagers. I remember saying that I thought I had made lots of mistakes when Marcy was a teenager, and you reminded me that I certainly didn't think they were mistakes at the time. So, you see, I'm still fighting *self-blame* and *self-doubt!* But what I do think is that we, as parents, have to pay attention to ourselves, to our kids, to what we know about them; we have to stay important in their lives. I guess you would say we have to stay **connected.** And Jim and I wanted to . . . want to. I also think the educational system has to work with us to help kids not feel so pressured to respond to certain "specifications" about how the culture thinks they need to be. I know Marcy struggled with that, and Jim and I did, too. We wanted the best for her, so we thought she had to do things in certain well-prescribed ways. We could have used some help from the schools! Unfortunately, they cooperated with those "prescriptions." I also remember, after we had taken some steps to help Marcy escape a bad situation, that you asked us if we would be interested in "protesting" some of those cultural specifications—the ones that say kids need to become separate and independent in certain ways, need to "leave" their homes and families. We certainly found out that the pressures for Marcy to move out and be on her own weren't helpful; they ended up alienating us from each other. So, yes, we are interested in protesting, and I'm saying this to invite other parents (and other teenagers) to join us in protesting.

VICKI: Protesting that "separation" metaphor? You mean "dissing separation?"

GINNY: Yes, definitely.

VICKI: Thanks. Sounds like **confidence** (rather than **self-doubt**) is operating here!

GINNY: (*Smiling*) I think so.

CHAPTER 10

Making Ourselves Up
Moving beyond Gender Discourse

SUGAR AND SPICE
AND EVERYTHING NICE—OH, REALLY?
Reveries and Conversations

Angie

Angie was 12 and she was angry. She was also vociferous, loud, and nonstop. Her parents had encouraged her to have opinions of her own and to express them. This fit her dad's growing-up family and didn't fit her mom's growing-up family. In Dad's family, the children (all sons) were brought up to stand up for and assert themselves, to fight for what they believed in against all odds. So they did; and it made sense to him, even in a family of two daughters, to promote the same behavior. In Mom's family, the children (all daughters) were to be demure and defer; they were put down for having differing opinions, and punished for straying from rigid family mores. Mom had had troubles in her teenage years, eventually leaving her family at a young age to get married. It made sense to her to raise her family in exactly the opposite manner to the way in which she had been raised. However, because she had only experienced what it was like in an authoritarian family, she had no idea of how a daughter who was raised differently might look.

Angie complained about everything: about how she was treated differently from her 10-year-old sister; about how her parents never listened to her point of view; about how her dad was "macho" and her mom didn't stand up to him; about how she got told to do everything and wasn't allowed to do anything;

about how her teachers didn't call on her and didn't agree with her. She had a finely tuned sense of justice. Her parents complained that she wouldn't do anything she was asked; that she was rude and disrespectful to them; that she fought with and was unkind to her sister; and that she was getting into trouble at school, including skipping classes. The ensuing conflict led to increased anger on Angie's part and increased frustration on her parents' part. The parents began to believe that there was something wrong with their parenting, and to question the decision they had made to bring up their children to have and express their own ideas.

Eventually, Angie was in danger of getting kicked out of school. Mom said, "She got mad at one of the teachers, so she stopped going to his class. She'd have to go to another school, and I don't want her there; she wouldn't know anyone." Angie responded, "He wouldn't listen to me. I even went up to him after class, and he told me I had been rude, so to go away."

One time they went with some friends of the family to a miniature speedway, where people race cars around a track. Angie couldn't go in one of the cars because she didn't have a license. She said it was okay with her, she'd just watch. Dad said she was pouting, so his response was "Okay, if you're going to act like that, then we're leaving!" "Like what?" she said. She got angry, yelled at him, and stormed off. "You embarrassed me in front of everyone!"

Brushing Hair

Mom's reverie was interrupted by Angie's plaintive whine. "So why do *I* have to go there? I won't know *any*one!"

"Well, I suppose you don't have to if you don't want to. I would think it might be interesting to you." She continued slowly brushing her daughter's long hair, glad that Angie still liked that kind of closeness.

"What could possibly be interesting about being with a bunch of families who are probably all screwed up?"

"Why would you say that?"

"They had to go to therapy, didn't they?"

Mom laughed, "Sure, and so did we, but we weren't 'screwed up.' We just had to find a way to make room for everybody's ideas—including yours, sweetheart."

Angie tried not to laugh, then responded, "But I'm still getting into trouble at school, and you're still not standing up for yourself."

Mom winced as she said, "We're working on that—both, I mean. That letter we sent your teachers, you know, the one we all worked on with our therapist, I had hoped that would give you some room for having your own ideas."

"Well, yes, sometimes the teachers seem more respectful."

"And is that helping you also respond with respect to them?"

"Geez, Mom!"

"Okay, okay, I know it's a two-way street; I was just thinking about your end of it."

"And what about you, Mom, *your* end of the street?"

"You mean my standing up for myself? It's hard to have been married for 15 years, right out of high school. Our society didn't much support my having my own life. We sort of did what your dad wanted, and he didn't really know how to see things differently, either. I'll tell you, Angie, it was an eye-opener to me to begin to realize that not only was it important for you to 'have a voice' and keep it, but also that I had lost mine and wanted to reclaim it. This therapy was good for me, too. I know you might not see yet how it is good for me *and* how it is going better for your dad and me, but it is . . . "

"Okay, I'll go to this get-together. Did you say there will be two other families? And will Dad be there?"

"Two other families, yes. Dad is coming later—after work. And, Angie . . . thanks."

Carrol

Carrol was 11. She thought she would probably always be 11. She wasn't going to be able to go anywhere or do anything; she had already had most of her privileges taken away from her. She didn't see any friends except at school. Her little brother was a pest and didn't understand at all how it was. Her mother just didn't get it. And her dad—sometimes he was funny and fun, but other times he was a real pig. Her teachers were a lost cause; they didn't get it either. Locked into 11.

Her feelings were almost palpable. Sometimes they were like butterflies caught in her insides, her stomach, her throat, her head. She was skittish, jumpy, unsettled. No wonder her parents had no idea what she was going to do next. She couldn't land. She didn't even know where she was. Other times her feelings were bundled up, stuffed together, tightly bound, and fossilized into a huge, round, smooth rock, which had settled somewhere where her heart should be. It felt cold, hard, impenetrable. Then it would shrink into a small stone and float up to her throat and get lodged there, silencing her; no voice could come out, could squeak around the sides of the polished stone. Until, suddenly, out it crashed, broken into tiny, sharp, dangerous fragments, like shrapnel flying into whatever bodies were in the way.

She knew her parents thought she would never shut up—that she was always talking, interrupting, not listening. She resented their always telling her what to do. Even more, she resented their always thinking they were right. She had a point of view, too. Why couldn't they listen to her? So why not argue? She had nothing to lose. They weren't listening anyway; they had already taken things away. It didn't matter. What mattered was that she had ideas, and she wanted her parents to hear them.

So she stormed off, slammed her door, yelled at them. Tears came to her eyes, but she wiped them away quickly. "Don't tell me what I think!" "Don't tell me what to do!" "I know!"

There were moments when her mom would look at her quizzically: "What is she thinking?" Sometimes they could even talk. Her mom agreed with her that her teachers should call on her more; just because she always had her hand up didn't mean they should ignore her. Other times her mom would just shake her head when Carrol stormed off in anger. Once, Carrol remembered, her mom followed her to her room, came in quietly, and just sat down. She didn't say anything. She just sat. That was good.

Carrol also remembered other moments with her Dad. He would argue with her, but at least it was an argument; she even felt like he gave her point of view some credence. But he was always right. (She knew he wasn't. Why did he have to pretend to be?) But at least the arguments meant he was there. When they weren't fighting, she could sometimes sit with him and watch TV; she'd sit down on the couch, sit next to him. He didn't move. That was good.

But they were so stupid. Her mom would say to others that she raised her daughter to have her own point of view. And then she didn't want to even hear it. Her dad would get into his macho stuff and strut around like the king of the hill. So she'd yell at him, and he'd tell her to watch herself. Didn't they know she was 11?

Mom didn't have a clue. It just didn't make sense to her at all. Her own growing-up family had felt so free-flowing; her mother was so open and giving. They had grown up like free spirits, flower children. Maybe that's why she wanted to provide a little more structure for her kids—but, try as she might, she still "gave in" and let her kids have their way. She was there for them, always available and accessible, at their beck and call. And in return the children were fun-loving and fun to be with; they, too, were free spirits. But in school . . . at least there they should toe the line. After all, it was important to "fit in." But they should be able to have their own minds, their own opinions, and make some decisions for themselves. This was becoming a dilemma.

Carrol had seemed to change when she got to middle school. Mom wondered what had happened. It didn't seem to make sense. Carrol was so loud, so angry; she would never sit still and have a conversation, and she wouldn't listen at all. She just stormed off. How did it turn out this way?

Making Cookies

"Can we make chocolate chip ones?" Carrol asked.

"Sure," responded Mom. "I think we should make something you'll like." She wondered how this meeting would go for Carrol. Only recently did she seem able to talk to anyone without lots of anger and nastiness coming out of her mouth.

"I know what you're thinking," quipped Carrol.

"What?"

"You're wondering how this is going to go and if I will keep my mouth shut."

"No, no," Mom said. "I don't *want* you to keep your mouth shut. If nothing else, what *I* learned in therapy is how important it is for you to stay in touch with what you want, what you think, what you believe. Remember? And if we—your dad and I—can stay close to your wanting to talk about what you are experiencing, then maybe you'll hold on to what you know, to your own relationship with yourself."

"Wow, is that what you got out of therapy? I didn't get all that!" answered Carrol. "I just got that it was okay for me to stick with my ideas. That's hard, though. Do you think those other girls at this meeting will be able to talk about this stuff? I mean, so many kids at school don't get it. They just go about their prissy, stuck-up little ways."

Mom scowled, then said, "I know this isn't easy, Carrol. It scares me a little. Because, you know I grew up with my own sense of who I was, what I wanted; and my mom, your grandmother, supported that. But I always felt like I didn't fit. Then I married your father, and that made me legitimate, I suppose. But, you know I'm not happy, and we—your father and I—are struggling to come to terms with that. So I guess I don't see this as an easy road."

"What does it all mean? How am I supposed to be?" Carrol cried. "I can't just give in. But I don't always want to have to be screaming and angry either. It seems so unfair!"

Jamie

Jamie was 13. She remembered being 10. She was on top of the world then. The years before had been tough—especially since she was seven, when her parents split. She'd stayed with her mom and felt close to her, but her mom was always so busy, out there with her friends, out there with her new business. Jamie felt alone a lot. Sure, she was encouraged to be herself, to speak her thoughts; she felt really comfortable, and liked, and included—by her mom's friends. But school was something else. Somehow, making friends with kids her own age was hard. She didn't seem to fit, except that one year in the fifth grade, when she was 10: She'd had a best friend for almost a year. Starting junior high was a shock, though; she slipped to outcast status again. All those cliques, none for her . . .

She wanted to be an actress, but her teacher said that was an unrealistic career choice.

She hated gym class, because she had asthma, and running got it to act up. Her teacher gave her a D because she didn't run the mile in the prescribed time.

She tried everything to fit in, then gave up and withdrew to loneliness. Even her friend from fifth grade had joined a clique and hardly talked to her.

Now it seemed that her only friends were her mom's friends. They listened to her, gave her space, allowed her to state her opinion, had discussions with her. One of her mom's friends even asked her once, "How are you managing to hold on to your own ideas? Sometimes the junior high school experience makes that hard for girls to do."

Jamie wondered about that question. She guessed she was holding on to her own ideas—in spite of her teachers seeming not to value her, and the stupid rules, and gym, and her awful math class. But the hard part was not having friends, so she answered, "It's easy to hold on to your own ideas when you don't have anyone to talk to."

Reviving Jamie

As Mom made herself a cup of coffee, she thought about what Jamie had said the other evening. It really hadn't been an answer to her friend's question, but it was probably what Jamie's experience was right now. She wondered how to talk about this with her daughter. Remembering how much they both valued their conversations together, she went to Jamie's bedroom and knocked on the door.

"Jamie, are you awake? I want to show you something."

"What?" snarled Jamie.

"No big deal. I just wanted to show you an invitation we got for a get-together." Mom suspected that this meeting would be a chance for Jamie to see that others her age had similar feelings, also felt squelched, and maybe experienced anger or hurt or some sort of stifling.

Jamie shuffled out of her bedroom, looking disheveled and bleary-eyed. "What now?"

Mom held on to her belief that this was just first-thing-in-the-morning blues, and not about her. "Can we talk? We're invited to a gathering with a couple of other families. The purpose is to share our experiences of 'losing one's voice' as a young teenage girl."

"What are you mumbling about?"

"Okay, loosen up, Jamie. Why don't you take some time to wake up, and then we can have this discussion." Mom began to realize that this was getting off to a bad start. Plus, she knew better: *She* had trouble focusing first thing in the morning, too.

Jamie looked at her mom to see whether she was serious. "Okay. That's okay. I can listen. What do you mean, 'losing my voice'?"

Maybe she can have this conversation after all, Mom thought. "Well, there have been some studies, some research, you know, about young girls—how they get bombarded with cultural ideas about how to be, especially when they reach junior high, and sometimes it gets them to sort of stop knowing what they know."

"Wait, wait, you're making no sense. You're mumbling again. I don't get it."

"I guess maybe we should go to this meeting and talk about it there," sighed Mom.

"Mom," Jamie interjected, "how come you decided to have a relationship with a woman instead of getting married again?"

"What? Where did that come from?"

"I don't know. It just popped into my head. I mean, other kids' parents, when they get divorced, they lots of times get married again. I mean, I wouldn't want a stepfather. Yuk!" Jamie paused, then added hesitantly, "I'm not so sure I like *her* much either . . . "

"Oh, Jamie," responded Mom. "Is this about you and me, or about you, or about my lifestyle, or what?"

"I don't know," came the plaintive cry. Jamie sat in silence for a minute, then said, "Maybe it's about 'losing my voice.'" Then she laughed heartily.

"You're putting me on." Then Mom started to laugh, too. "All kidding aside, Jamie, it may be about 'voice.' You see, I have found that it is sometimes hard to be the kind of woman I want to be in the world, to assert what I want, to follow my own wishes, to speak my own thoughts. Some men, but not all men, would respect that. However, bigger than that, the culture seems divided about how to handle it. You know sexuality itself is a construction. Maybe the notions of homosexuality and heterosexuality are just inventions anyway . . . "

"You're losing me again," sighed Jamie.

"Can we keep having this discussion?" Mom asked. "I mean, maybe not now, but from now on, at other times. I think how *you* keep *your* voice is very important. And I don't think there's any one right way. But I do think talking about it might help us both get clearer."

"Okay. I think I want some breakfast now. Do we have to go to that meeting?"

Mom laughed. "Well, maybe, maybe not. Let's eat first."

Do You Hear What I Hear?

"We asked you here this evening because *we* have some ideas that we want to get *your* ideas about. Over the past three or four years, we have become increasingly interested in how young girls, like the three of you here, are influenced by the larger cultural society and how those influences shape the way you think about yourselves and the way you relate to yourselves, your family, and your friends, as you grow from childhood to adulthood. Of course, we are also interested in how parents respond or react to, cooperate with, or challenge these cultural influences. What we are talking about is something we have addressed with all of you in the therapy room; we've talked about it as 'voice' or 'your own ideas' or your 'self-narrative.' But we also know that these influences we are talking about are invisible and only noticeable in their effects, like the complaints you all showed up with in therapy—**anger, defiance,** and **giving up.** So we'd like to revisit our therapy with you by showing old movies—no, actually by showing pieces of videotape from our work together, and then get your comments. What we want to do is make visible the influences that are silencing young girls, but we also want to discuss with you the strategies you developed as families, and how these strategies may have looked different for you girls, your mothers, and your fathers. Could we roll the first tape?"

"Oh, Angie's dad will be a little late. Could you start with someone else's?"

"No problem. How about we start with yours, Jamie? You and your mom are here, right?"

"Okay, I guess," responded Jamie.

"This one is with you by yourself. Here we go."

Jamie[1]

THERAPIST: So what's your response when your teachers don't seem to acknowledge your point of view?

JAMIE: What do you mean?

THERAPIST: Well, like when your gym teacher won't listen to you when you say your asthma is kicking up, or when your math teacher makes fun of your questions.

JAMIE: It's just not fair!

THERAPIST: So what's your response? Is it more anger or sadness or a kind of silencing or what?

JAMIE: I'm not sure. I don't know.

THERAPIST: Would it surprise you to hear that this is the same answer I get from other girls your age?

JAMIE: I guess not.

THERAPIST: So it's kind of a *not knowing?*

JAMIE: Well, maybe. I mean, what good is it going to do? When I try to say something, no one listens. So I just give up.

THERAPIST: So it's a *giving up?*

JAMIE: Yeah.

THERAPIST: What effect do you think this *giving up* has on you?

JAMIE: What do you mean?

THERAPIST: I mean, does this *giving up* silence you, make you sad, isolate you, what?

[1]This is a fictional interview.

JAMIE: Oh, it silences me, all right. Except when I'm at home. And then my mom gets it all.

THERAPIST: How do you mean?

JAMIE: I tell her.

THERAPIST: So the *giving up* doesn't follow you home?

JAMIE: No, not at all. But it doesn't help.

THERAPIST: Explain.

JAMIE: Well, it doesn't help at school. I still don't have any friends.

THERAPIST: So the *giving up* silences you at school, but not at home. It sounds like the *giving up* also isolates you at school.

JAMIE: Yeah.

"Well, it makes me angry," Mom interrupted. They stopped the tape and turned the lights back on.

"Say more."

"I don't like what happens there, but I feel powerless. The few times I've tried to talk to the principal or written letters to the teachers, they have sort of put me off. It's almost demeaning."

"But at least I know you support me, Mom," interjected Jamie. "It was helpful for me to watch this tape. I mean, I could see that *giving up* wasn't exactly helping me, but I didn't know what else to do."

"Could we show just one more bit of tape?"

"Sure."

THERAPIST: Do you think any other kids your age are affected in this way?

JAMIE: They don't seem to be. They just go along with it. Except for the rebellious ones.

THERAPIST: What do you mean?

JAMIE: Some girls are just defiant.

THERAPIST: So there are three categories: *giving up, defiance,* and *going along?*

JAMIE: I guess.

THERAPIST: It's kind of a dilemma, isn't it?

JAMIE: That's just what my mom says!

Jamie laughed. She had forgotten this conversation. Then she said, "Maybe that's why I don't have any friends."

Mom asked, "How do you mean? Because you don't just go along?"

"We wondered that, too. In fact, we suspect that is the case. But what we also wondered is this: What strategies have you two developed to keep from giving in to **giving up?** That's a funny way to say it!"

Mom responded, "I think continuing to talk has helped. Also, Jamie knows that *I* haven't given up. Plus, I encourage her (and my friends do too) to keep her voice, to say what she believes, to be however she wants to be."

"Yeah, but that doesn't make it any easier to not have any friends," Jamie added.

"It does sound like **giving up** hasn't gotten you to give up on yourself or to give yourself up," the therapists said. "I also wonder if it would be helpful for you to hear that the older girls and young women we know who have kept their 'voice' seem much less apt to be influenced by **self-doubt** or **evaluation.**"

"I guess so," said Jamie.

"That sounds really interesting. Maybe we could discuss that some more, Jamie. I think I might have some of that experience myself—not giving myself up or giving up on myself." Mom smiled and added knowingly, "Plus, I have found that over time, there are other young women with similar experiences—persons who can become your friends."

"Well," Angie blurted out, "I know something about what you're saying."

"How about we look at your tape next? I notice your dad is here now."

"Okay, good," answered Angie. "Yes," chimed in Mom and Dad.

Angie, Mom, and Dad[2]

Angie was sitting on the edge of the couch, her feet up in her dad's lap, who was at the other end. Mom was sitting on a chair to Angie's left.

THERAPIST: Let me ask you one more question, okay?

ANGIE: Me?

THERAPIST: Do you think that your dad could hear what you said?

ANGIE: You'd have to ask him. Maybe he heard, but it won't last too long.

THERAPIST: So, he took you seriously?

ANGIE: (*To Dad*) Don't look at me like that.

THERAPIST: So the **frustration** tells you what? That he's not taking you seriously?

ANGIE: Exactly.

THERAPIST: Can I ask you a question, Gene [Dad]?

[2]This transcript is based on composite interviews and has been highly fictionalized.

DAD: Sure.

THERAPIST: When you notice what you call *upset* on Angie's part, how does that affect you?

DAD: It upsets *me*. I think she's too loud and noisy, and I don't have any idea what to do.

THERAPIST: So then what?

DAD: I try to get her to quiet down, and then I try to find out what the trouble is.

THERAPIST: Do you think that is when Angie experiences what she calls *frustration?*

DAD: Well, probably.

MOM: I understand that. It's what she tells me happens at school, too. Her teachers don't understand her, and that leads to *frustration* and gets her to act angry. That's when they call me or her dad and tell us that she's defiant.

THERAPIST: So what do you understand about that?

MOM: Sometimes it's hard for her (and me, too) to be able to say what we want or say what we're thinking and to believe that others hear us. Sometimes we think we have to get really angry before anyone will pay attention.

THERAPIST: So that's the *upset* Gene is talking about—the *anger?*

MOM: Yes, but you know we've been trying an experiment lately.

THERAPIST: Yes, I'm interested in hearing about it. Will you tell me about it?

MOM: Of course. We—Gene and I—have been trying to listen to Angie, to what she says she wants, and letting her know what we're hearing. That way, the *anger* doesn't take over and the *frustration* doesn't get going so easily.

ANGIE: Yeah, and then I can do things without them always telling me what to do and how to do it.

DAD: Well, it works better for me, too, because I resent having to control things, control her. What we are working for is an independent adult. When I get accused by my daughter of interfering in her life, it's a reaction to something. And that's when I think something has gone too far.

ANGIE: How come *you* get to decide what has gone too far?

THERAPIST: (*To Angie*) Hold on a second. Gene, it sounds like you are trying to pay attention to what your daughter is saying and not get into **controlling.**

DAD: Right. I'd rather do that.

MOM: And I'd rather help Angie be clear about what she wants, because I understand how sometimes she can't be clear.

THERAPIST: Like sometimes the **anger** and **frustration** tell her no one gets what she's saying?

MOM: Right.

ANGIE: Well, they don't!

THERAPIST: Okay, Angie, I can see that's what happens for you. How do you find yourself being clear about what you want without the **anger** and **frustration** taking over?

ANGIE: Well, I don't always. I mean, they have to give me a chance.

THERAPIST: So you think that the **anger** and **frustration** have less of a chance to take over if you experience your parents doing the listening they say they're trying to do?

"Well, this is an eye-opener for me," Dad interjected. "I have very little patience with **anger** in this family. So, watching this session again, I can tell that's what I need to fight—the impatience."

"You know, after this session, I found that I could hear Angie's desires and ideas much better than before. I don't know why that was . . . Of course, I didn't always agree with her, but I didn't find myself so conflicted as I had," Mom added.

"How do you think you overcame that conflict?" asked the therapists. "We're asking that because we believe that it's mothers of daughters who most help them keep their 'voice,' and we were paying attention here to how you seemed to understand her experience from a woman's point of view."

Mom answered, "What was happening for her somehow resonated with my experience, even though I responded really differently as a young teenager, and even differently as an adult woman. But I believe she has a right to her own ideas, as do I. And I also believe Gene will appreciate that—will be able to hang in there and have the patience to hear her."

"Kind of a sense of 'entitlement,' would you say?" the therapists asked.

"For Angie?" responded Mom. "Yes, definitely. And it's good to see that."

"Me, too," said Dad. "I must admit, I have a hard time with her, but this tells me I could see it differently."

"What do you mean, Dad?" asked Angie, somewhat distrustfully. "How would you act if you 'saw it differently'?"

"Maybe you've got me there, Angie," retorted Dad. "I guess I'll have to wait and see."

"But, Gene," said Mom. "You know what 'entitlement' means. You've got it. How would it be for you to notice Angie has got it, too?"

"Yeah, Dad," joined Angie. "And what if Mom had it, too?"

"Hey," said Dad. "Okay, okay. I'll watch it."

At that point the therapists entered the conversation, suggesting that they move on to the next tape. "So what if we see what is next on the agenda?"

Carrol, Mom, and Dad[3]

Carrol was snuggled close to Mom, who had her arm around her. Dad was sitting in a nearby chair, while Danny, the younger brother, was fidgeting in another chair to Dad's left.

THERAPIST: So Carrol, what are you thinking the problem is in this family?

CARROL: It's just so *unfair*!

THERAPIST: "Unfair." What is this *unfairness*?

CARROL: I didn't say "unfairness"! I said everything is unfair; they're unfair, my teachers are unfair. They don't treat me right.

THERAPIST: Okay. So say some more about how things are "unfair." What does it look like?

CARROL: It looks awful. They make me practice the piano every day and clean up their messes. They don't make Danny do *anything*!

THERAPIST: So you feel "made" to do things? And this experience seems "unfair"?

CARROL: Yeah, well, it is!

THERAPIST: What about at school?

CARROL: They don't call on me, and I always have my hand up. So then I just call out, and they tell me to be quiet, to behave myself. Sometimes they put my name on the board and I have to stay after school. And I'm just giving them their stupid answers!

THERAPIST: So this is what you mean by "unfair" at school?

CARROL: Well, yes. Don't you get it?!

THERAPIST: I think so. Would it be at all helpful if I told you that I can see how it seems "unfair"?

[3]This fictional transcript is a composite based on several interviews with families struggling with **unfairness.**

CARROL: So?

THERAPIST: But what I'm curious about is how this **unfairness** affects you.

CARROL: What does *that* mean?

THERAPIST: Well, what happens when you experience **unfairness**? Does it get you to be angry or to say angry things, or does it instead get you to be quiet and withdraw, or maybe does it get you to be sad, or none of these things, or lots of these things?

CARROL: I'm just mad!

THERAPIST: So when that **anger** takes over, does it help you or does it make the **unfairness** get bigger?

CARROL: You're talking in puzzles.

THERAPIST: Let me try again. When **anger** gets the better of you, is that helpful or not helpful?

CARROL: Well, it doesn't work.

THERAPIST: Do you mean it doesn't make the **unfairness** go away?

CARROL: I guess.

MOM: I want to say something here.

THERAPIST: Sure, go ahead.

MOM: Sometimes Carrol and I can talk, and I understand how she feels "put upon" or "not understood," and I want to make that okay for her.

THERAPIST: Have you found a way to make that okay for her? I know, from what you've told me, that sometimes you have some conflict about that. You want her to stand her ground, to say what she means, but you also have some worries about her making it in the world.

MOM: I mean, my mother let us girls say what we thought, and I guess we didn't turn out so bad. I just want Carrol to "fit in."

THERAPIST: What would that mean—to "fit in"?

MOM: I guess be like other girls her age.

CARROL: Mom! How boring!

"Can we talk about this discussion for a minute?" asked the therapists.

"Absolutely," answered Mom. "I'm realizing here—maybe for the first time, maybe again—that I was asking something of Carrol that I hadn't even done myself: to 'fit in.' And when I said it wasn't so bad, I realized I *liked* the upbringing I had. Where my problem started was when I tried to 'fit in.' Why would I want my daughter to do that?"

"What are you saying, Mom?" Carrol said. "That it's okay to be the way I am?"

"What I'm saying, Carrol, is that it's okay to be you. I don't always think all that *anger* is okay, but I know I'll do my part to understand your point of view."

"Me, too," chimed in Dad. "I can't say I'm getting all of this, but you need to know I want to. I'm interested in you. I just don't get why you're so upset over what seems trivial to me."

"You see," said Carrol, "he just doesn't understand!"

"Can you see that he wants to?" asked Mom.

"I don't know."

"Well, maybe this is a good time for us to take a break," the therapists added. It is sounding, at least to us, that all of you have similar things you are struggling with and thinking about, and we think you have special knowledges about those things that you can share with each other. But first we'd like to invite you to listen in on our conversation, because we have some students who want to raise some questions."

A Conversation about "Voice"

STUDENT: Right you are! Here's a question for you—you seem to be focusing on what you are calling "voice." What does that mean? And what is the point here of all these mother–daughter discussions?

VICKI: We hoped it would become evident! We are following Carol Gilligan's ideas and research [Gilligan, 1982, 1990], which indicate that young girls, particularly in early adolescence, tend to "lose their voice," to "not know what they know." In other words, there seems to be a profound shift in the lives of young girls at about middle school age: They go from being easygoing and fun-loving to responding in what seem to be socially prescribed ways—that is, prescribed for how persons gendered female are supposed to respond. Many of the data of these prescriptions are transmitted through educational systems, but they are also passed down by families—by mothers and fathers who have had a lifetime of being in a relationship to the world and to each other in gender-specific ways.

STUDENT: So I noticed that most of what you talk about here focuses on daughters and mothers. What about fathers? They are seeming fairly peripheral. How do they enter in here?

VICKI: What we have found in our work with women—individually, in couples, and as mothers in families—is that they too are suffering the effects of having "lost their voice" in early adolescence. We suspect that this loss of voice is something they are struggling with in their lives, so when they come into the therapy room, we try to "unmask" some of the gender specifications for women. However, we also believe that women's loss of voice has major effects on their daughters (and sons) that somehow play into—or inadvertently cooperate with—their daughters' own experience in their early teenage years. It's not that we want to exclude mother–son relationships or father–daughter relationships; we simply wonder whether the first step in "having a voice" or "holding on to one's voice" might not be through the mother–daughter connection.

STUDENT: So what you are saying here is that daughters might be more apt to keep their voice, to be in the world in their own preferred ways, to "know they can author their own lives"—as you have said elsewhere—if their mothers not only recognize their daughters' voice, but also reclaim their own voice?

VICKI: Well said.

STUDENT: What about fathers, then?

VICKI: We keep having this discussion with each other and with fathers in families and husbands in couples, and we believe that showing respect and listening seem to be the most helpful stances for men in families to take. Our own experience with each other, and in our relationships with others in our lives, is that men need to take the first step toward opening space for women to bring forth their own ideas. And that step may be a "backing up," a waiting, a position that shows interest and respect for others' ideas. When this step is taken in conjunction with women, as wives and as mothers (particularly as we are showing here), stepping forward with their own thoughts, ideas, values—having a voice—then we think this creates a context that promotes personal agency, that promotes young girls' holding on to their voice.

FROGS AND SNAILS
AND PUPPY DOG TAILS—NOT REALLY!
What Are You Thinking, Anyway?

Larry

Larry's dad didn't know what to think. What was going on in Larry's head? He was a terrific kid, played a great first base, took apart the car and put it back together, didn't want to mow the lawn, knew every airplane that had ever been made, and was lots of fun to hang out with. But the stealing . . . why was that happening? When he asked Larry about it, Larry just shrugged and said he wanted whatever the item was, even though sometimes it was dumb stuff. Dad kept thinking, "He's a lot like I was at that age. But I never got into stealing. What is all this about, anyway?"

Then he remembered . . . he wasn't much of a "thinker" when he was Larry's age, either, and not much of a talker. He did the same old stuff, not reflecting on life, just following the plan. It had seemed to work for him. He was well trained to pursue what he wanted, and also well trained to figure that out. So when he decided to become an apprentice in a body shop when he was just out of high school, it was okay with his parents. And he'd been pretty successful. His marriage hadn't worked out, but then nothing was perfect. "When did I start to really think about my life?" Dad asked himself. "Maybe not until recently. Maybe not until we started into therapy when we all got worried about Larry's stealing."

Larry was 12 and spaced out. Whatever happened, happened. Life was okay mostly, though sometimes he was really unsettled and didn't know why. But what the heck. He couldn't do anything about it, anyway. His folks lived in separate houses. They both had gotten remarried. He couldn't care less. Thinking about it was too much trouble. In fact, he couldn't even think about thinking about it. He didn't much like school. The teachers were mean. His friends were okay; nobody better was around. He flitted from one thing to the next—whatever caught his eye. Sometimes he'd take things. He didn't know why. It was just there, so he took it.

That first day they all went to therapy, he sure didn't want to go. Then that stupid therapist wanted *everybody* there—even his stupid stepfather, plus that weird person his dad had gotten married to and her dumb daughter. He didn't want to cry when they all talked about how they worried about him, how much they loved him. The tears just came to his eyes. And then the therapist said she could see how much his family cared about him. Geez. How stupid!

Why didn't they just leave him alone? He'd be grown up in a little while, then he could drive, have a girlfriend, get a job, move out, be on his own. Then he could do what he wanted. Right? His dad had a good job; he ran his own body shop. Maybe he'd work for him, take over the shop when his dad retired. Or if he couldn't stand that, he'd just go live with some friends. They could make it. Lots of kids did. To heck with them all!

Hanging Out

"I'm sure glad you decided to hang out here with me today," Dad said, as he and Larry got ready to open up the shop for the Saturday morning customers.

"Didn't have nuthin' else to do," Larry grunted.

Dad started to think about how to help Larry think, then thought maybe he would just talk to him. "So what do you think about working here?" he asked.

"Whaddya mean?"

"Well, you're 12, so I thought you might have started thinking about what you'd like to do, and maybe working here would be one of those things."

"I dunno."

Dead end, thought Dad. I'll try something else . . . or maybe not, maybe pursue this a little bit. Asking Larry what he thinks—that's what I learned to do in therapy . . .

"So do you like working here, or not?"

Larry took a long look at him, then said, "It's okay."

"It's okay," repeated Dad. "Better than some of the other stuff you do, or worse?"

"Better, I guess," mumbled Larry.

"So are you just answering 'cause I'm asking, or are you thinking about this?"

"I'm thinking about it, I'm thinking about it," Larry said in exasperation.

Dad laughed. "Okay, okay. I just don't want you to go on 'automatic' like you used to. Remember?"

"Yeah, I 'member," he mumbled. Then he looked up from the car he had been exploring, looked straight at his dad, and said, "I bet you're talking about the stealing again, aren't you?"

"No, I wasn't thinking about that so much," answered Dad. "I was thinking about helping you get out of that **nonthinking** that we used to talk about in therapy."

"Oh, that," Larry said. "I haven't thought about that much." He laughed.

"Remember that conversation . . . when you really first turned it around?" asked Dad.

Larry's Turnaround[4]

THERAPIST: What does this mean, that your mom and dad are interested in having a party for you? Does this mean that there has been a kind of turnaround in your life?

LARRY: Yeah.

THERAPIST: Tell me about that, Larry. What's the turnaround?

LARRY: I don't know. It's just been better lately, I guess. I don't know . . .

THERAPIST: So the turnaround has to do with that there's been less . . . there hasn't been any recurrence of those **stealing habits,** right?

LARRY: No, no **stealing.**

---

[4]Much of this transcript has appeared previously in Dickerson and Zimmerman (1993), although the context here is different and the point made about **nonthinking** as a problem boys often struggle with is new.

THERAPIST: So tell me about that. How is that happening?

LARRY: I don't know.

THERAPIST: No idea?

LARRY: No.

THERAPIST: Well, I'm going to remind you about how long I've known you—it's not even two months since I first met you. Not even two months, and there has been no recurrence of these problems.

LARRY: Yeah.

THERAPIST: Doesn't this sound pretty amazing to you?

LARRY: I just haven't had it.

THERAPIST: Just haven't had it? So does that mean if the *stealing habits* started to sneak up on you, would you be able to fight them off?

LARRY: I don't know.

THERAPIST: What do you think?

LARRY: I don't know.

THERAPIST: Would you be interested in fighting them off?

LARRY: Yeah.

THERAPIST: You would? I would have guessed that. Why would you be interested in fighting them off? How would it be helpful to you?

LARRY: Pretty helpful. You know, I don't like feeling it in the first place, but sometimes it's just going to happen.

THERAPIST: Yeah, it's funny how trouble gets into somebody's life; it just sort of happens. But you're not much interested in these bad habits' continuing, are you?

LARRY: Yeah.

THERAPIST: So you'd be interested in fighting them off?

LARRY: Yeah.

THERAPIST: Larry, what do you think it is about you as a person that you aren't much interested in these bad habits continuing?

LARRY: I don't know. I just don't want them, because they got me in trouble.

"So, remember, Larry," said Dad. "At first you couldn't answer these questions much. Mostly, it was 'I don't know.' "

"Well, yeah, but that therapist sure kept after me to come up with something. The funny thing, though, was that I didn't feel pressured. I think she knew I really *didn't know* at first. She was just trying to get me to think about it. I remember the last conversation we had."

Larry and Thinking

THERAPIST: So was that the old *sneakiness* habit coming back?

LARRY: Yeah, kind of. But I don't think it was anything like a *sneakiness* habit. You know, it was just like . . . I didn't do it, like, because it was . . . 'cause I just felt I had to do it. It was like I did it because I *thought* about it.

THERAPIST: So, it wasn't because . . . although it looks like *sneakiness* . . .

LARRY: It looks like the old *sneakiness* . . .

THERAPIST: It looked like the old *sneakiness,* but it wasn't, because you *thought* about it?

LARRY: Yeah. (*Nods*)

THERAPIST: It wasn't that *nonthinking.* You were worried that you'd be punished in a way that you didn't think was right, so it was more of a decision, even though you can see now it wasn't a helpful decision?

LARRY: Yeah. (*Nods more vigorously*)

THERAPIST: So if this kind of thing were to happen again, would it be fair to say you would *think* about it, and then make a decision?

LARRY: Oh, yeah.

"So, see, Dad," said Larry. "I know how to *think!*"

Dad chuckled. "Okay, son. I remember that conversation, too. Don't forget, I was right there listening in. So just keep me posted, all right? Otherwise, I worry."

"Well, I'm not going to be perfect, you know," mumbled Larry, as he went back to polishing the car he had been working on.

Dad looked long and hard at him, finally saying, "We'll just have to keep working at it—both of us."

"Right, Dad."

Then, remembering something, Dad said, "You know that letter, the one you sent to that other kid, when our therapist suggested you might have some 'special knowledge' to pass on? She wondered if maybe *nonthinking* and a *noncaring* were somehow similar, and she asked if you would write about your struggles and your successes to—what was his name—Bret?"

"Yeah. It wasn't much of a letter."

"You don't think so? Well, Bret seemed to like it."

"I guess."[5]

---

[5]This letter is fictional, although clients do sometimes write letters to other clients.

Dear Bret,

My name is Larry. I'm 12 years old and I'm in sixth grade. I've had troubles with stealing and stuff, but I've stopped that now. We think it's because I started "thinking" about my life and about what's important to me. Our therapist told us that you were having troubles, too. I just wanted to wish you "Good luck" and to say that it might be helpful to think about what you want. It sure helped me.

Your friend,
Larry

P.S. My therapist helped me with this letter, but it's what I think!

To Care or Not To Care

Bret[6]

Jerry, Bret's dad, wondered how his son had gotten sucked in. What was it? God, he seemed so young, only 13, and having to put up with all that bullshit. Maybe it only made sense *because* he was so young, and free smokes and beer (and probably drugs too) and those girlie magazines were all just too much to say "no" to at his age. Jerry blamed himself some; after all, he was in the middle of a career change, going—really—toward something he wanted for himself, teaching instead of working in a big computer company. And, after all, they *had* discussed it as a family, and everyone agreed it was for the best. But what about the fallout: the time he didn't have to spend with his family, going to school, working an extra job, his wife taking on extra work? Did it really matter, doing what worked for you in your life when you had these other responsibilities? His son. He was important. How had all these changes affected him? Jerry blamed himself a lot. Even though Bret said it wasn't that. One thing he knew . . . he did have some responsibility for his family, his wife, his kids . . . but what did it mean?

He remembered that first therapy session, when Bret said there wasn't anything wrong with his family. He was glad to hear that. In fact, as he looked back on the whole therapy experience, there was a consistent message from Bret—that he thought his family listened to him. How important was that? Pretty important. So maybe it wasn't about him, about his choices. For sure, the therapist had focused on their resources and strengths and what worked for them and what they really wanted; that had helped him (and Jane) remember that they had already utilized some good ideas, and maybe they could pay attention

---

[6]Bret is this young man's real name. Although his story has been somewhat fictionalized, the transcript provided later is from an actual session. We've agreed that this makes him the coauthor of this part of the chapter.

to what those ideas and choices were. As parents they *did* make a difference, and paying attention to how they made things work did have better effects on all their family relationships. Plus, Bret got himself out of that bad situation he was in—and he did it himself! So, thinking back, maybe they had done an okay job. But, there was still that nagging feeling—how was it that Bret seemed to just "not care" about stuff? Had *he*, Jerry, been like that when he was 13? Was there something about being 13 and being a male child in this world, this culture? Maybe so . . . seemed like the therapist thought so . . .

Bret "couldn't care less." Life just rolled along, like roller-blading, which he loved to do. Too bad he didn't have more time for it. But then there were all those other things going on. School sucked . . . his teacher didn't care about him anyway. His older brother was a jock and wouldn't understand. His parents were okay. He liked them okay. And he had friends. But, man, what a "turn-on" it had been, to get free drugs and smokes and beer and hang out with the guys. *This* was what life must be about, this was being a *man*! But it turned out pretty bad. It didn't feel right, what Matt did . . . it felt wrong. He was glad his friend Joe called the cops. Then he got why it felt bad to him. It felt like a violation. And the cops got it. And his parents got it. And the therapist got it. But the aftereffects felt pretty terrible. He started wondering what was wrong about everything . . . school . . . the world . . . friends . . . family . . . life . . . things just didn't matter much after that. It was pretty confusing. His parents were upset. He had no idea what made sense. Maybe he could just hang out and it would all go away. Maybe . . .

Working It Out

"Remember when we talked about that philosophy, Bret, the philosophy of commitment?" Jerry asked.

"Oh, yeah. Whose idea was that, anyway?"

"Well, it seemed like you must have said it, or me or your mom. I mean, I'm bringing it up, because it seems counter to the **noncaring** we had talked about. Commitment means that you care."

"I guess."

"Oh, come on, Bret," Jerry pleaded. "Are we making this up here?"

"Nah. I just don't want to talk about it," said Bret.

"To quote a line . . . 'If not now, when?' "

"What?"

"Never mind. You wouldn't get it."

"Try me!"

"Okay. The point here is that we *need* to talk about it. This **noncaring** stuff continues to be present in your life. It's getting you to do things that makes your mom and me think that you don't mean that line about commitment, about how you care about your family, about how you know we're listening to you. It makes us think you really *don't care*! And that worries me, because the way the therapist has talked about this, you have taken big steps to overcome **noncaring,** and I guess I just don't see it. But I want to." Jerry finally stopped, realizing he was probably overwhelming Bret at this point.

Bret looked bewildered, chewing on his fingernail, then said, "Well, if that's what you think . . . "

"Oh, come on! You know what I'm talking about! You really got things to work for you for a while. Think about that! *How* did you do it?" Jerry pleaded.

"Are you trying to get me to talk?" Bret asked.

"I'm trying to get you to *think*," responded Jerry. "You know," he added, "I know something about this. I didn't think much about my life, my choices, what I wanted, until a couple of years ago. Remember when I finally decided to chuck the corporate world and go back to school and do what I *really* wanted? It wasn't too long ago, but I was in my mid-30s. I really wish I could have thought about that when I was *your* age. And not just about what I wanted to do career-wise, but what my life would look like, my responsibilities for relationships, my life partner, my kids."

"Okay, okay, Dad," Bret said. "Calm down. Give it a rest."

"Do you get this at all?"

"Well, does it fit **caring** instead of **noncaring, thinking** about things instead of a **couldn't-care-less** attitude?" Bret asked.

Jerry laughed. "I guess you get *some* of it!"

"So what are you driving at?" said Bret. "Do you think I'm not getting something? That I should be acting differently? What's the deal?"

"I don't know," Jerry responded. "When you don't talk to us, I don't know *what* you're thinking, or *if* you're thinking. That worries me."

"You want me to talk to you? Is that what you want?"

"What a novel idea!"

"Oh, come on! What do you mean?" Bret said.

"I'm kidding. The idea that you might be interested in what I want amuses me."

"So . . . ?"

"I want to know what's happening in that brain of yours," Jerry said.

"Well," Bret reminded him, "would it help if I replayed that tape from a few months ago? You seemed to think I was thinking and caring then."

"Yeah, refresh my memory," laughed Jerry.

Jerry, Jane, and Bret

THERAPIST: So, Jerry, what are you seeing in the last couple of weeks that you're seeing as going in a good direction?

JERRY: I see Bret focusing his energies mostly on more fun activities, on things that aren't really going to get him in trouble. He's enjoying himself again. He's a little bit more relaxed. He's not as uptight.

THERAPIST: Yes, I see that in here, too.

JERRY: And he listens more.

THERAPIST: I'm always curious about this. How can parents tell that their kids are listening?

JERRY: You can tell, especially when I'm talking with Bret, and he's listening and doesn't yell back and get emotional and upset . . . the temper tantrums have stopped. Jane and I talk a lot and try to reach an agreement, and we try to give him some privileges back. We see a more caring, listening individual.

THERAPIST: So it sounds like some flexibility on your part, giving some privileges back.

JERRY: Well, Bret's behavior was really good. And when you love somebody, you give in a little. Well, it wasn't really giving in . . . he earned it.

THERAPIST: So when you love somebody, it sounds like you were looking for something to appreciate.

JERRY: Well, it has become noticeable.

THERAPIST: What do you think it is about you that helped Bret to be more caring, more responsible?

JERRY: I don't think it was totally me; it was a combination of Jane and me and Bret. We all had to give in a little bit and give. It's amazing what that can start doing.

THERAPIST: It seems like everybody has to make efforts at the same time, but sometimes in families it seems like parents have to make the move first. So was that your experience, that you both took the first step?

JERRY: Yeah, well, Jane was really big on that. He's just a little kid; we have to do it first.

BRET: I'm a little kid?

JERRY: Well, compared to me, you're little.

THERAPIST: How old are you, 13? So maybe you're acting even bigger than 13. What do you think?

JERRY: Right now he is.

THERAPIST: So, Jerry, you took your cue from Jane in this.

JERRY: Well, I was being kind of stubborn, and somebody had to take the first step.

THERAPIST: Is **stubbornness** one of the things that gets you sometimes?

JERRY: (*Jerry and Jane both laugh*) I was watching myself do it and was "catching myself in the act."

THERAPIST: What did you think . . . when you gave up the **stubbornness?**

JERRY: Flexibility is a good thing. You have to listen. Kids can be right, too.

THERAPIST: So you think it's that flexibility that allowed you to hear Jane talking about taking the first step?

JERRY: I don't know exactly what it was, but I remembered that I'm older and more responsible.

THERAPIST: What do you think it was that allowed you to hear that?

JERRY: Well, we listen to each other.

THERAPIST: Sounds like "listening" is big in your family.

JERRY and JANE: Sometimes!

JERRY: We all know that we're not perfect. We're wiser to listen. We might learn something.

THERAPIST: So (*Writing*) . . . "Take the first step," and "We listen to each other." What do you think is operating now that is helping you all to stay on the right track—continuing to listen, continuing to be flexible, Bret continuing to show a more caring version of himself?

JERRY: All of us are starting to work together, so to speak. The ball is starting to roll, and it's happening more. Not that there aren't ups and downs. But the ups are increasing.

THERAPIST: If you were to say what qualities this family might have recaptured that this incident had taken away from you, what qualities would you say they were?

JERRY: I think the caring for each other.

THERAPIST: So the **caring** is overcoming the **noncaring.** Would you say it is your best weapon?

JANE: Uh-huh!

THERAPIST: So could you say a word or two about how you show caring to one another?

JERRY: How do we show caring? Pretty much hugs. We say, "I love you." Our kids say, "Bye, I love you," when they walk out the door. I think that's really good. It keeps things going.

JANE: It's also being there for each other, helping each other out.

JERRY: And Bret was gone all day today, but he called to tell us where he was, because he knew we were coming here. That shows a lot of caring and responsibility. He got on a pay phone and called us.

JANE: He seems happier.

THERAPIST: (*To Bret*) Do you think you are going in a more caring direction?

BRET: Yeah.

THERAPIST: If *noncaring* or *anger* came back in your life, do you have some idea about what you might do to fight against it?

BRET: I'm not sure.

THERAPIST: Do you have some confidence that you could fight it?

BRET: Yeah.

THERAPIST: How did you get that confidence? Did it come back with the caring?

BRET: Yeah.

THERAPIST: So you're not interested in the *noncaring* coming back?

BRET: No, it's stupid.

"So, see, Dad," Bret said. "Remember how *you* had confidence in me?"
"And you had some in yourself, too!"

The Authors Speak

Our decision to show fathers and sons conversing here (and mothers and daughters earlier) is not intended to exclude the other parent; nor does it have to do with men training men "to be a man." We also do not want to exclude other family forms. (See Weingarten, 1994, 1996, for work that addresses and challenges conventional thinking in both these cases.) Rather, what we believe is that mothers and daughters and fathers and sons all can join to challenge dominant discourses about women (their experience of subjugation and of losing their voice) and about men (their experience of "just doing it" without reflection). Also, in this last transcript, we hope that it became noticeable that although we only showed the portion with the father (and a little with the son), the parents were clearly acting together as a team—and listening to each other! Perhaps this family's special knowledge ("We listen to each other") is something we all could learn from. We could apply it in its specifics to helping girls hold on to their voice and boys catch up to thinking and caring.

We would like to add that we agree with Michael White (1992) that a boy's relationship with his mother is an important source of learning and should be embraced. Mothers can offer a picture of various ways to be that the dominant culture tries to discourage in men. In our experience, the mother–son relationship needs support, because the culture tries to encourage women to separate themselves from boys in early adolescence. At the same time, boys often begin to engage in disrespectful habits toward their mothers, perhaps beginning to practice how they are being encouraged as men to respond to women. We find that confronting this with a family, by asking the boy whether this behavior really fits his picture of how he wants to treat someone he cares about, is useful and very effective. This is particularly so if the boy is younger than 15 or 16. After that age, more work is required to help young men separate from these disrespectful habits, as boys' culture is generally very active in supporting these dominant notions of masculinity.

We can likewise make a similar argument for the father–daughter relationship. As the father of girls, I (Jeff) feel I can play an important role in encouraging a sense of voice with my daughters. I hope that I will be able to put aside any dominant-culture-shaped male reactions as they begin to assert themselves in what *they* want as they get older. As a daughter, I (Vicki) experienced my relationship with my father as one in which he encouraged my having my own ideas, and supported me in this regard—at a time when girls growing up had severely limited options. For girls to hold on to what they know, to speak their voice, and to have their fathers support them in ways that usually only boys are supported will continue to counter the dominant culture's more "usual" ways that girls are encouraged to be.

We end this chapter and this section hoping that you, our readers, have enjoyed your time with these clients. We plan to pull this all together in the next section, extending our conversation to include our students, and finally letting you know again what we hope for you in this experience.

PART III

Bringing It All
Back Home

CHAPTER 11

When Students Talk
A Different Experience
of Training and Supervision

The Authors Speak

Listen to our students . . .

DAY 1

I'm Linda. I'm not sure when I decided to take the plunge and sign up for Vicki and Jeff's intensive.[1] I had gone to some workshops in their Narrative Workshop Series, had read a few articles, and had tried to comprehend Michael White and David Epston's 1990 book. All of this was done in an attempt to get caught up with my students. As a clinician and supervisor at a community mental health agency, I work with lots of interns from the surrounding graduate programs. Many of them are coming in with narrative ideas, having been exposed to narrative thinking and practice in classes that Vicki and Jeff teach in the universities in the area. I was finding that the interns' ideas didn't fit very well within my frame of reference, which was basically a systems approach with a developmental theory background. However, I was also finding their ideas somewhat intriguing. They were nonpathologizing, respectful of the

---

[1]We offer week-long intensives in narrative therapy during the summer months at our training center, Bay Area Family Therapy Training Associates.

client, full of curiosity, and somehow challenging of oppressive practices. This represented a position that I pride myself on taking. However, I was noticing that narrative work seemed to reflect these ideas more clearly. But I am getting ahead of my story.

Starting Out

I was a little nervous. There were 10 of us in the intensive, some I had heard of, others I didn't know at all. We must have all looked a little scared. But I figured that at least I'd get caught up on the theory. Some of what I had read was so confusing, so dense. The terms were unfamiliar to me: "discourse," "deconstruction," "gender specifications," "subjugating practices." I felt like I needed a glossary. And "externalizing"—I wasn't at all sure how that worked; it seemed like a useful technique, but so what? Vicki and Jeff suggested we do a quick introduction—our names, where we were from—and said that part of the rest of the day's work would include a longer introduction. As we went around the room, it was interesting: There were people from as far away as Tennessee and Minnesota and Canada, as well as us local folks; there were a couple of intern therapists, and also some very experienced clinicians, trained in various approaches. Jeff and Vicki gave a quick overview of the week, saying that the day would start with a narrative interview (whatever that meant), and the rest of the week would include some live interviews with clients, an opportunity for all of us to be members of a reflecting team, and a series of exercises to help us experience a way of thinking and get some practice in the work. It was sounding overwhelming to me. I was wishing I could fade into the woodwork, and now it seemed like I would have to participate actively. Well, I was the one who had decided to come here. I might as well bite the bullet and make it happen.

A Narrative Interview

Vicki and Jeff started by saying they were going to ask each of us some questions—things like "What was it about the narrative approach that appealed to us?" and "What was it about our life experience that attracted us to this way of thinking?" and "What did we hope to come away with in this week?" They also organized us into two groups, one of which would act as a reflecting team for the people in the first round of interviews. The directions for the people on the reflecting team were to pay attention to the "preferred developments" for each interviewee, and then to raise questions about those developments. Jeff and Vicki said they'd help. This was pretty confusing so far. I was thinking they should just start the interviews, and then maybe it would be clearer. One of the women who was a therapist in a residential treatment center volunteered to be interviewed first. She responded to the opening questions by saying that she . . . well, I'll let her words speak for themselves.[2]

JILL: In my life I have taken an activist position, seeing myself as someone who wanted to be an agent of social change. I have also positioned myself within the feminist critique, so continuing to notice oppressive practices and to bring forth voices of liberation has been important to me.

JEFF: How do you see this "activist position" and situating yourself within the "feminist critique" as having to do with narrative ideas?

JILL: I understand narrative as a way of viewing persons and problems differently. I'm not sure I could put into words how it does that. That's why I'm here. I really want to understand more about locating problems in their sociopolitical context.

VICKI: What do you think it is about you as a person or about your life experience that contributes to your interest in narrative?

JILL: Well, I'm not sure. Maybe it has to do with an experience in which I continually felt that my ideas, and my mother's ideas, were valued. And I noticed that this wasn't generally the case in the world. So I began to question how people's experience gets constructed. I see narrative therapy as also doing that—you know, challenging dominant discourse.

The interview continued in this vein for a few more minutes. I began to relax, thinking this was really interesting, even though Jill was using some of those words I wasn't sure I understood. I also began to wonder how I might answer similar questions. I was noticing that it wasn't as hard as I thought it might be to pick up preferred developments. It certainly seemed that Jill was pleased with her way of thinking, and I began to be curious about what I heard her say about how her thinking had evolved toward narrative ideas. However, again I am getting ahead of myself. I was in the first group, so I decided to go next.

LINDA: I'm really attracted to what I think is narrative "theory," although I'm not sure I could say what that theory is. What I do know is that it is respectful of the client—that this approach is one that believes that clients have their own answers.

JEFF: Could you say more about how you came to this position yourself?

LINDA: Well, I'm not sure I know. Actually, I've always struggled to "fit in." I experienced a lot of pressure in my life to do that, and it has

---

[2]All of these transcripts are fictionalized.

been hard for me to resist that pressure. Maybe that's why I want to be respectful of others.

JEFF: Resistance is an important value to you?

LINDA: I guess you could say that.

JEFF: What qualities do you think you have as a person that have contributed to your interest in resisting certain societal pressures?

LINDA: Well, I'm not sure I know. I know that I connect a lot with the teenagers I work with. I love the renegades and the resisters.

JEFF: Would you say that one quality you might have is a "strong will"? I say that, because in my experience with women who are resisting *evaluation,* they talk about their strong-mindedness, their strength of will.

LINDA: (*Laughing*) That fits for me.

VICKI: Jeff, can I ask you a question? You said something to Linda about why you were suggesting a certain quality. I know we call that "situating" your question. Will you say something about how that is important?

JEFF: Well, by situating, I was saying where my thinking was coming from. I had come up with a possibility that may or may not fit for Linda. In order to create a "reflexive" position for her—one in which she could consider whether or not this idea fit for her—I said something about what my experience was that supported this possibility.

VICKI: And we are going to ask members of the reflecting team to do the same thing. (*Turning to the group*) You all might pay attention to how we try to do that and help each other do that. When we ask a question, we will often say why we are asking it, from our experience, or our fantasy, or our own philosophies.

My mind was reeling. I was learning something about myself that I quite liked, while at the same time I was learning about a way of asking questions that opened spaces for people to consider what was preferred by them. How could this all go on simultaneously? I was feeling great by the end of my interview. At the same time, I was wanting to sit back and watch and listen to the other interviews so that I could consider what was happening. I also could hardly wait for the questions of the reflecting team.

The Reflecting Team: A First Go-Round

The interviews of the first group (five of us) had taken a couple of hours. The other five (the reflecting team) then went into the mirrored room, while those of us who had been interviewed observed. We were asked to pay attention to what was helpful or not helpful among the comments and questions to be raised. Vicki stayed with us, while Jeff went into the room with the reflecting team. He started by saying:

JEFF: I'm here to help you all. Mostly, what I will do is ask you to "situate" your questions. If you would like, I can also help you take what you are noticing and put it into a question. So does anybody have any questions for anyone? We should probably focus on one person at a time.

LARRY: Well, I have a question for Linda. I heard her say something about answers coming from within, or that clients have their own answers. I wondered where she got that idea and how it was a helpful one for her to hold on to as a therapist.

JEFF: Is there something from your personal experience that tells you it might be helpful for Linda to be able to know about that?

LARRY: Well, I use a lot of guided imagery in my work, so I guess I believe that clients have answers, too, or I wouldn't work that way.

JEFF: So perhaps you are wondering how that idea is helpful to Linda in the way she works with clients?

LARRY: Yeah, that, too.

SHARON: I found myself admiring what I saw as a certain rebelliousness, which seems counter to a prescription to "fit in." I wondered, as Linda moved toward more of a "rebel" position in her life, how she might create a community that would support that position.

JEFF: How is it that the notion of "rebelliousness" stood out for you, and why do you think it is important for Linda to think about creating a community of support?

SHARON: Well, I'm a rebel, I guess, and sometimes I find that people around me don't think very highly of that rebellious quality, so I struggle myself with finding support.

JEFF: So you think that thinking about the structure of that community might be helpful to Linda—who would be in that community, how would she know like-minded persons, and so on?

SHARON: Definitely.

MARY: I wondered about what future areas of resistance Linda might find for herself and how she would use her strong will to appreciate the resistance.

JEFF: Are you thinking about how she would use her strong will for herself?

MARY: Oh, yes! I say that because in my own life, the strong will was taken over from me in the past by practices of "fitting in" and "going along with"—not unlike what Linda said. So to consider where I might use my strong will to fight for what *I* want has been really helpful!

Can you imagine what this was like? To sit behind the mirror and listen to persons raising questions for me about my life, my preferences? I felt like a fly on the wall, a mouse in the corner: I was eavesdropping on a conversation about *me*! But the best thing of all is that it didn't matter if it fit or not, because *I* got to decide. For example, that thing about "rebelliousness" didn't really fit, because I couldn't see myself going that far. But it did help to think about creating a community of support. The biggest thing that stuck out for me was using my strong will for myself. I commented on that when we switched places with the team.

VICKI: I'm curious what fit for you all. What was helpful or not helpful?

LINDA: I loved it! It was just like being a fly on the wall. I remember once when I was a teenager and went to camp, they had a weird process where the camp counselor met with a group of kids and sent one of the kids away while the rest talked about that person. We never got to hear what was said, and we never got any feedback from it. It felt awful. This was such a different experience. People were so respect-ful. They asked questions, which helped me think about what I had said, and even what I hadn't said but was a raising of possibilities.

VICKI: Anything in particular you want to comment on? It might be helpful for the team to hear which of their questions fit best for you or if any missed the point. This way, they can understand better how what they say has real effects on their clients.

LINDA: Oh, okay. It wasn't too helpful when Sharon mentioned "rebel-liousness," because I hadn't talked about myself that way at all. I don't see myself like that. But I did hear that she was coming from her own perspective there.

VICKI: You mean when she situated her question?

LINDA: Yeah! It was helpful to me, however, when she talked about creating a community of support, because I think I've always been fearful that if I didn't "fit in" there wouldn't be anybody who would like me.

VICKI: So it seemed possible to you that you could create a community of like-minded people?

LINDA: Yes, definitely. I also liked it a lot when I heard the question about my using my strong will for myself.

VICKI: Rather than *pressure* taking it and using it against you?

LINDA: Yeah.

The rest of the day went like this. It felt like time stood still. It was so rich and powerful. We all got to experience it. I was exhausted by the end of the day, but it was work well worth it. Then Vicki and Jeff gave us three articles to read [Dickerson & Zimmerman, 1992, 1993; Dickerson, Zimmerman, & Berndt, 1994]. (They actually had sent us two articles [Zimmerman & Dickerson, 1994b, 1995] before the week started to get us going on the theory.) The three articles had to do with adolescents, because the case the next day was going to be with a young woman, and then Jeff was going to see a family on Wednesday. They said tomorrow they'd start with questions about the reading or questions in general, and then we'd see a live interview. What a day!

The Authors Speak

We have evolved our intensives toward providing experiences for attendees. In the past, we did didactic presentations and spent a great deal of time on theoretical discussions. Despite my (Jeff's) enjoyment of this, and despite its being my preferred learning style, we both (Jeff and Vicki) realized that this wasn't true for most people. It was easy to get lost in these conversations, and we noticed that abstract ideas seemed to relate little to people's experience. We also realized that narrative therapy is a therapy of experience, and that teaching it must therefore involve creating experience as well. To stay in a propositional domain (ideas, thoughts, theories, etc.) when teaching a therapy of experience began to make little sense. Yes, to do this work you need a coherent conceptual and theoretical framework. But how best to get it? There are books and articles that address the theory, and yet we have gotten feedback from many people that they don't "get it" that way. We imagine that they are saying it is difficult to enter into these writings with their experience. What we hope to do in our training is to create experiences that the trainees can then connect to a conceptual framework. In other words, we use the experiences to help generate alternative knowledges, much of which will come from the trainees' new conclusions. Clearly, this is similar to client work—in which we notice experiences in a person's life that aren't being attended to, and we ask questions to provoke meaning. Working with clients in this manner is a focus on experience, which becomes the "stuff" of new narratives. Once people have experience of alternative possibilities or knowledges, they begin to fill in the new narratives themselves by attending to different experiences and by making new meaning of their experiences. For trainees, this may mean going back to the reading and seeing whether it now makes more sense. The direction goes from experience to theory. When we talk about why we have written the preceding chapters the way we have, this is what is influencing us. We hope this book has created an experience for you, our readers, that is more evocative of your own experience then it might have been if we had presented the material didactically.

Now for the specifics up to this point. What better way to start out a training in narrative therapy than to create a personal experi-ence for each attendee of what it is like to be interviewed in this manner and to have one's own life thought about from this perspec-tive? It also provides an opportunity for the two of us to ask a wide variety of narrative questions in context, as opposed to just reviewing a list of possibilities with the group. When we do the second set of interviews (after the first group is finished), we often stop and label the questions—why they are so labeled, why we picked this particu-lar question, and what we hope the question might be accomplishing. Thus, attendees have the experience of how preferred developments in their lives might be responded to (and the effects of this process); an experience of how questions might be used (and many examples of questions); and a sense of what it is like to have an audience of other professionals respond to these developments.

Using a reflecting team on the first day is a new development for us. We were a bit nervous about it, as *fear* told us that professionals, without training, would pathologize or ask interpretive questions or connect what was being said to the theories they carried around about people or families. We decided to try it anyway, knowing that one of us would be with the team to keep the direction of questions going toward preferred developments. Our experience also told us that when comments on the team are situated, then the person whose life is being spoken about has a greater opportunity to choose whether the comments fit for him or her. If the comments or questions seem to come from a position of truth or greater knowledge and are left unsituated, this is often what is concluded, particularly if the person speaking is one who has been assigned a position of power or authority within the culture. I (Jeff) often tell beginning teams that if their comments or questions seem to come from a pathologizing theory or from normative social judgments, I will ask them to situate it ex-tremely in their own fantasies. One training possibility that emerges from this process is that the persons experiencing the reflecting team can let the team members know what effect their questions have had, and they will do this more directly than many clients will. One thing we have learned in doing this is to instruct team members that the experience of the person whose story they are raising questions about is privileged (just as the clients' experience is privileged in therapy), and that any negative effects are to be understood and responsibility

for them taken by the questioner—rather than analyzed or interpreted. A reflecting team guideline, handed out after the experience,
serves as a useful summary.

DAY 2

Hi! My name is Philip. I'm going to pick up the narrative at this point,
mostly so you'll get both gendered views. Linda suggested I give you an
overview of the live client interviews, rather than just jumping into how
the second day started. I thought that was a good idea—wish I'd thought
of it myself—so most of what I'm going to say next is a result of Linda's
and my discussion. We couldn't believe how Jeff and Vicki could get such
a wide variety of interviews scheduled. Obviously you can't show everything, and maybe what they brought forth in the interviews is really what
the narrative approach is about, but nonetheless . . . The first interview
was with a young woman (aged 23, I think) who had been struggling with
anxiety and the *pressures* that lots of young people face in terms of what
to do, how to live their lives, how to decide. Vicki worked with her, and
I'll talk more about that shortly. Then on the third day, Jeff saw a young
woman (in her middle teens) who was struggling with *bulimia.* They gave
us a useful article to read about that [Zimmerman & Dickerson, 1994a],
and the interview was really helpful. The same afternoon, Jeff also saw a
family with two young boys, 11 and 15. It was a first-session interview, so
we got to see a lot about problem construction and how to do that in a
family setting. Then on the fourth day, Vicki saw a couple (more articles
for us to read [Zimmerman & Dickerson, 1993a, 1993b])—one that
represented a "blended" family, in which some of the problems centered
around dealing with the children from the husband's first marriage. The
great thing about that interview was that it brought out problems of
violence and its effects—in this case, the emotional abuse that the wife
was suffering from the adolescent son, and the husband's responsibility
in regard to that. I learned some important things to pay attention to
from this case: entitlement; violence and its effects; responsibility; men's
appreciation of women's experience. It was powerful.

So, back to our narrative. You might wonder how we had time to do
anything but see interviews and be on reflecting teams. Actually, that
might have been enough in some ways; however, as I look back at the
week, I think that it wouldn't have all hung together so well without the
exercises. These created an experience for me that affected my thinking
surprisingly. We started the second day with some questions from the
reading or any questions we had from the prior day's experience. What
Vicki and Jeff mostly did was simply record our questions, indicating that

they thought most would be answered in the course of the week. An example was "How do you decide what to externalize?", which they said would probably be answered with the live interviews. Another example was "What is the difference between landscape-of-action and landscape-of-consciousness questions?" They actually had interrupted the interview process occasionally the previous day and pointed out the kind of question they were asking, but they said we would get a chance to do more of this in an exercise later in the week. Another interesting question had to do with "Is narrative therapy a systems therapy?" They said "No," and again they thought the exercises would help us see this.[3] I would have liked a more theoretical conversation, but understood Jeff and Vicki's intent to keep this training experience-based. There were some clarification questions from the reading, and some discussion of what certain passages meant; here again, this could easily have led to more thorough theoretical discussions, but we had a client coming, so I'll talk about that next. One other thing happened here: Vicki and Jeff also gave us a handout about reflecting teams, reviewing the process.[4] Because we had been on teams the day before, they didn't go over it much with us except to remember to watch for "unique outcomes" and "preferred developments" as we observed the interview.

I had read a draft of Chapter 6 of this book, so I had some idea of how a narrative approach can be powerful in working with persons struggling with *anxiety,* but it was more powerful seeing it in action. It was remarkable that this was only Vicki's 10th session with this young woman. The problem was severe, and there had been many developments. What was helpful was hearing the review of the work, which I gathered Jeff and Vicki typically do when they see a client with a reflecting team. They catch us up to the work in the client's presence; it seems to me that this must also have a helpful effect on the client, who can thus notice his or her own progress in front of an audience. In this case the problem was *anxiety,* but Vicki and Annie (the client) had called it the *second-guessing voice.* That seemed like an interesting name, so we asked Vicki about it later, and she said it came out of an early discussion with Annie. The name seemed very helpful, because it clearly had effects of *anxiety* and *anger,* both of which could be looked at separately in terms of further effects. But calling the problem the *second-guessing voice* also

---

[3]In addition to the exercises described here, there is another one we sometimes use (see Dickerson & Zimmerman, 1995).

[4]See Appendix A for this handout. It is a combination, revision, and recreation of other handouts we have seen—specifically, one Michael White has distributed at the Dulwich Centre, and also one that our colleague John Neal devised for the MRI Narrative Therapy Externship.

showed how the culture was encouraging the problem through *pressures* Annie was experiencing in regard to "growing up" (i.e., what young people call "having a life," including an education, a career, a relation-ship—and having all these things in highly specified ways). I guess this was what was most helpful in seeing this client first, because we came to understand how "externalizing" has to do with capturing the client's experience, but in a way that also captures the sociopolitical specifica-tions. (I can't believe I'm talking like this.)

It was also a helpful case to have a first experience (not counting the first day) of being on a reflecting team—with a client. There were lots of developments that we could raise questions about and that Jeff could help us situate. Also, Annie was pleased with the process and commented on our remarks in ways that let us know how helpful a reflecting team can be. We asked her and Vicki whether we could include a little of the transcript of the reflecting team and Annie's remarks here.

Annie's Voice

Reflecting Team for Annie

TEAM MEMBER 1 (TM$_1$): There was a phrase that Annie used—"non-action realization." It made me wonder about what qualities Annie has that allows her to use the "nonaction realization" in situations where the *anxiety* is trying to get her to use her "bad bag of tools." I was particularly struck by the "nonaction" part of the phrase, think-ing about situations where it is sometimes helpful to "not act." For myself, being someone who has to fix things and "act," that was an interesting phrase for me—so I was wondering about Annie's ability to access that.

TM$_2$: As a "piggyback" off that, another phrase I was interested in was that she realized she was beginning to "trust less" her emotional state as being forever. I think that's a neat thing to realize, and I'd be interested in the steps it took to get there—just as a personal curiosity, because that has taken me a long time to figure out. So, what are the steps . . .

TM$_3$: She was talking about her strengths versus *anxiety's* strengths . . . as she has let go of *anxiety's* grip, what of her own strength has she put in its place? What new dialogue . . .

JEFF: You mean what is she saying to herself?

TM$_3$: More, I wonder, how does she access her strength? Is it by saying it to herself? Or is it by a memory? How, in the face of this huge emotion, does she access that memory?

JEFF: Oh, I see, like how does she access that knowledge?

TM$_3$: Right.

JEFF: And why were you interested?

TM$_3$: Because for me that would be a really hard thing to do—to access that knowledge in the face of the huge emotion, the old pattern.

TM$_4$: I was intrigued by how her view of strength seems to be evolving. She talked about how previously she saw strength as "I can take it," "I can handle it," "I can stick with it," sort of to prove she was strong. Now she seems to have moved to feeling sometimes it's stronger to "not do." I wonder, a year from now, how she imagines it might go from here. I'm interested because I'm trying to evolve toward these other definitions that are really counter to our culture and counter to how we've been brought up to think.

JEFF: Are you interested in—if she continued in this direction, what specific ways that might look? And that's fitting your own attempts as well?

TM$_4$: Yes, and I was also intrigued by her tools. One was a "mindless focusing" and the other was "nonaction realization."

[Later:]

JEFF: I have a question for the women in the room. I hear from a lot of women that focusing on what a woman needs and wants, rather than focusing on what others or what the world says that women should focus on, is quite a hard shift, and I noticed that Annie had taken some important steps in that direction. I was curious if the women in the room would say something about that shift—its difficulties, its usefulness potentially—from your own experience.

TM$_1$: Sort of being able to listen to one's own voice and not being overwhelmed by those other voices?

TM$_4$: Well, for myself there's always this constant dialogue that if I'm doing something for myself, then it must be selfish or self-centered. So I have to wonder what are the benefits of sticking with that. But it is always a dialogue.

JEFF: How do you deal with how **guilt** gets thrown in the way by men who might be oblivious to what women want, by parents, by kids who want what they want? How do you hold on to your wants in the face of those strong invitations to give them up?

TM$_2$: I have in mind a "fighter"—like Peter Pan. It actually comes into my mind that someone comes in to help me—it's actually part of me, but I still think of her as coming in to help me. I visualize it, and I've had to practice it, but it helps.

TM₁: For me, what's really important is my support group, my team. When I'm feeling overwhelmed by **guilt** and **shoulds** and feeling **not okay** and giving in to all those voices and demands and expectations, I have a group of friends and people that I can turn to where I can create a space for my own voice to get stronger again. So that's important for me. The emotional feeling I get that they care about me silences the **guilt** long enough that I can hear my own voice.

JEFF: I have one more question. I was paying attention to this list, this rather long list, that got developed in here in Vicki's conversation with Annie. A lot of developments have occurred, like she's able to give herself permission to do what she wants—to take care of herself emotionally in these phone conversations, rather than feel like she has to take care of the person on the phone. She's able to resist the "you should be strong enough to take care of others" voice; she feels stronger actually if she takes care of herself (I thought that was way beyond a 23-year-old realization). Also, she was easing up on herself; she was not stuck in one way of emotionally responding; she sees that things will go away, that she doesn't have to fight so hard, that she can let go; she has thrown out these bad tools; she has discovered these "nonaction realizations" (which I thought was another thing that was way ahead of a 23-year-old realization); she wants to pull away and has some ideas about how to handle some tough situations with her parents (even though they're hard to do, she has some ideas about how to do it); and she has confidence building and know-how in the end of things. I guess my question is—you know, my reaction as a man is that I don't know what to make of those things completely—so I'm curious: For the women in the room, would you say those were small steps along the way, big steps, medium steps? I'm sitting here imagining that this was more than what might be usual for a 23-year-old, but I don't have the experience that the women might have, so I'm curious. Where would you put those developments?

TM₁: *Big* steps.

TM₃: *Huge* steps.

JEFF: Like . . . what?

TM₂: Like age?

JEFF: Yes, like where did you run into taking those steps?

TM₂: I'm not sure I've gotten them all yet. Maybe like late 30s, early 40s.

TM₁: Yes, certainly some of them mid-30s, and some of them I'm still struggling with personally in my 40s.

JEFF: That was my sense, but I didn't want to guess . . .

Annie's Response

VICKI: So what in particular was interesting to you, or helpful to you, or not helpful?

ANNIE: It seems a question that kept arising was, when I'm feeling a lot of things, how do I access my mind? It seems like it came up a lot. And it comes up a lot with you. And it's a question you keep asking and it's hard to answer, because it's hard to get back to that space. So I just think it's interesting that it comes up, and I think it's really an important question.

VICKI: Uh-huh . . . Why do you think it's an important question?

ANNIE: Because it's that transition that everyone needs to work on. It's something that can save you.

VICKI: Like knowing about it—what you access, what you do—would be a helpful thing, because you're more apt to access it, you think?

ANNIE: Yeah, you could make a career out of it! Write it down on a piece of paper.

VICKI: (*Laughing*) You could write a book!

ANNIE: Yes. Do this! It's kind of like the miracle that saves you . . .

[Later:]

ANNIE: It was also helpful to me to hear how I can do this better now than before. I have ideas, and I have all the stuff around it.

VICKI: When you figure this out and you market it and sell it, would you test it first on this group and on me?

ANNIE: (*Laughs*) Well, maybe it's just me.

VICKI: It probably is somewhat idiosyncratic to you, but I suspect you might know some things that would be helpful to others, to women especially.

ANNIE: That was one of the other things that was really great to hear—I'm as smart as a 40-year-old! (*Smiles*) That was a good way to end it.

VICKI: (*Laughs*)

ANNIE: Because we've talked a lot about being a woman, and being weighted down by *pressures,* feeling like nothing I was doing was right, and the *guilt* and stuff.

VICKI: Yeah, those *expectations* hang out.

Well, there was more, but this seems like a lot to digest in retrospect. So let me summarize. Several things became clear to me:

1. I could understand better what got "externalized" and why.
2. I understood the power of the reflecting team—how it "thick-ened" a preferred story for a client, serving both as an audience and as a process for opening reflexive space for the client.
3. I saw why situating one's question is so important: It allows the client to pick and choose what fits for him or her.
4. I began to notice what Jeff and Vicki were noticing with their clients—how they picked up the "gaps"; how they focused on antiproblem strategies; how they pursued preferred develop-ments; and how they remained transparent to the client (and to us) about why they were asking what they were asking, doing what they were doing. I also noticed how they brought in the sociopolitical dimension, paying attention to gender, specifically with Annie—*her* voice, rather than how the culture often en-courages women to be in ways that are not helpful to them. And, finally, I observed how they pay attention to race and ethnicity; in this case, Jeff realized how it might be important to Annie, as a young Asian-American woman, to be seen and respected as someone older and wiser than her chronological age.

In short, this was a good case to start with. I wondered what was in store for the afternoon.

The Problem Exercise[5]

We started the afternoon with Jeff and Vicki suggesting we think about a problem that we could "play" and that we could interview. We weren't sure what they meant. They then said that it might be helpful if we picked a problem that we had some experience with—not just with clients, but personally. Everyone looked around nervously. Someone said, "How

[5]This exercise was originally designed by Sallyann Roth and David Epston (1996). We use our own variation. We have found it the single most helpful exercise for helping trainees appreciate the epistemological shift that we believe the narrative approach represents.

about *procrastination?*" We all laughed and commented that many of us had experience with that problem, but then we decided it wasn't probably something clients would be dealing with in therapy. "How about a bigger problem, a well-known one—like *depression* or *anxiety?*" someone said. Vicki agreed that such a problem might be better, as long as we stayed with our experience of how the problem attacked us personally. She said something about how the mental health culture has taken people's experience (say, of sadness) and turned it into this thing we now all commonly refer to as *depression.* I wasn't sure what she meant by that, but we all agreed to try *depression.* Vicki said she would like to play the problem, because she thought she had some experience with it, and she asked a couple of us to join her. Jeff would join the rest of the group in questioning *depression.* I wanted to try my hand at being the problem, but I wasn't sure I had a lot of experience with *depression* as such. Vicki commented that this particular problem seems to look a little different with men, but it would probably be helpful to have both versions. One of the other women in the group also joined us.

Someone started with this question "Could you describe yourself to us?" I had no idea what to say. Vicki responded, "Well, I take on different descriptions for different people, but often people say they experience me as a big, black, heavy blob that oozes into everything and takes over their lives." Wow. "How do you do that?" another person asked. No one said anything for a minute. Then the other trainee said, "I hang out all the time and just wait for the opportunity to get into people's lives." Vicki added, "I am extremely subtle and sneaky; I lie in wait, and when things seem to go a little awry for people, I'm there. I get them to feel really bad. I sometimes get them to blame themselves." So then Jeff asked, "What do you get people to tell themselves?"

It went on like this for a while. I thought I wouldn't be able to respond. I tried once. I said, "Well, I feel really terrible, like my life is going to end," and Vicki asked me, "Are you talking from the perspective of *depression* or from the perspective of someone who is experiencing *depression?*" I shook my head. I couldn't quite get it. What was I supposed to do? Jeff prompted, "You sound a little like a person who is feeling 'depressed.' Could you try it again and see if you could speak *as depression?*" "Okay, okay," I said. "I make people feel like their lives are going to end, like they might not want to live any more." "Great," Jeff said. "You've got it now." (This isn't so easy. We had to act like the problem is a real thing. I realized how comfortable I had been with the notion that the problem was me—or a part of me. Who said the problem was me?) After a while, the questions got even harder. They were asking how I (as *depression*) acted differentially on men and on women. They wanted to know whether there was a particular age group I worked on. They were interested in what things from the culture supported my existence. They were curious about the various effects I had on people's lives. I (as Philip) began to realize how powerful I (as *depression*) was and how the culture of therapy has really thickened this problem. I (as Philip) was ready to stop this exercise.

When we all talked about it afterward, the two of us who had been *depression* (along with Vicki) said how difficult it was at first to stay in the role of the problem, but how helpful it became as we really began to experience the problem as separate from people. The rest of the group (those who had been involved in asking the questions) commented on the rich variety of questions they felt they could ask as they became more and more curious about this problem, how it operates on people, and what it uses from the culture to get so powerful. We decided to do it one more time in the whole group, with other people being the problem; then we went into two groups of five and did a couple of rounds, so everyone would have an experience of being the problem.

I can't tell you how exactly it became clear to me, but I realized then what it meant to say that narrative therapy sees problems as residing in the meaning people give to their experience—meaning that is encouraged by cultural discourses. I was pretty weary at this point. We had an hour left in the afternoon, so we started another exercise. But I'm going to bow out here. Linda will describe it with the next day's activities.

The Authors Speak

We'd like to comment on a number of different aspects that Philip attended to on this day. First, we'll address our choice in "not answering" questions. (Actually, I [Jeff] can't resist answering *some* questions, and I [Vicki] prefer to stay with nondidactic experiences. We agree that maybe it is, as Eddie put it in Chapter 7, a "gender thing.") Our preference for a narrative metaphor leads us away from what Bruner (1986) has called a propositional domain of thought and into a narrative one. Questions that lead to didactic or theoretical discussions tend to expand and take up time and space in the training. One effect is that many people are left out, as they do not relate well to these types of conversations. Instead, we like to take notes on what our attendees are asking about, and to look for opportunities to come back to the questions when we are doing an exercise or seeing a live interview. These questions help us know what to attend to and what to label for the attendees. This also helps us pace our comments along the lines of their experience.

We believe that teaching this work involves creating exercises/experiences for the attendees personally, as well as modeling/experiencing the work via live interviews. Without the live

BRINGING IT ALL BACK HOME

interviews, students have no real picture of the process. We appreciate Michael White's (1989–1990) comments about watching and imitating, and agree with him (referring to Geertz, 1986) that "it is in the copying that we originate." This has certainly been our personal experience. The opportunity to watch experienced narrative therapists do the work helps trainees notice some of the possibilities. As this also involves participating on a reflecting team, an opportunity is created to ask questions and see what effect they have on the rest of the team and on the client. Since the two of us usually work together, one of us can then do the interview and the other can assist the reflecting team. We question the team members about their questions, asking them to situate them, as we have discussed previously. We also help them formulate questions on the spot (if they want help). We do this by soliciting the observations they want to ask about and then helping them turn their comments into questions. With very inexperienced participants, or those coming from very different perspectives, we may carefully interview the team members about developments we noticed and ask whether they noticed them too. Did these developments stand out for them, and if so, why? This allows them to respond along the lines of the guidelines we have developed. For clients who agree to participate in this process, we provide videotapes for them so that they can review the sessions at home if they wish. They are approached collaboratively, even as part of the teaching; we encourage them to comment on the team's comments, both for their own benefit and for that of the team. Each client is invited to stay when a session is finished, to hear our discussion with the attendees about the interview. We offer no information about clients unless they are present, and any review that we do in front of them is subject to their editorial comments.

As we have mentioned in footnote 5, our experience is that the problem exercise provides a context that often becomes a turning point in people's understanding of the ideas we are teaching. The direct experience of the shift from the problem's being a person or existing in a person to the problem's being separate from a person and shaped by the various discourses that influence a person seems invaluable. Without it people don't really seem to "get" the difference. We also use this exercise to begin to "unmask" the invisible constructions that shape our experience. These include gender, race, social class, and heterosexual dominance, as well as constructions that come from psychology and the so-called social sciences. For therapists, these may involve professional specifications such as "You, the therapist, are solely responsible for the client to get better," and "The work is done between you and the client(s) only." These specifications shape therapists' experience and constrain their behavior; this further contributes to "problems" that affect therapists' attitudes toward their work. When we do the problem exercise with therapists about such problems as *evaluation* and *overresponsibility,* then these problems tell us how they use professional specifications to operate on therapists. This is similar to how *depression* may use performance expectations for men in the culture or how *anxiety* may tell someone of a lower social class, "You must be inadequate. You won't be able to perform like others." We also use this exercise to help people notice more behavioral tactics that problems employ, how problems get hold of relationships and pit people against each other, what problems get people to conclude, and so on. Finally, we are most enthusiastic at the opportunity this exercise provides to help "unmask" the cultural context that supports problems.

DAY 3

Hi, Linda here. We started the next exercise at the end of the second day, partly because we had time, but partly because it flowed really well from what we had just done. We met briefly and talked about "effects" questions, and then we went into small groups (three or four people per group) and asked "effects" questions of someone who was experiencing a problem. We were asked to present an already externalized problem. This was the first part of a two-part exercise that we did at separate times, but they fit together in a structured interview process that Vicki and Jeff described to us.

Structure and Sample Questions for a Narrative Interview[6]

After having done the problem exercise, it was fairly easy to ask "effects" questions of people who were experiencing a problem. I volunteered to be the one interviewed, because I had a fairly circumscribed problem that I thought I could present in an already externalized way. It was *frustra-tion*—mostly about how I was getting caught in difficult situations at work. When the trainees in our group began to question me, it didn't seem much different from how I've experienced other interviews, because at first they weren't using externalizing language. They'd say things like "When do you most get frustrated?" or "Do you get more frustrated in

[6]See Appendix B.

some situations than in others?" Part of my job as the interviewee was to let people know the effects their questions were having on me. I wasn't shy about saying that their questions were making me feel "frustrated"! I told them they weren't acting like the problem was the problem. Finally, someone said, "How is *frustration* affecting you?" That was pretty straightforward, and it clearly shifted things. Then someone else picked up the ball: "What does *frustration* tell you about yourself, about others?" "How does it direct your actions? What does it get you to do?" Now it was happening. I told them so, and it felt pretty good to me. So that's how we ended the second day.

We had a handout from Vicki and Jeff on some candidate interview questions. I think that's what helped people get into it in the "effects" questions exercise—they tried variations of the sample questions. We reviewed the exercise on the morning of the third day, and then Jeff and Vicki asked us to go into another exercise in which we would ask "reauthoring" questions. We looked at the possibilities: "landscape-of-action" questions, "landscape-of-consciousness" questions that access "unique outcomes," and other questions that promote "reflexivity" and "circulation." Then we tried it. They said we could do it any way we wanted—go back into the same groups or not, ask reauthoring questions based on the problem we had asked "effects" questions about the day before, or ask somebody reauthoring questions about developments in her or his life. They said there didn't seem to be any one way that was best, but we should pick what fit for us. (This is what I keep remembering from the whole week. Jeff and Vicki were so consistent in teaching us the way they said they thought about things. From my family systems background, I remembered this is called "isomorphism.")

In this exercise I decided to try my hand at questioning. We took the option of asking reauthoring questions of one of the trainees, who wanted to talk about a recent development in his life—one of "coming out of *shyness*." Because we had already been asking reauthoring questions in reflecting team work, this seemed to go fairly well. What extended the richness of the exercise for me was to experiment with many different types of questions. (You may want to reread Chapters 3 through 5 in this book for a review of the questions. Chapters 1 and 2 may also be helpful if you want another look at the thinking behind the work. I know that reading this material was helpful for me, especially after we did the problem exercise.) Anyway, my favorite questions are the "experience-of-experience" ones, maybe because they really opened up space for me when they were asked. For example, we asked Charlie (the guy coming out of *shyness*), "Who in your life, who perhaps may have known you growing up, would be *least* surprised at this development?" He thought for a minute, then laughed and said, "Well, my second-grade teacher wouldn't be at all surprised. She probably would have labeled me ADHD! In fact, she would have been *more* surprised if she had seen the *shyness* of the last few years. I believe she'd be pleased if she could see me now." That led to other questions: "What would she be pleased about?" "What would you want her to see?" "Who else would see that now?" "How would you let others know that *shyness* is no longer influencing you, but that you are deciding for yourself how you want to be?" We were getting it now, and it was becoming lots of fun.

The client who came in the late morning was a 15-year-old girl (Susan) Jeff had been working with, who was struggling with *bulimia.* He reviewed with her the power of *bulimia* and the effects on her of isolation and lack of confidence, among other things. Then his interview proceeded to explore the small steps she was taking in an anti-*bulimic* direction. Rather than explore this case here, I refer you to Chapter 6, where Karen talks about her work in regaining her own power ("Karen Power") in her fight against *bulimia.* The work with Susan was similar. Also, one of the pluses we experienced in this intensive was that we got to write a team letter to Susan later in the week; it summarizes what we observed, as well as our reflecting team responses. We reproduce that letter here.

Letter to Susan

Dear Susan:

The team wanted to write this letter to you to summarize our reflections on your developments, which you shared with us last week.

We were struck by *bulimia*'s power to get you to grow down and not up. You said that it has been using its power to take away *your* life goals and replace them with *its* goals for you—to waste away and die, to keep you controlled by it and by others, and to isolate you. When we heard you say that to keep you believing that you are fat when you are really thin, *bulimia* jerks your strings like a puppet, we wondered whether this was a discovery that might be helpful to other young women. You also said that by keeping you worried about how you look, *bulimia* keeps you tense. Do you think other women in the culture deal with the same tension? They all see the same bare-stomach ads in the magazines that you do. How do you think other young women in your life deal with this tension? What would you say to younger women, like your cousin Rachel, about this?

Given this, can you imagine *bulimia*'s distress when you came up with the title "Fighting to Be Your Own Self"? This led us to wonder what specific developments you were paying attention to when you came up with this title. Some of the things that stood out for us were noticing and stating your own ideas about medications. How did you take this stand? How were you able to know what your body was telling you about this? This seemed important, because our experience is that *bulimia* stops one from knowing what one's body wants. It is like the woman whose letter you took home. She said, "*Anorexia* makes me want to . . . punish my body instead of respecting and caring for it."

Another development that stood out for us was how you were able to pay attention to what pleased you and not just what pleased others. You were able to wear the clothes you wanted and not the clothes *bulimia* wanted. You even said, "I don't care what people think of me," and "Who cares what I look like?" You said your friends who count will like you for who you are and not what you look like. How are you able to know that your opinions and your friends' opinions count more than *bulimia's* opinions? What else might be different as you please yourself more and *bulimia* less? We also noticed that you were having fun again, at work and at dance class. You really seemed to love what you were doing and to take pride in doing it. How is what *you* love different from what *bulimia* loves? What do you think will happen to *bulimia* as you keep going in this direction of fun and enjoyment instead of torture and control and restrictions (like Bridget referred to in the tape)?[7]

You seem to feel strongly that a woman's appearance ought to be pleasing to her and not subject to men's standards of appearance for a woman. We wondered what future standards might be created for yourself and others (like Rachel or Jeff's daughters) if you and your mother teamed up against the standards that support *bulimia.* We were imagining that the connection between you and your mother and between the women in the Anti-Anorexia/Anti-Bulimia League might be the kind of fortress all women could use to support themselves against male dominant versions that don't fit for most women. With this connection as a fortress, *anorexia* and *bulimia's* power is greatly weakened.

We would like to be caught up on any further developments, and would like your permission for Jeff to share these with us. Would you also be willing for us to have a copy of this letter to share with other young women who are just starting their battle with *anorexia* and *bulimia?* What you have learned could be helpful to them.

Yours anti-anorexically and anti-bulimically,

Jeff and the Team

An Initial Session

The day seemed full already. We ate a late lunch, and then Jeff had an initial session scheduled with a family for 2:00. What was so helpful about this session—I think Philip already commented on this—was that we had the

---

[7]This refers to a tape from David Epston's Anti-Anorexia/Anti-Bulimia League archives.

opportunity to see how a problem gets constructed. We also saw Jeff do something that he and Vicki had talked about, something they do when they work with families: They usually ask the young persons in the family to go first. This gives children and teenagers the opportunity to talk about the problem from their perspective, rather than just reacting to what the parents say is the problem. Also, in this case, the 15-year-old boy described his experience in a way that his parents had not heard before—undoubtedly because of the serious and respectful way Jeff talked with him, as well as the work done to separate him from the problem. I realized how different it was to talk with someone without being influenced by causal theories that might affect the conversation. What emerged was a real appreciation of the boy's experience. First he talked about his problems at school with peer relationships and how that had the effect of *withdrawal* on him; then he described how his parents' work (they both traveled a lot in their work) got him into a place of missing them and feeling gypped. The effects of that were *intense anger* and *frustration,* which got between him and his parents and led to loneliness and more *withdrawal,* and finally to emotional distance or what Jeff called *apartness,* which affected the whole family. It was also interesting to me—to all of us—that in what seemed like a very short period of time, Jeff had a chance to talk with each member of the family, find that they all were affected by *apartness, and* elicit some "unique outcomes" as well. That also gave the reflecting team some material to raise questions about. The family had talked about a "tickle" and a "ball fight," which were ways they had developed to overcome *apartness,* so we raised questions about these and about the other connecting things they did together and their desire to be close.

Later—actually the next morning, but I'm going to talk about this instead of Philip, because it fits here (entitlement, you know!)—we did some more talking about how Jeff came up with that particular construction of the problem. He could have stayed with *withdrawal* for the teenager, especially as it referred to his peer relationships, but also to his relationship with his parents. Or he could have focused on *intense anger* and *frustration* and how these got between the teenager and his parents. What was helpful about moving it to a relationship problem—*apartness*—was that it captured more of everyone's experience. Also, *intense anger* and *frustration* could then be thought of as the "tools" of *apartness* or the habits it encouraged. The family could be left with this question: "What kind of connection do you want?" Another interesting thing about observing this case was that the work also clearly showed the thinking that Vicki and Jeff have been doing in regard to "dissing separation" and paying attention to a desire for "connection" in families. More and more, this way of thinking and working was looking like all of a piece to me. I was beginning to get it.

The Authors Speak

Asking trainees to practice with one another in small groups seems to have several positive effects. *Evaluation* can interfere less because the teachers aren't watching. The participants can share the effects of the questions they ask. They also can help one another come up with questions, and this lessens the pressure. And they can talk about their general experience of the training in a smaller group context. Given that constructing the problem can be the most difficult skill (and a very important one) to develop, beginning with a problem already partially defined helps move the process along. Similarly, in the reauthoring exercise, beginning with some "developments"— either presented by the person being interviewed or left over from the "effects" exercise—allows for a starting point of asking questions without having to find unique outcomes. The focus in either case stays on asking questions, which, for some trainees, is a relatively new experience. For those more familiar with questions as the process of therapy, asking them from the point of view we have been discussing is different from asking questions to fill in hypotheses that exist in the therapist's head.

Linda has commented on her interest in experience-of-experience questions. Michael White (1995b) noted that these questions bring relationships into the therapy room. They also have the potential to involve the actual people in a client's life more directly. This can be done by bringing others into a therapy session, by having the client mobilize help from them outside of therapy, or by bringing them in through the client's imagination.

It seems really useful to us in a training setting to bring in clients at different stages of their work. It is our experience that at first, clients further along in therapy allow the trainees to practice reauthoring questions in a context where the problem isn't as present. Later, it seems more useful to include a beginning session to give students a view of problem construction. On Day 4, following this session, we do more work with our students directly on problem construction.

DAY 4

My turn again (Philip). Although Linda stole my thunder talking about our opening discussion, let me say that it was a perfect way for us to start out the day. As it turns out, what we did next was an exercise in constructing the problem. Vicki and Jeff said that this tends to be the more difficult thing to do, which is why they start us out asking "effects" questions and then "reauthoring" questions around an already external- ized problem. Also, by this time, we had an idea of how to think about the problem in its sociopolitical context—that is, to think about how the problem is encouraged by certain cultural discourses.

Problem Construction Exercise

We did this first in a large group so that everyone could experience the process and also so that we could have Jeff and Vicki assist us (although I must say that they mostly sat back and let us try it). Once in a while, they helped us rephrase a question or suggested that we stay with a candidate for the externalized problem or with one line of questioning a little longer. They also helped us continue to use externalizing language as we were working toward a construction of the problem. More often, they stopped the process and asked the "client" about the effects of the conversation or about what path the person saw as useful.

Linda volunteered to present a problem she was dealing with in her life. It turned out to be quite helpful, because she started with something that we began to see as an effect of the problem; then we moved to a bigger description; and finally we incorporated the cultural (and gen- dered) influence. But let me be more specific. She started with the problem as **boredom** at work. We struggled with asking questions using externalizing language, and for a while it just seemed to be going around in circles. Finally, she used words like "should" and "doubt," like she *should* be more interested in what she was doing, and beginning to *doubt* that this work was for her or that she was any good at it. One of our members picked up on this as the **shoulds** and **doubts** and asked how they were affecting her. Looking back at the process, I think that we might have been able to go further with these constructions, but someone else jumped in with **job dissatisfaction** as the problem, and Linda picked up on it. I found that what I wanted to do was jump quickly to the times when **job dissatisfaction** wasn't around or when it affected her less, but after checking with Linda about how the interview was going, Jeff and Vicki suggested that we look more at the effects of the problem before we did that. I think their thinking was that we might not have come up with an externalization that captured enough of Linda's experience, or with one that picked up the "discourse" that was affecting her.

I learned many useful things from doing this exercise. One was to list the effects of the problem as a way of continuing to use externalizing language and to promote more separation from the problem. Another was to stay open to the thought that the construction of the problem could evolve. Anyway, what we finally got to were *overresponsibility* and *evaluation* as the problems influencing Linda, telling her she "should" do more and getting her to "doubt" whether she was any good at her work; of course the effect of all that was *job dissatisfaction.* So the *shoulds* and *doubts* could have been helpful, but the exercise itself let us see (1) that the exact name we give to the problem isn't as important as how it gets co-constructed by the client and the therapist; (2) how important it is in problem contruction to capture cultural context; and (3) how important it is for the therapist to stay tuned in to what the client's report is of her or his experience. We did, by the way, pick up a unique outcome or two. As Vicki and Jeff have said earlier, they do tend to "pop out" as the person engages in an externalizing conversation and experiences more "space" and thus more possibilities.

Interview with a Couple: Gender and Violence

Vicki had scheduled a session with a couple for us to observe that afternoon. We talked a bit before they came in about how to think about constructing problems when working with a couple. (Chapter 7 of this book gives a description of this process and the thinking behind it.) At any rate, we knew to pay attention to pattern and to each person's end of the pattern. We also were cued to think about how each member of the couple was influenced by gender training.

When the couple came in Vicki reviewed the work, saying that they had worked together at three separate intervals over the last couple of years. This was a second marriage for the husband, his first wife having died of cancer; he had two children from that marriage, a daughter (currently 23) and a son (19). A recurring difficulty for this couple was the relationship with the 19-year-old son (who would not come to therapy); in particular, he was emotionally abusive toward his father's wife. The effect this had on the spouses' relationship was that she experienced a great deal of *hurt* and *pain,* as well as *fear* for her safety and for her emotional well-being. This *fear* told her that her husband must not care for her enough or understand her *pain,* because he, in her eyes, was doing nothing (at least nothing that worked) to lessen the abuse. He, on the other hand, was also affected by *fear*—in this case, a *fear* that he might lose his son forever if he took too strong a stand. This *fear* was based on his belief that he had not done a good job of parenting the son or of establishing the kind of relationship with him that he wanted. The *fear* kept him from working to create the connection he desired, and also pushed him instead to try to "solve" the problem, to "fix" things, which he did by making checklists for his son to fill out (the son ignored these).

What was helpful for me (Philip), as a man, was to see how Vicki was working with the husband to help him appreciate his wife's *pain* and to take responsibility for his participation, even though it was inadvertent, in his son's "violent behavior" toward his wife. Vicki concurrently worked with the wife on her standing up for herself in the face of the *fear* and *pain.* I wondered how I could do this work on my own, especially after the reflecting team got together and I saw how powerful a team can be in this regard.

What the team did, after raising questions about steps this husband and wife had taken more toward what they wanted, was to have a brief discussion about violence in relationships. One person raised a question for the wife about how standing up for herself against *fear* might also be a sign of commitment to the relationship. Another asked how the husband thought about his responsibility to let his son know about what actions and language might have the effect of *hurt* and *fear* on women. Also, how could he (as a man, husband, father) begin to appreciate what *violence* was for women, how they experienced it? Although this was a bit of a departure from what we had done previously on reflecting teams, it was within the realm of curiosity and of exploring what might be questions for the spouses to ask themselves. (Vicki actually wrote us a letter three weeks after the intensive, letting us know the longer-term effects this discussion had had on the couple. The wife moved out temporarily, making clear to her husband her commitment to the relationship, but also moving herself into a place of emotional safety. And the husband began to battle his "out-of-control" feelings so that he could notice ways of connecting with his son. His thought was that from this place of connection, he could then have a discussion with him about how to treat others. Both husband and wife were explicit about their desire to stay in relationship with each other.)

The Authors Speak

We use the problem construction exercise in our small-group training sessions and in consultation groups. We can repeat the process for each participant, if the group finds it useful. One member presents an experience that he or she is calling a problem. Then one of the other members can start a line of questioning. Others can join in but not start a new line of questioning until the group has completed the first one. Our own position varies. We may ask why a question is being asked, if this is not obvious. Usually such a question is coming more from the participant's head than from the interaction with the "client." We sometimes help frame a question in a manner more consistent with a narrative metaphor. We may stop and have a reflective conversation with the person who posed the question. We often ask the "client" to discuss the effects of the question or line of questions. Are the questions useful? Do they have pathologizing effects? If several different possibilities arise, we ask which one seems most interesting to the "client." We rarely jump in to pursue a line of questioning, believing that it is more helpful to trainees to develop their own styles, and more helpful also if we engage the "client" in conversation to deconstruct the process. At the end, after the group has constructed a problem, everyone (except the client) has a reflective conversation, focusing on the unique outcomes that inevitably pop out.

The live session on Day 4 that Philip has described represented a difficult situation—how to confront issues of *fear* and *violence* and still stay in pace with the clients. A team approach allows for more possibilities in this case than the usual therapist–client situation does. For example, from entry points of unique outcomes (i.e., by starting with developments they have managed), the team can work backward to these issues. For example, we noticed the efforts the husband had made to treat his wife respectfully—how he stood up to certain specifications that often affect some men and support them in ignoring their wives' experience. We wondered who taught this man about respect, and who he thought should teach this to his son. Another possibility for a team is to have the male and female team members situate their respective questions in a context of gender in a way that might relate to the clients' experience. We find that interesting possibilities for team conversations can arise while the team stays in tune with clients' experience.

DAY 5

I (Linda) get to wrap this up, even though it gives me one more day than Philip—but Day 5 was really only half a day (entitlement again, but not too much—right?). Vicki and Jeff suggested that there were many possibilities for spending the next three hours. One was to have a heavy-duty theoretical discussion—something they both said they would enjoy, even though their experience was that most people didn't learn as well in this mode. (Jeff said something about not wanting to give an intensive that he wouldn't want to participate in; I think he meant that he likes to talk about theoretical ideas.) Another was to write a team letter to Susan summarizing her work with Jeff and her battle against **bulimia**. As you already know, that was one of the options we took. A third was for all of us to interview Vicki and Jeff in the way that they interviewed us on the first day—an intriguing idea. Yet another option was for them to ask us reauthoring questions about our developments over the week, although they said that this might take up the whole time. And a fifth was for us to participate in a typical case consultation, such as they do in their consultation groups. They also wanted to spend some time having a conversation with us about what was helpful or not helpful in the week, but they could do that with us over lunch (which they provided). We all decided on the second option (writing the letter) and the fifth (doing a case consultation).

Philip wanted to present a case. Jeff and Vicki asked that half of the group act as a reflecting team. What we were to pay attention to were Philip's preferred developments as a therapist working with this particular case. This already was a different way to think about consultation. The other four were to observe the process and perhaps make "metacomments" (whatever those are) about what occurred. Philip then proceeded to tell us about his work with an individual male, whom he had seen weekly over the course of two years. His experience was that they had made some progress, but his client continued to complain that no progress was being made. What Vicki and Jeff began to do seemed so different to me, so novel, that it took a minute to catch what was going on. In fact, what they were doing was exactly what I had seen them do with clients: They asked Philip what *effect* this experience had on him. What this question accomplished was that it allowed Philip to begin to notice how the effects of struggling with the client continued to contribute to the struggle, making it difficult for him to access his own ideas, his own therapeutic skills. This process took case consultation to a new level. No longer were we all sitting around telling someone else how to do it better. (It also occurred to me: Isn't that what we have done to clients all along?) At any rate, they continued to explore the effects of the struggle and to notice further effects, until sufficient space was created between Philip and the problem that he began to notice his own good work and better ideas. The work of the reflecting team then became fairly straightforward.

This experience was empowering for all of us. We could see how respectful it was of the therapist; in this case, it allowed Philip to reclaim preferred ways of working. At the same time, there was still space available to introduce new ideas and new thoughts, although these frequently came from the therapist's own set of stored resources. It was a helpful experience for me as a supervisor, and I began to ponder how to be this way with the interns in my agency.

We stopped for lunch, all of us aware that we were now at the end of our journey—at least this phase of it. We spent some time with Jeff and Vicki letting them know what was helpful to us or not helpful. They wanted to hear both, and it was clear that they wanted to continually fine-tune how this intensive would go, so that it could be most helpful to participants.

The Authors Speak

We've already commented on our experience that theoretical conversations are only useful to some. This group chose not to engage in a theoretical discussion. Inviting them to interview us was another way of indicating that we participate in this process as people, and that we would be happy to share our experience and developments as well.

The case consultation Linda has described illustrates how we do supervision, whether on a one-to-one basis with a supervisee or in a group. It mirrors what we do with clients. Through this process, consulting therapists usually notice new possibilities—ways of working they have previously pursued with other clients, or even options that exist with the client they are presenting but that they are currently not following through on. When we see therapists getting off their preferred course, we understand it as an effect of the problem. We suspect that you, too, have been affected by a problem that has overtaken a client. We certainly have! When this happens, we stop doing things that we know are useful and that we know we do with other clients. In only a very small number of cases does this have anything to do with the effects of the therapist's own previous experience—and when it does, this usually feels different. We think the notion of countertransference is consistent with the therapy model it comes from: It pathologizes the therapist to explain what is happening, just as such a model pathologizes clients to explain problems. We believe, instead, that problems are powerful and can disrupt the efforts of very good therapists.

At any rate, we believe that this kind of consultation interview is useful. We may ask how the problem is affecting the therapist. We may ask what the therapist would like to see happening, and in what ways it is or isn't. We wonder how the problem is stopping the therapist from doing what he or she would like. We notice unique outcomes in the work or in relationships with other clients. After going through this process, we ask whether the therapist would like to ask us any specific questions about what he or she is doing. Often, at this point, there are no questions. Therapists who are at more of a beginning stage may ask a question or two about a possible direction. Having them ask the questions keeps the process paced to their experience (instead of our making suggestions and volunteering information in areas that may or may not make sense to them).

Very occasionally, we may raise a question about the larger cultural context.

In live supervision we may do a very short interview, like the one just described, before the client arrives. We also ask whether the therapist would like us to come in after about 10 minutes for a reflection (we do this routinely in the early training of therapists). This is a conversation between one of us and the therapist about the direction she or he is going in. The therapist can ask questions as well. There are no call-ins, but the therapist can call for an early reflection or minireflection if he or she feels it is useful. After the interview, the reflecting team's questions, and the client's comments in response to the team, one of us comes in to interview the therapist and the team. (See Chapter 5.) This also provides an opportunity to notice the developments in the therapist's work and respond to them (e.g., "This question stood out for me, and I wondered . . .). After the client leaves, a minireauthoring interview, connected to the brief one held before the session, can occur with the therapist.

This Is the End

In a final discussion with attendees about what was and was not helpful, we find that we continue to learn new ways of thinking about how to engage people in the process of learning about narrative. As we have said at the very beginning, things are never the same, and we continue to be interested in how to invite participants to experience what we consider a new way of thinking. We hope we have engaged you in this process in ways that are consistent with these ideas, and that you have enjoyed these adventures in narrative therapy.

EPILOGUE

Eyes of the World

The Authors Speak—One Last Time

As a way of ending this book, we asked a colleague, John Neal, to interview us about our experience of writing it. Our conversation follows.

JOHN: So now that you've written this book, and written it in the way you have, what kinds of thoughts are you left with?

JEFF: Will people get into the flow of it? Will it work for them? It's not the usual academic book.

VICKI: Will anybody actually buy it? (*Laughing*) Will they persevere through it?

JEFF: Will they be able to digest something academic that's presented in a more everyday, people-type way? When people don't have their academic hats on, they are more likely to engage in this type of speaking (and perhaps writing). Will it be okay that we didn't speak (write) in a very academic voice?

JOHN: I noticed that the two of you seemed to be having a lot of fun. How do you think the readers will relate to your playfulness?

VICKI: Well, I've enjoyed writing it. It has been fun. I think if people could enter into it with a sense of having fun, it might be really interesting and useful.

JEFF: We've talked about this. I don't think we could have done it any other way. The playfulness speaks to how we are in our work, in our lives. If we don't live our lives according to a professionalism that is traditionally defined, and we don't do a therapy that is traditionally defined, why would we want to write that way?

VICKI: Also, we found that we couldn't write the "old" didactic ways as easily any more. If you've noticed, all the middle chapters on doing the work are situated in our own experience.

JEFF: Yes, we tried to separate out a traditional teaching voice from a theoretical voice from an "authors speak" voice where we situated our work, but some of it is still mixed in together.

JOHN: How did you stumble on this idea—problems talk . . .

VICKI: I remember a conversation we had about a movie we had seen, which got me to remember some other experiences I have had in developing multimedia presentations.

JEFF: It got us to think about different lenses, seeing things not through a traditional lens—opening up multiple lenses. I think the problem talking preceded that, though.

VICKI: I remember how we stumbled on it—it was at a workshop we gave in southern California in 1993, and Melissa [Griffith] asked us a question—she asked how we thought about the problem in the room.

JEFF: Yes, I remember now. I said I thought about it like that little slimy green monster from *Ghostbusters*. We then started to talk about the problem that way.

VICKI: And to think about it that way. That's when I started thinking about the problem as being somewhere else in the room, away from the clients—like in a plant. This also affected the way we started teaching and doing workshops together.

JOHN: Are you saying that the kinds of questions people asked is what got you thinking this way?

VICKI: That was part of it, and also watching how people were learning, paying attention to what was working for people.

JEFF: And how the idea spoke to us about ourselves—being free from having to live up to any specifications, questioning whether they're useful. Not accepting them as "givens"—just like we would with our clients. Not accepting that there is a "given" way to think about anything, including writing a book.

VICKI: Right, and about writing it a certain way.

JOHN: So you went inside this metaphor and then the book came out of it?

JEFF: That would be a way to look at it. That's not the way we thought about it at the time, but yes, that's what we did.

VICKI: Maybe it speaks more to how we were doing that already.

JEFF: We were beginning to live our lives inside those ideas more, and then everything became consistent with that.

VICKI: And the book became a vehicle to continue to do that.

JEFF: Also, a piece of input that encouraged us to write this way is that a lot of people were saying that they read all this stuff and they didn't "get it." Why would we want to write a book in the same format that people aren't "getting," and that doesn't fit the way the work is anyway? So that influenced us, too.

JOHN: What have you learned from writing the book the way you have? How has it affected you to have done it this way?

JEFF: Well, I know it is consistent with my personal evolution—how I think about things, how I am personally in the world. Writing this book confirmed this process.

VICKI: And I think it served as our audience. It became a reflexive experience in continuing to appreciate this way of thinking and how it has transformed our lives, as well as remind us of why this work fits for us personally.

JOHN: Is there anything in particular that you want people to get out of reading this book?

VICKI: Well, there are lots of things, if you mean in a specific way—like privileging the client's experience, for example. That's critical. And also that people can think about and challenge specifications for how to live their lives.

JEFF: More generally, perhaps, we hope they begin to experience themselves differently and experience themselves in relation to their clients differently. To repeat what we have said often in this book, we wanted to invite people into a way of thinking that we find is almost impossible to get just by talking about it. So we hope what we did worked.

JOHN: Is there anything you would want me to ask you that we haven't touched on?

JEFF: Just to thank people for reading it, if they've gotten this far. And to say we'd be really open to hearing what they have to say about what parts worked for them, if they want to write us or let us know some way.

VICKI: Yes, definitely. Thanks for this interview, John. And thanks for reading, readers.

Afterword

KARL TOMM

I am delighted to have had the opportunity to offer some reflections on this fascinating book. Reading it, I felt as if I were engaged in a series of stimulating conversations with a variety of interesting persons, including a number of "virtual" persons in the guise of theoretical perspectives, like "Otto Freudian," and problems, like the "Red Devil." In the spirit of this playful style, I would like to introduce you to Narra Tiva and Bringit Forther. Imagine the following conversation between Bringit and Narra upon finishing this book:

BRINGIT FORTHER: Narra, it was simply wonderful to get to know you so much better through these pages! I've heard so much about you over the last few years, but I must admit I found you a bit elusive. It seems to me that Vicki and Jeff have given you a much clearer form by writing this book. How was it for you, to be taken into their hands and presented in this way?

NARRA TIVA: I just loved it! I could feel myself coming alive and developing a fuller identity. I felt as if I was being born into the world. I have more "substance" than ever before.

BRINGIT: But you've been around for some time now. In what way is this birth, or rebirth, if you like, different?

NARRA: I think it's the way in which Vicki and Jeff were able to mold me gently at different points and then back off together with the reader and take a look at what they'd done. By bringing in different voices and allowing a back-and-forth conversation of speaking and listening to take place, there seemed to be much more space for reflection, and I felt myself growing in this reflective space.

BRINGIT: Yes, that's how I experienced it as well. In most books, the author speaks in a continuous stream and the reader is invited into a stance of passive listening. A reader could, of course, deliberately stop at any time to reflect, but when the authors encourage this it helps a lot! By deliberately bringing out other voices in the text and introducing a process of turn taking in speech, like breathing in and breathing out, the invitations to reflection in this book are more frequent and the space to reflect in is greater. And what seems so important to me is that this reflection adds a third dimension to the two-dimensional surface of the medium of print.

NARRA: Yes, I felt more space to breathe, to expand my chest, to spread my wings . . .

BRINGIT: Is it fair for me to be more direct and ask you to define who or what you actually are, Narra?

NARRA: Sure. Hmm . . . let me think, . . . how can I say this?

BRINGIT: Are you a theory? A frame of reference? An ideology? A method of therapy? A collection of practices?

NARRA: I suppose I could be any of those things, but my preference is to be a way of being in the world.

BRINGIT: Are you implying you could be different things to different people?

NARRA: Yes. Some therapists embrace me as a theory to explain what therapy is all about. They can become quite excited and enthusiastic about me. Sometimes they talk as if they know all about me, but they don't actually share my preferred way of being.

BRINGIT: Are you referring to narrative therapy enthusiasts who become groupies and criticize other ways of thinking and practicing in therapy?

NARRA: Yes. It embarrasses me quite a bit sometimes. I realize they're just finding their own way, but they participate in creating the same kind of oppressive culture among therapists that they are trying to deconstruct among members of families or larger communities.

BRINGIT: It must be difficult to challenge oppressive practices without oppressing others oneself.

NARRA: It certainly is, especially when a therapist tries to apply narrative methods without externalizing. It is so important to separate problematic patterns of thought, feeling, or action from individuals before challenging them. This is why I enjoyed Vicki and Jeff's method of personifying problems and giving them voices as if they were separate persons.

BRINGIT: It's a lot easier to punch a problem without hurting anyone when you can visualize it as separate from everyone! (*Chuckles*)

NARRA: Yes, I like to see therapists keeping their externalizing "scalpel" sharp so that they can cut cleanly when they do "surgery" on the noxious aspects of a person's identity.

BRINGIT: One of the things I've been wondering about, Narra, is the degree to which your success relies on therapists' internalizing your way of being in the world as well as engaging in these externalizing and restorying practices.

NARRA: Yes, this is something I expect will emerge more fully in the future as various authors who give me life add to my identity.

BRINGIT: I noticed that Vicki and Jeff acknowledged at the beginning of this book that they were writing within a cultural context and probably could not see what they themselves were immersed in. This acknowledgment made me feel warmth for them because it offered me as a reader the space to imagine other future developments. (*Pause*) Would you say that it is desirable for therapists to open themselves to receive and to internalize you within themselves? Would this make it easier for them to enter your way of being in the world?

NARRA: Yes, I think such internalizing processes are invisible in the present status of the field. However, Vicki and Jeff described some extremely useful internalizing exercises in the last section of this book, on training. They make it easy for me to make an appearance in the lives of their trainees.

BRINGIT: When your full shape eventually becomes crystal clear, we'll be able to see all your moles as well!

NARRA: That's okay with me. I'm not devoted to perfection. Being good enough in contributing to healing and wellness is just fine. . . . By the way, Bringit, are you prepared to make an appearance yet? Who are you?

BRINGIT: This is your day, Narra, not mine.

NARRA: Come on, Bringit. Give us an inkling of where you're coming from. I'm sure Vicki and Jeff wouldn't mind.

BRINGIT: (*Shyly*) Well, I must admit that I have internalized a lot of your ways of thinking and practicing, Narra, but I like to keep a little closer to my body and not be fully taken into the text of stories. I'm also still very interested in context and patterns of interaction, like Virginia Batesonian. I get a little frightened sometimes when Jerome Foucaultian gets all wound up.

NARRA: I know what you mean. Jerome can be pretty powerful, but fortunately we're on the same side, and have even become close friends. . . . "Bringit Forther." An interesting name. Where did you get it?

BRINGIT: Well, it has to do with how we make distinctions and the ways in which they emerge in our conversations. For instance, we distinguish and actively "bring forth" specific entities, qualities, relationships, et cetera, as we interact and speak. We each have our own personal initiative and responsibility as well as biomedical and sociocultural limitations that affect how and what we bring forth.

NARRA: Just a minute! Slow down there. What exactly are you trying to say?

BRINGIT: I know it's confusing for me to describe myself without giving an adequate background. Maybe it's best to leave this for another book.

NARRA: Okay! It's nice to have something to look forward to.

BRINGIT: Just one more comment, Narra, before we end. I especially appreciated the way Vicki and Jeff emphasized the degree to which you pay attention to the client's experience. This was an enormous relief to me. I've often had the impression that narrative therapists can become so immersed in the story that they put it above the client's actual experience. Indeed, your emphasis on experience made me realize that we might be more closely related than I'd thought!

NARRA: Well, that's good to hear. Given the pervasiveness of oppressive practices out there, I need all the friends I can get!

APPENDIX A

Reflecting Team Guidelines

A. What to pay attention to

1. During the interview (30–40 minutes), team members notice the client's preferred developments, or what might occur as "unique outcomes" or contradictions to the problem story. These can be thought of as entry points into an alternative meaning. Team members can listen for these possibilities, even if they are not explicitly elicited by the therapist.
2. The team can be curious about these developments, how they might have occurred, or what about the client's lived experience might have contributed to these contradictions or preferences.
3. Team members can wonder about these contradictions (unique outcomes) by asking both landscape-of-consciousness and landscape-of-action questions:

   a. Are those unique outcomes preferred? Why or why not?
   b. Do they have a history? A future ? If so, what is it?
   c. What different attitudes have they brought forth for the client, toward others?
   d. Who else might be aware of these contradictions or preferred developments (in the past, present, or future)?
   e. What different actions or behaviors have occurred in response to these events?

4. Team members should realize that these events or ideas have probably been neglected, not attended to, by the client. (They can remind themselves that they are asking "reauthoring" questions.)

5. Team members can also recall that they are helping the client make meaning in response to preferred developments; they are not simply noticing or commenting on "positives."

B. How to respond

1. Team members (three to six) interview one another for 10–15 minutes. One member asks a question—from his or her curiosity about the preferred developments he or she has noticed.
2. Each question can reflect some interest in both the occurrence and the history of the unique outcome, as well as the possible future.
3. Team members "situate" each remark; that is, they indicate what about their own personal experience, education, or thinking has informed each question. If a team member does not "situate" a question, then another member can ask the questioner to do so.
4. If a member makes a comment rather than poses a question, another member can respond by asking what question this comment might evoke.

C. Transparency

1. By "situating" each question, the team members make it apparent that their remarks are not necessarily right or helpful for the client, because they come primarily from the team members' own experience or ideas.
2. Situating a remark may also include why a team member thinks the comment may be helpful to the client—even though the client may not experience it that way.

D. Reflexivity

1. The reflecting team's musings become similar to an "overheard conversation" on which clients can "reflect," picking those remarks and questions that have most meaning for them and that best fit their experience.
2. The reflecting team can also be thought of as an audience to a client's preferred story.

APPENDIX B

Structure and Sample Questions for a Narrative Interview

Problem construction and externalizing questions

- Think of the problem as a thing, and talk about it as an active agent in a person's life.
- Think about the culture's role in the formation of the problem.
- Come to some agreement with the client about what to call the problem.
- Use externalizing language even if you are not sure what to call the problem.

Examples

1. What would you call the problem that is most affecting you?
2. What's your main experience when this problem is around? What are you noticing?
3. Do you think it is more **self-doubt** or **evaluation**?

"Effects" questions

- Continue and thicken the construction of the problem, and extend the field of influence of the problem. (In an interview, these questions overlap with the first set of questions—and also with the next set, deconstructing questions.)

- Sometimes an "effect" of the problem more clearly captures the client's experience and can then become the agreed-upon externalized problem.
- Explore all aspects of the client's experience:
  - Attitudes, behaviors (include reciprocal pattern).
  - In life: school, work, social life, recreation.
  - In relationships: family, friends, intimate others.
  - The client's attitude toward himself or herself (personal story).

Examples

1. How does the problem direct you? What does it get you to do?
2. What does the problem steal from you? What enjoyment has it taken from you?
3. What kinds of things does it tell you?
4. What does it tell you about yourself? About your spouse [mother, father, etc.]?
5. When *self-doubt* attacks you, how does it get you not to trust your own ideas?

Deconstructing questions

- Think about directly challenging personal and cultural stories that have contributed to the evolution of the problem. (These challenges are implicit in "effects" questions.)
- Extend the field of influence to the margins where personal preferences may be hiding.

Examples

1. How do you think *self-doubt* uses *evaluation* of how women [men] are supposed to be to strengthen its position?
2. Do you think *self-doubt* has attacked others in your family or your friends, or only you?
3. When *self-doubt* made an appearance in your life, how did it take over?
4. What kinds of training techniques does *self-doubt* use to bolster its position?

Restorying questions: Entry points

- Notice "gaps" or contradictions to the problem story (unique outcomes)—past, present, or future.
- Notice what comes up in the telling of the problem story—on the periphery. Ask about it. These can then become entry points to a possible more preferred story.
- It is important to ask whether unique outcomes are preferred or not.

Examples

1. Since *self-doubt* didn't seem to make an appearance in your life until you were 12, what pleased you about yourself before that time?
2. Did you have a struggle with *self-doubt* before you made this appointment and came here? How did you win that battle?
3. Are there some relationships in which *self-doubt* finds it harder to get a foothold? Why do you think that is?
4. When you do more what you want and are not so paralyzed by *self-doubt*, how do you do that?
5. Are you pleased when you can decide what you want without *self-doubt* tricking you?

Restorying questions: Landscape of action

- Draw attention in detail to behaviors and events that are more preferred by the client.
- Elicit sequences of events to bring forth a sense of agency for the client, that is, what led up to the preferred behavior, what he or she did to prepare for the action, and so on.
- Locate events in history, going backward to possible precursors and forward to future possibilities ("future-looking-back questions").
- These questions "thicken" the plot line.

Examples

1. When *self-doubt* tried to get you not to show up today, how did you handle it?
2. Was there any special preparation you did to get yourself ready to fight off *self-doubt*?
3. What strategies do you know about that *self-doubt* may have tried to steal away from you, but that you called upon in the past and that you can also use now?
4. As you win more battles against *self-doubt*, how will your life look in the future?
5. Five years from now, as you look back, what steps do you think you will have taken to embrace *self-acceptance* in your life rather than *self-doubt*?

Restorying questions: Landscape of consciousness

- Ask about intentions, desires, preferences, values, beliefs.
- Focus on commitment to preferred ways of being.
- Ask "experience-of-experience" questions to create a reflexive position.
- These questions are asked in a back-and-forth process with landscape-of-action questions.

Examples

1. As you see yourself winning more and more battles against *self-doubt*, how are you thinking of yourself as a person? What do these victories tell you?
2. Is this something you have known about yourself for a long time? Does it fit a certain philosophy of life that you might have?
3. If I were to tell others about your successes, how do you think I might describe you?

Reauthoring context: Reflexivity and circulation

- Name the counterplot.
- Bring forth appreciation for the new story from family, friends, others.
- Circulate the story to a wider audience.
- Continue to create a reflexive position for the client.

Examples

1. As you put *self-doubt* behind you, what might you call this new path you are taking in life?
2. Now that you have made this commitment to yourself, who else would celebrate it with you?
3. As your husband [wife, son, etc.] continues to notice your new happiness with yourself, what might he [she] be pleased about, both for you and for your relationship?
4. If your mother [father, etc.] could be here now, what would she [he] be able to comment on about your strengths in beating *self-doubt* and your present and future commitment to yourself?
5. What do you know about your own victories that you might be willing to share with others who are having similar struggles?

References

Anderson, H., Goolishian, H., & Winderman, L. (1986). Problem determined systems: Towards a transformation in family therapy. *Journal of Strategic and Systemic Therapies, 5*, 1–14.

Anderson, W. T. (1990). *Reality isn't what it used to be*. New York: Harper & Row.

Brown, L., & Gilligan, C. (1992). *Meeting at the crossroads*. Cambridge, MA: Harvard University Press.

Bruner, J. (1986). *Actual minds, possible worlds*. Cambridge, MA: Harvard University Press.

Bruner, J. (1990). *Acts of meaning*. Cambridge, MA: Harvard University Press.

Derrida, J. (1981). *Positions*. Chicago: University of Chicago Press.

Derrida, J. (1991). In P. Kamfuf (Ed.), *A Derrida reader: Between the blinds*. New York: Columbia University Press.

Dickerson, V. C., & Zimmerman, J. L. (1992). Families with adolescents: Escaping problem lifestyles. *Family Process, 31*, 351–363.

Dickerson, V. C., & Zimmerman, J. L. (1993). A narrative approach to families with adolescents. In S. Friedman (Ed.), *The new language of change: Constructive collaboration in psychotherapy*. New York: Guilford Press.

Dickerson, V. C., & Zimmerman, J. L. (1995). A constructionist exercise in anti-pathologizing. *Journal of Systemic Therapies, 14*, 33–45.

Dickerson, V. C., Zimmerman, J. L., & Berndt, L. (1994). Challenging developmental "truths": Separating from separation. *Dulwich Centre Newsletter, 4*, 2–12.

Epston, D. (1993, March 9–10). *Narrative therapy with children*. Workshop given at Bay Area Family Therapy, Cupertino, CA.

Epston, D. (1994, February 10–11). *The Anti-Anorexia League: Resistance and counter-practices*. Workshop given at Bay Area Family Therapy, Cupertino, CA.

308 References

Foucault, M. (1979). *Discipline and punish: The birth of the prison*. Harmondsworth, England: Penguin Books.

Foucault, M. (1980). *Power knowledge: Selected interviews and other writings*. New York: Pantheon Books.

Foucault, M. (1984a). *The history of sexuality*. Harmondsworth, England: Penguin Books.

Foucault, M. (1984b). The subject and power. In H. Dreyfus & P. Rabinow (Eds.), *Michel Foucault: Beyond*. Chicago: University of Chicago Press.

Gaines, A. (1992). From DSM-I to III-R: Voices of self, mastery and the other. A cultural constructivist reading of U.S. psychiatric classification. *Social Science and Medicine, 35*(1), 3–24.

Gergen, K. (1985). The social constructionist movement in modern psychology. *American Psychologist, 40*, 266–275.

Gergen, K. (1991). *The saturated self: Dilemmas of identity in contemporary life*. New York: Basic Books.

Geertz, C. (1986). Making experiences, authoring selves. In V. Turner & E. Bruner (Eds.), *The anthropology of experience*. Chicago: University of Illinois Press.

Gilligan, C. (1982). *In a different voice: Psychological theory and women's development*. Cambridge, MA: Harvard University Press.

Gilligan, C. (1990). Joining the resistance: Psychology, politics, girls and women. *Michigan Quarterly Review, 29*, 501–536.

Gottman, J. L. (1994). Why marriages fail. *Family Therapy Networker, 18*(3), 41–48.

Gremillion, H. (1992). Psychiatry as social ordering: Anorexia nervosa, a paradigm. *Social Science and Medicine, 35*(1), 57–71.

Hare-Mustin, R. T. (1994). Discourses in the mirrored room: A postmodern analysis of therapy. *Family Process, 33*, 19–35.

Jenkins, A. (1990). *Invitations to responsibility*. Adelaide, South Australia: Dulwich Centre Publications.

Madigan, S. (1994). Body politics. *Family Therapy Networker, 18*(6), 27.

Madigan, S. (1996). Undermining the problem in the privatization of problems in persons: Considering the socio-political and cultural context in the externalizing of internalized problem conversations. *Journal of Systemic Therapies, 15*, 47–62.

Myerhoff, B. (1982). Life history among the elderly: Performance, visibility and remembering. In J. Ruby (Ed.), *A crack in the mirror: Reflexive perspectives in anthropology*. Philadelphia: University of Pennsylvania Press.

Neal, J. (1996). *Revising the influence of men's culture in narrative couples therapy*. Unpublished manuscript.

Roth, S., & Epston, D. (1996). Developing externalizing conversations: An exercise. *Journal of Systemic Therapies, 15*, 5–12.

Selvini-Palazzoli, M., Boscolo, L., Cecchin, G., & Prata, G. (1980). Hypothesizing–circularity–neutrality. *Family Process, 19*, 73–85.

Turner, V. (1969). *The ritual process*. Ithaca, NY: Cornell University Press.

van Gennep, A. (1960). *The rites of passage*. Chicago: University of Chicago Press.

Weingarten, K. (1991). The discourses of intimacy: Adding a social construc-tionist and feminist view. *Family Process, 30,* 285–305.

Weingarten, K. (1994). *The mother's voice: Strengthening intimacy in families.* New York: Harcourt Brace & Co.

Weingarten, K. (Ed.). (1996). *Cultural resistance: Challenging beliefs about men, women, and therapy.* New York: The Haworth Press.

White, M. (1984). Pseudo-encopresis: From avalanche to victory, from vicious to virtuous cycles. *Family Systems Medicine, 2*(2), 150–160.

White, M. (1985). Fear busting and monster taming: An approach to the fears of young children. *Dulwich Centre Review,* pp. 29–34.

White, M. (1988, Winter). The process of questioning: A therapy of literary merit? *Dulwich Centre Newsletter,* pp. 8–14.

White, M. (1989–1990, Summer). Family therapy training and supervision in a world of experience and narrative. *Dulwich Centre Newsletter,* pp. 27–38.

White, M. (1991). Deconstruction and therapy. *Dulwich Centre Newsletter, 3,* 21–40.

White, M. (1992). Men's culture, the men's movement and the constitution of men's lives. *Dulwich Centre Newsletter, 3 & 4,* 33–52.

White, M. (1995a). *Re-authoring lives: Interviews and essays.* Adelaide, South Australia: Dulwich Centre Publications.

White, M. (1995b, September 13, 14). *The life of the therapist: Inspiration in narrative therapy.* Workshop given at Bay Area Family Therapy, Cupertino, CA.

White, M., & Epston, D. (1990). *Narrative means to therapeutic ends.* New York: Norton.

Zimmerman, J. L., & Dickerson, V. C. (1993a). Bringing forth the restraining influence of pattern and relationship discourse in couple's therapy. In S. Gilligan & R. Price (Eds.), *Therapeutic conversations.* New York: Norton.

Zimmerman, J. L., & Dickerson, V. C. (1993b). Separating couples from restrain-ing patterns and the relationship discourse that supports them. *Journal of Marital and Family Therapy, 19,* 403–413.

Zimmerman, J. L., & Dickerson, V. C. (1994a). Tales of the body thief: Exter-nalizing and deconstructing eating problems. In M. F. Hoyt (Ed.), *Construc-tive therapies.* New York: Guilford Press.

Zimmerman, J. L., & Dickerson, V. C. (1994b). Using a narrative metaphor: Implications for theory and clinical practice. *Family Process, 33,* 233–246.

Zimmerman, J. L., & Dickerson, V. C. (1995). Narrative therapy and the work of Michael White. In M. Elkaim (Ed.), *Panorama des thérapies familiales.* Paris: Editions du Seuil.

Index